Bile Acids
in
Gastroenterology

Bile Acids
in
Gastroenterology

Edited by

L. Barbara
R.H. Dowling
A.F. Hofmann
E. Roda

*Proceedings of an International Symposium held at Cortina d'Ampezzo,
Italy, 17–20th March 1982*

British Library Cataloguing in Publication Data

Bile acids in gastroenterology: proceedings
of an international symposium held in Cortina
d'Ampezzo, Italy, 17–20th March 1982.
1. Bile acids—Metabolism—Congress
I. Barbara, Luigi
612'.35   QP752.B54

Library of Congress Cataloguing in Publication Data

Main entry under title:

Bile acids in gastroenterology.
    Includes bibliographical references and index.
    1. Bile acids—Congresses.   I. Barbara, L. (Luigi)
        [DNLM: 1. Bile acids and salts—Congresses.
    2. Gastroenterology—Congresses. WI 703 B5975 1982]
QP752.B54B55   1983   612'.35   83-7965

ISBN 978-94-011-7771-9   ISBN 978-94-011-7769-6 (eBook)
DOI 10.1007/978-94-011-7769-6

Copyright © 1983 Springer Science+Business Media Dordrecht
Originally published by MTP Press Limited in 1983
Softcover reprint of the hardcover 1st edition 1983

Phototypesetting by Georgia Origination, Liverpool

Contents

List of Contributors

D. ALVARO
Cattedra di Gastroenterologia II
Università di Roma
Viale dell'Università 37
00161 Rome, Italy

M. ANGELICO
Cattedra di Gastroenterologia II
Università di Roma
Viale dell'Università 37
00161 Rome, Italy

F. A. ATTILI
Cattedra di Fisipatologia Digestiva
Università di L'Aquila
Via Verdi, 67100 L'Aquila
Italy

W. F. BALISTRERI
Division of Pediatric Gastroenterology
Children's Hospital Research Foundation
Elland and Bethesda Avenues
Cincinnati, Ohio 45229, USA

W. M. BELKNAP
Division of Pediatric Gastroenterology
Children's Hospital Research Foundation
Elland and Bethesda Avenues
Cincinnati, Ohio 45229, USA

K. von BERGMANN
Medizinische Universitätsklinik Bonn
D–5300 Bonn–Venusberg
FRG

A. L. BLUM
Department of Medicine
Triemli Hospital
Birmensdorferstrasse 497
CH–8063 Zurich
Switzerland

L. CAPOCACCIA
Cattedra di Gastroenterologia II
Università di Roma
Viale dell'Università 37
00161 Rome, Italy

M. C. CAREY
Department of Medicine
Harvard Medical School
Division of Gastroenterology
Brigham and Women's Hospital
75 Francis Street
Boston, Massachusetts 02115, USA

N. CARULLI
Clinica Medica I
Università di Modena
Policlinico – Via del Pozzo 71
41100 Modena, Italy

V. S. CHADWICK
Gastroenterology Unit
Department of Medicine
Royal Postgraduate Medical School
Ducane Road
London W12 0HS, UK

E. CORAZZIARI
Cattedra di Gastroenterologia
Clinica Medica II
Viale del Policlinico
00100 Roma, Italy

S. A. CUMMINGS
Division of Gastroenterology
Department of Medicine
University of California at San Diego
225 Dickinson St.
San Diego
California 92103
USA

A. DE SANTIS
Cattedra di Gastroenterologia II
Università di Roma
Viale dell'Università 37
Rome, Italy

S. ERLINGER
Service d'Hépatologie et Unité de Recherches
de Physiopathologie
Hépatique (INSERM U-24)
Hôpital Beaujon
92118, Clichy Cedex, France

C. J. FIMMEL
Department of Medicine
Triemli Hospital
Birmensdorferstrasse 497
CH-8063 Zurich
Switzerland

J. E. HEUBI
Division of Pediatric Gastroenterology
Children's Hospital Research Foundation
Elland and Bethesda Avenues
Cincinnati, Ohio 45229, USA

N. F. LA RUSSO
Department of Medicine
Division of Gastroenterology
Mayo Medical School
Rochester MA 55901, USA

G. A. MANNES
Department of Internal Medicine II
Klinikum Groshadern
University of Munich
D-8000 Munich 70
West Germany

M. MARIN
Cattedra di Gastroenterologia II
Università di Roma
Viale dell'Università 37
00161 Rome, Italy

E. DE MASI
IV Clinica Chirurgica
Viale del Policlinico
00100 Roma
Italy

P. N. MATON
Gastroenterology Unit
Department of Medicine
Royal Postgraduate Medical School
Ducane Road
London W12 0HS

G. PAUMGARTNER
Department of Internal Medicine II
Klinikum Groshadern
University of Munich
D-8000 Munich 70
West Germany

M. PONZ DE LEON
Clinica Medica I
Università di Modena
Policlinico – Via del Pozzo 71
41100 Modena, Italy

A. RODA
Istituto di Scienze Chimiche
Facoltà di Farmacia
Univerità di Bologna
Via S. Donato 15
40100 Bologna, Italy

A. C. SELDEN
Gastroenterology Unit
Department of Medicine
Royal Postgraduate Medical School
Ducane Road
London W12 0HS

K. D. R. SETCHELL
Division of Clinical Chemistry
Clinical Research Centre
Harrow, Middlesex HA1 3UJ
UK

F. STELLARD
Department of Internal Medicine II
Klinikum Groshadern
University of Munich
D-8000 Munich 70
West Germany

F. J. SUCHY
Division of Pediatric Gastroenterology
Children's Hospital Research Foundation
Elland and Bethesda Avenue
Cincinnati, Ohio 45229, USA

A. TORSOLI
Cattedra di Gastroenterologia
Clinica Medica II
Viale del Policlinico, 00100, Roma,
Italy

F. ZIRONI
Clinica Medica I
Università di Modena
Policlinico – Via del Pozzo, 71
41100 Modena, Italy

Preface

Over the past 10 years there has been a veritable explosion of knowledge in bile acid research. Those working in this area are fortunate to meet their colleagues from time to time at International Meetings which are often held in attractive parts of the world. The 7th International Symposium on bile acids 'Bile Acids in Gastroenterology' was no exception. It took place in Cortina d'Ampezzo in the heart of the Italian Dolomites, from 17th–20th March 1982. This meeting was organised by a Scientific Committee, with representatives from Italy, the United States and Great Britain, in collaboration with the Italian Society of Gastroenterology. The format of the meeting was somewhat different from that of previous years. In addition to the free communications (verbal and poster presentations) which characterise many scientific meetings, there was also an Advanced Postgraduate Course on bile acids given by a distinguished international panel of experts. Their contributions form the basis for this timely volume which should be of interest both to basic scientists and to clinical investigators alike.

The editors are indebted to Dr Gian Germano Giuliani, Gipharmex SpA, Milano, whose generous support made the meeting possible. They also thank Mr P. M. Lister, Managing Editor, MTP Press Limited and Mrs Veronica Cesari, Italian Society of Gastroenterology for help with the publication of these proceedings.

R. Herman Dowling

1
Liquid–solid extraction, lipophilic gel chromatography and capillary column gas chromatography in the analysis of bile acids from biological samples

K. D. R. SETCHELL

INTRODUCTION

Most of the methods currently employed for the determination of bile acids in biological samples require some form of initial extraction procedure. Techniques which are generally available include the following:

(1) Liquid–liquid partition.
(2) Protein precipitation.
(3) Liquid–solid extraction – anion exchange resins, neutral polystyrene polymers of Amberlite XAD and reverse-phase octadecylsilane-bonded silica.
(4) Liquid–gel extraction – Lipidex 1000.

The complexity in the composition of bile acids in biological samples renders liquid–liquid partition extraction techniques less suitable since these require the use of polar solvents or the addition of an ion-pair reagent to obtain quantitative recoveries of all classes of bile acids[1,2]. Liquid–solid extraction techniques were introduced, and methods were described for the extraction of bile acids using the anion exchange resin Amberlyst A-26[3] and the neutral resins of Amberlite XAD-2[4] and XAD-7[5]. These neutral resins, although revolutionizing the extraction stage, did have drawbacks, one of which was the poor recovery of polar sulphated bile acids[6]. This was recently explained from the finding that this neutral resin possessed weak anion exchange properties, which accounted for the irreversible adsorption of acidic steroids and the inability to obtain quantitative recoveries when the resin was eluted with neutral alcoholic solvents[7]. Furthermore – irrespective of whether a column procedure, for which the sample flow rate is critical[8], or a batch method[5] is employed – the numbers of samples which can be extracted are limited.

As a consequence of the considerable time required to extract bile acids from large numbers of samples, the trend in bile acid methodology over the last decade has been towards practical simplicity with the introduction of radioimmunoassays[9-13], enzyme immunoassay[14] and fluorimetric methods[15-20]. One of the dangers in oversimplifying assay designs, however, is the difficulty in interpreting the data obtained, since the effects of non-specific interference due to the complexity of the biological matrix is increasingly dependent upon the specificity of the 'end-point' determination.

Outlined below are recently developed liquid–solid and liquid–gel extraction techniques which have considerably increased the ease and speed of quantitatively extracting bile acids from biological samples and which are consequently applicable to more routine applications of bile acid measurement.

LIQUID–SOLID EXTRACTION OF BILE ACIDS

One of the most exciting developments in extraction techniques has been the introduction of reverse-phase octadecylsilane-bonded silica cartridges which have dramatically increased the speed of quantitatively extracting polar compounds from aqueous solutions. These cartridges, of which several types are now commercially available, were applied initially to the extraction of neutral steroids from urine[21,22] and serum[7,22] and have more recently been applied to the extraction of bile acids from a variety of biological samples[23-26].

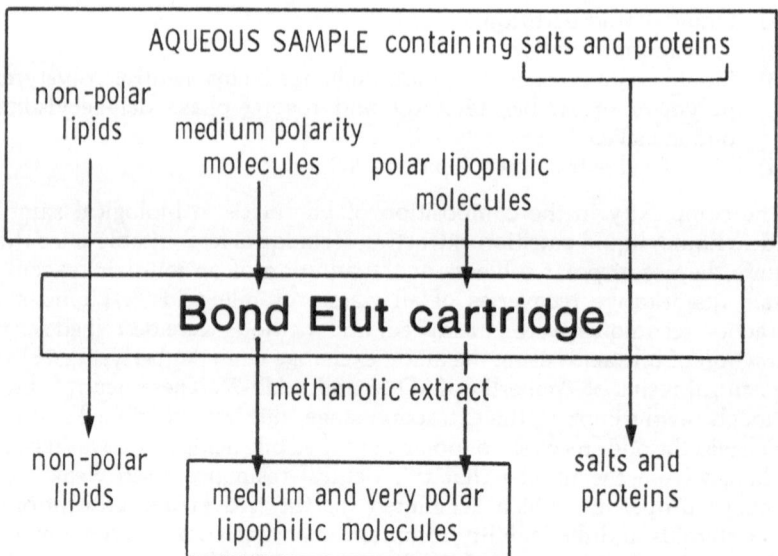

Figure 1.1 Principal characteristics of reverse-phase octadecylsilane-bonded silica cartridges

2

Reverse-phase octadecylsilane-bonded silica cartridges behave as polar adsorbents (Figure 1.1) and consequently will only extract, from aqueous solutions, lipophilic molecules of medium and high polarity. Salts and proteins together with non-polar lipids pass directly through the cartridge and are discarded.

For the quantitative extraction of bile acids from serum samples, the main problem to overcome is their strong binding to serum proteins[27] and it is not sufficient merely to dilute the serum with water, which has been advocated[23]. When serum is diluted with water and passed through these cartridges, the recovery of unconjugated bile acids and bile acid sulphates in the methanolic eluant is poor (Table 1.1) and most of these bile acids are eluted in the aqueous phase[24]. The binding of bile acids to albumin can be decreased by increasing the pH and temperature[27] and with these considerations a method was developed in which the serum is diluted with 4 volumes of 0.1 mol/l sodium hydroxide and heated to 64 °C in a water bath before it is passed through the cartridge[24]. The recoveries of a variety of bile acids and their conjugates in the methanolic extract using two types of commercially available cartridges (Bond Elut, Analytichem International, Harbor City, California, USA obtained from Jones Chromatography, Llanbradach, Wales: and Sep-Pak-C_{18} Waters Associates, Milford MA, USA) are summarized in Table 1.1 and are reported in detail elsewhere[24].

Quantitative recoveries of very polar bile acids, e.g. the trisulphate conjugate of taurocholate, are obtained by this procedure since these reverse-phase octadecylsilane-bonded silica cartridges do not have the disadvantage of the weak ionic properties of the Amberlite XAD resins[7].

This liquid–solid extraction procedure takes only a few minutes to perform and by the use of a specially designed vacuum apparatus (Vac Elut, Analytichem International, California, USA) it is possible to extract simultaneously ten samples in approximately 5 minutes[24]. The capacity of these cartridges is high (about 0.2 mmol of bile acid/cartridge) and the ease and speed of the technique make it superior to other extraction techniques currently available. Since it can be semiautomated, it is suitable for large numbers of samples often encountered by laboratories performing routine immunoassay methods for serum bile acids. By the inclusion of this rapid extraction step the specificity of many radioimmunoassays, which is a function of non-specific binding or matrix interference[28], may be improved.

LIPOPHILIC GELS

The development of lipophilic gel chromatography has been pioneered over the last decade by the efforts of Professor Sjövall's group at the Karolinska Institute in Stockholm. Figure 1.2 shows the types of lipophilic gels which are now commercially available, all of which are based upon the cross-linked polysaccharide gel, Sephadex.

Sephadex LH-20 is a hydroxypropyl ether of Sephadex G-25 (Pharmacia Fine Chemicals, Uppsala, Sweden) and is a gel which readily swells in polar organic solvents, producing most commonly straight phase partition

3

Table 1.1 Mean (±SD) percentage recovery of a selection of radiolabelled bile acid and cholesterol which were added to serum and extracted using reverse-phase octadecylsilane-bonded silica cartridges

Conditions	Taurocholic	Glycocholic	Lithocholic	Cholic	Lithocholic-3-sulphate	Taurochenodeoxycholic-3-sulphate	Glycocholic-trisulphate	Cholesterol
1:1 dilution with water (Bond Elut)	81.8±4.6	80.2±1.6	25.6±7.1	76.1±3.4	7.9±3.5	—	—	—
1:4 dilution with 0.1 mol/l sodium hydroxide at 64 °C (Sep-Pak)	99.9±0.7	97.8±2.0	97.2±1.0	98.7±2.7	93.3±2.5	—	104.4±6.4	3.2±0.8
1:4 dilution with 0.1 mol/l sodium hydroxide at 64 °C (Bond Elut)	97.9±0.7	97.1±1.1	97.2±3.7	96.8±1.4	93.3±2.5	95.1±3.1	97.6±6.6	2.5±0.4

4

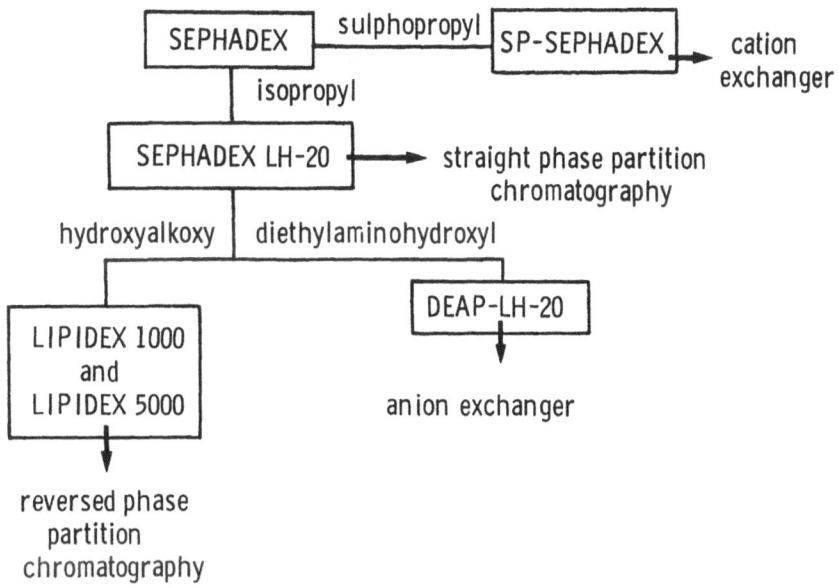

Figure 1.2 Types of commercially available lipophilic gels

chromatography systems. Methods for the separation of bile acids into conjugate groups based upon straight phase partition chromatography using Sephadex LH-20 have been described[8,29].

Diethylaminohydroxypropyl Sephadex LH-20 (DEAP-LH-20 or Lipidex-DEAP, Packard-Becker BV., Groningen, The Netherlands) is prepared from Sephadex LH-20 by the introduction of a diethylamine group after first preparing the chlorohydroxypropyl derivative[30,31]. This gel, which is a lipophilic anion exchanger, has been applied to the group fractionation of neutral steroids[32] and bile acids[8] based upon their mode of conjugation.

Lipidex 1000 and 5000 (Packard-Becker BV., Groningen, The Netherlands) are both derivatives of Sephadex which contain long-chain (C_{11}–C_{14}) hydroxyalkyl substituents[33]. These lipophilic gels consequently allow the use of miscible non-polar solvent systems and thus separations by reverse-phase partition chromatography are possible[33].

SP-Sephadex (Pharmacia Fine Chemicals, Uppsala, Sweden) is a cation-exchange gel in which sulphopropyl groups have been substituted into the polysaccharide matrix. This gel has ben used as an alternative to the cation exchange resin Amberlyst A-15[34–36].

LIQUID–GEL EXTRACTION OF UNCONJUGATED BILE ACIDS

The potential of the lipophilic gel, Lipidex 1000, for the extraction of un-conjugated bile acids and steroids from acidic aqueous solutions was first reported by Dyfverman and Sjövall[37,38]. The principal characteristics of Lipidex 1000 are illustrated in Figure 1.3. In contrast to reverse-phase

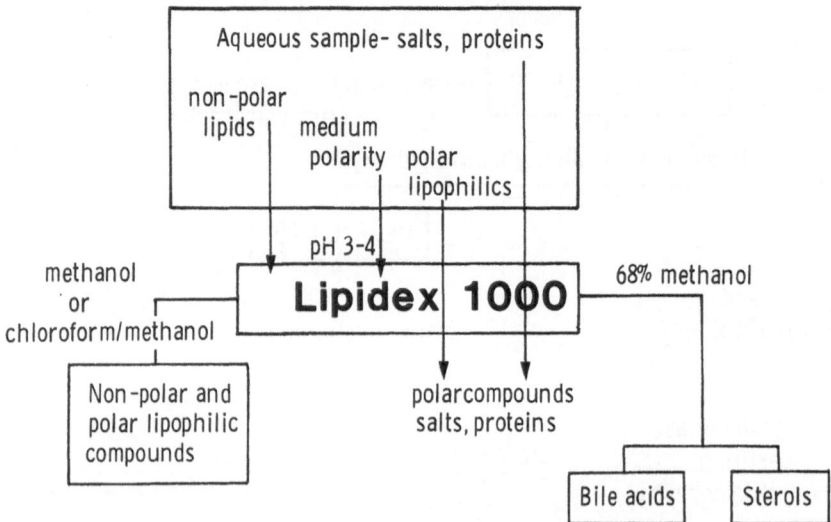

Figure 1.3 Principal characteristics of the lipophilic gel Lipidex 1000

octadecylsilane-bonded silica, this gel behaves as a non-polar adsorbent and extracts, from acidified aqueous solutions, only lipophilic molecules which are of non-polar and medium polarity characteristics. Polar lipids together with salts and proteins are excluded and discarded.

Unconjugated bile acids are quantitatively removed from acidic solutions and adsorbed to the gel[35,38] while the extraction of conjugated bile acids by this gel is not quantitative (Table 1.2). Taurine-conjugated bile acids and a large proportion of glycine conjugates pass directly through the gel bed in the acidic aqueous solution; however, it has been shown that by the inclusion of

Table 1.2 Percentage recovery of radiolabelled compounds which were added to a biological extract redissolved in acidic water and extracted by Lipidex 1000

	Lipidex 1000	
Compound	Aqueous	Methanol
Cholesterol	—	95.5
Palmitic acid	—	95.8
Lithocholic-ethyl ester	—	98.7
Lithocholic acid	—	98.4
Cholic acid	1.0	99.9
Glycocholic acid	3.0–32.0	68.0–96.4
Taurocholic acid	98.2	—
Lithocholic-sulphate	—	100.3

an ion-pair reagent the recovery of these conjugates can be increased[38] and this ion-pair effect most probably explains the variability in the recovery of glycocholate between different samples from the acidic solution (Table 1.2).

The method is rapid since the extraction efficiency is independent of the sample flow rate through the gel and the capacity of the gel is extremely high. Once adsorbed, bile acids can be quantitatively recovered in a single fraction by eluting the gel with 20 ml of methanol (Table 1.2). Alternatively, since the gel is lipophilic and non-polar, by increasing the polarity of the eluting solvent it is possible to perform reverse-phase partition chromatography and separate monohydroxy-sterols, which are retained on the gel, from the more polar bile acids[34,35]. This is a particularly useful advantage since it provides a method of removing any cholesterol which may be present in the sample and which would otherwise interfere in the subsequent gas chromatography or gas chromatography–mass spectrometry analysis of the bile acids[34].

Lipidex 1000 is an attractive alternative to liquid–liquid partitioning for the quantitative extraction of unconjugated bile acids from enzymatic and alkaline hydrolysates[34,35]. The aqueous samples only require the pH to be adjusted to between pH 3 and 4 with acetic acid or hydrochloric acid, after which they are rapidly percolated through a small column of Lipidex 1000. Furthermore, the use of inflammable and hazardous solvents is avoided and a relatively pure sample, free of monohydroxysterols, is obtained in a methanolic solution.

APPLICATIONS TO BIOLOGICAL SAMPLES

The extraction procedures using reverse-phase octadecylsilane-bonded silica cartridges and Lipidex 1000 are complementary and when combined with capillary column gas chromatography and mass spectrometry provide a powerful method for the analysis of bile acids from a variety of biological materials. Depending upon the analytical requirements, the flexibility of these techniques will allow a variety of analytical objectives to be met.

Analysis of serum bile acids

Figure 1.4 illustrates a general scheme for the qualitative and quantitative determination of bile acids in serum samples. After the quantitative extraction of bile acids using the Bond Elut cartridges[24] either an enzymatic hydrolysis with cholylglycine hydrolase[39,40] (a measure of total non-sulphated bile acids) or a combined solvolysis and alkaline hydrolysis (total serum bile acids) may be carried out. In either case the Lipidex 1000 gel is ideally suited to the quantitative extraction of unconjugated bile acids from the acidified aqueous hydrolysates and also provides a means of removing residual amounts of cholesterol or other sterols from the sample.

Figure 1.5 shows capillary column gas chromatographic profiles obtained for the total non-sulphated bile acids which are typical of a normal adult and a patient with primary biliary cirrhosis when the above analysis procedure is employed. Quantitative values for serum bile acids in normals and patients

7

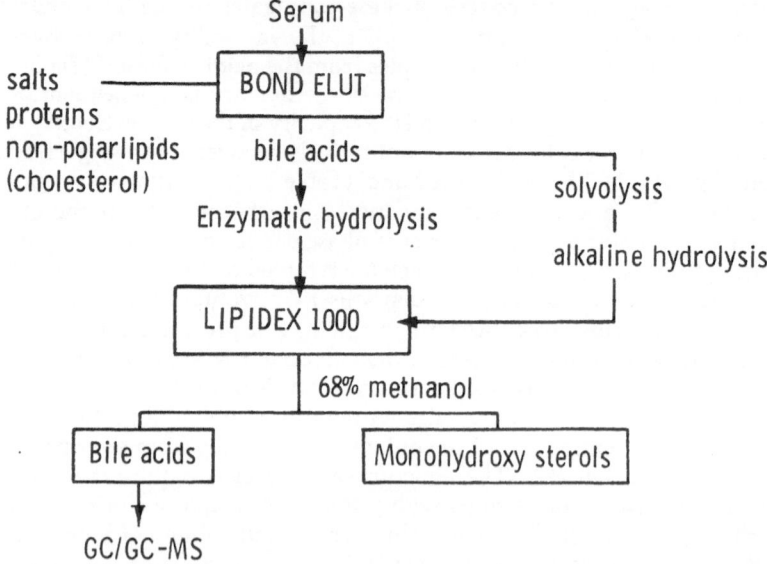

Figure 1.4 A general flexible scheme for the analysis of serum bile acids.
GC = Gas chromatography: MS = mass spectroscopy

with liver disease determined by this procedure are reported elsewhere[34].

Determination of unconjugated bile acids in serum

Studies using these analytical techniques have recently indicated the quantitative and qualitative importance of unconjugated bile acids in normal human serum[41,42]. With the exception of patients with stagnant-loop syndrome and bacterial overgrowths[43], the presence of unconjugated bile acids in serum has received little attention[44].

Unconjugated bile acids can be measured by gas chromatography[34] or gas chromatography–mass spectrometry[42] after their isolation using Lipidex 1000 and preparation of the methyl ester–trimethylsilyl ether derivatives (Figure 1.6).

The separate determination of unconjugated and conjugated bile acids is necessary in many metabolic studies, particularly those studying pharmacological loads of bile acids. Since Lipidex 1000 will extract a significant and variable amount of glycine-conjugated bile acids (Table 1.2), this method of isolating unconjugated bile acids is unsuitable if their determination is to be carried out using immunoassays which significantly cross-react with glycine conjugates. In this situation, a specific group separation of individual bile acids from serum extracts based on their mode of conjugation is possible using the anion exchange gel DEAP-LH-20 as described elsewhere[8,34,42].

Where an enzyme–fluorimetric method[15] is to be used for the measurement of bile acids in the individual fractions from the anion exchange gel, it is important to use SP-Sephadex and not Amberlyst A-15 resin for the essential

8

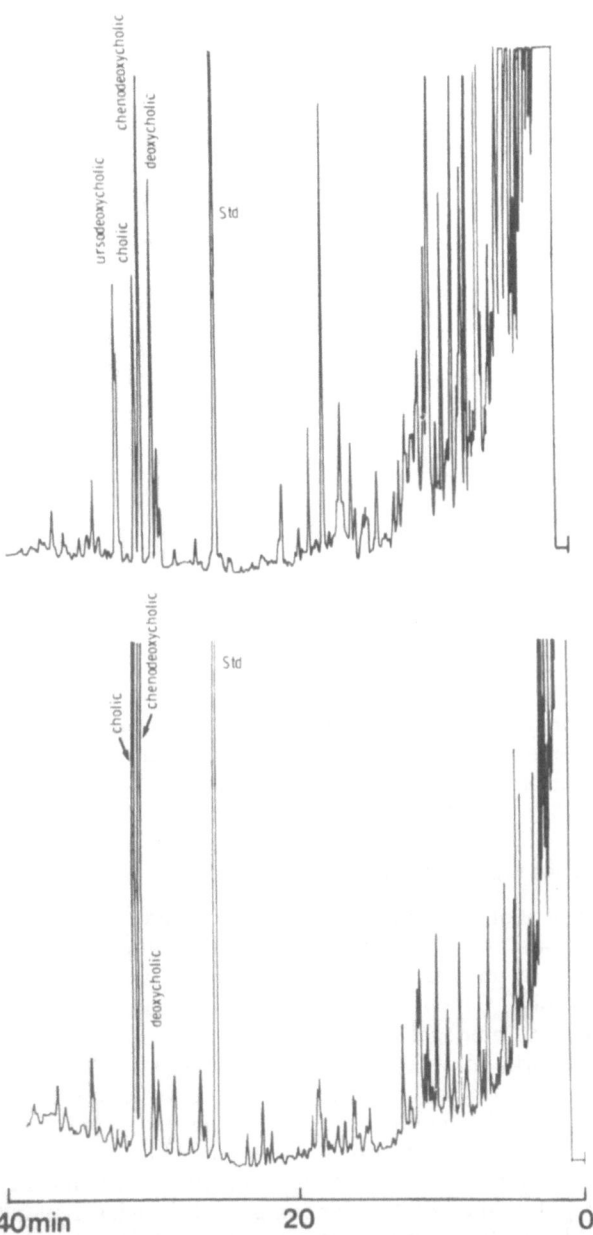

Figure 1.5 Capillary column gas chromatographic profiles indicating the principal non-sulphated bile acids in the serum of a normal adult (upper) and a patient with primary biliary cirrhosis (lower). Bile acids were analysed as their methyl ester-trimethylsilyl ethers on a 25 m glass capillary column coated with silicone OV-1 using temperature programmed operation from 225 °C to 285 °C with increments of 2 °C/min. Std=standard

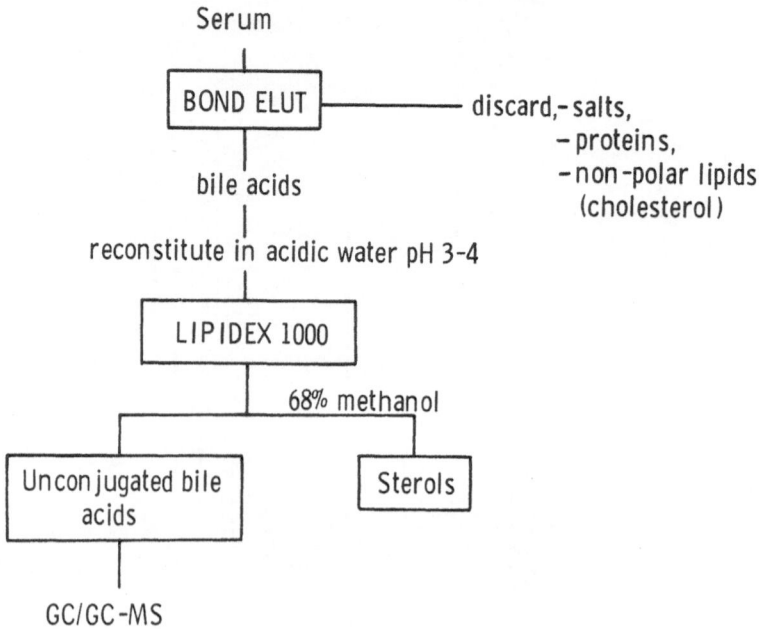

Figure 1.6 General scheme for a rapid extraction and isolation of unconjugated bile acids from serum. GC=Gas chromatography; MS=mass spectroscopy

cation exchange step before DEAP-LH-20 chromatography, since a considerable overestimation of the bile acid concentration occurs due to an unknown interference derived from the resin[36].

Measurement of faecal bile acids

The measurement of bile acids in faeces has received increased attention over the last few years, most probably because of the importance of cholesterol and bile acids in gastroenterological diseases such as colon cancer. An analytical method, which is described in detail elsewhere[35], utilizes these liquid–solid and liquid–gel extraction techniques in combination, for the desalting and partial purification of faecal extracts.

Bile acids and related compounds after extraction from faeces by sequential refluxing in alcohols are quantitatively extracted from an acidified aqueous solution by passage through a column of Lipidex 1000 followed by a Bond Elut cartridge. The Lipidex 1000 column, with its high capacity, adsorbs non-polar lipids while polar compounds which escape extraction are then trapped on the reversed-phase octadecylsilane-bonded silica. A quantitative recovery of all classes of compounds is possible by elution of both chromatographic materials with methanol. The combined extracts can be further purified and compounds separated into groups based upon the state of conjugation using the lipophilic gel DEAP-LH-20 and this method

10

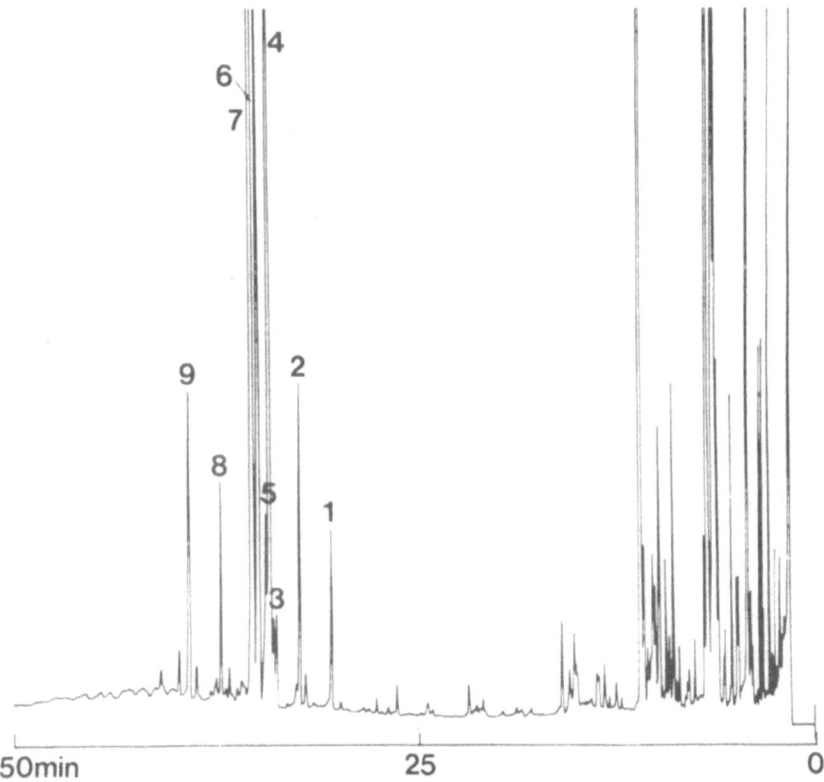

Figure 1.7 A capillary column gas chromatographic profile of the unconjugated bile acids excreted in the faeces of a patient with diarrhoea. Bile acids were extracted and purified by techniques using liquid–solid and liquid–gel extraction and isolated by lipophilic anion exchange chromatography[35]. Bile acids were analysed as their methyl ester–trimethylsilyl ethers on a capillary column coated with silicone OV-1. The principal bile acids identified by gas chromatography–mass spectrometry and the quantitative excretion are as follows: 1, coprostanol (internal standard) (0.7 mg/day); 2, lithocholic acid (10.9 mg/day); 3, 3β, 12α-dihydroxy-5β-cholanoic (3.1 mg/day); 4, deoxycholic acid (40.6 mg/day); 5, 3β, 7α, 12α-trihydroxy-5β-cholanoic (6.1 mg/day); 6, chenodeoxycholic acid (32.0 mg/day); 7, cholic acid (67.8 mg/day); 8, 7-oxo-3α-hydroxy-5β-cholanoic (13.1 mg/day); 9, 12-oxo-3α, 7α-dihydroxy-5β-cholanoic (31.4 mg/day)

therefore permits the separate determination of sterols and bile acids by gas chromatography.

A capillary column gas chromatographic profile of the unconjugated bile acid fraction from the faeces of a patient with chronic diarrhoea of unknown aetiology is shown in Figure 1.7 and illustrates the potential of this approach. The chromatogram is characterized by relatively large amounts of the primary bile acids cholic and chenodeoxycholic acids compared with the secondary bile acids, which predominate in normal subjects[35].

CAPILLARY COLUMN GAS CHROMATOGRAPHY

The gas chromatographic analysis of bile acids in biological extracts has always been complicated by the diversity in chemical structure of bile acids, the presence of interfering compounds and in certain types of samples the low concentrations of minor components. Many attempts have been made to overcome these problems, evidenced from the wide range of derivatives that have been examined and the various types of column packings which have been evaluated[45-50]. Ultimately, however, the gas chromatographic conditions chosen should depend upon the type and complexity of the bile acids in the biological extract, since at present no universal chromatography phase is available which is capable of separating the wide spectrum of primary and secondary bile acids.

With the advent of capillary column gas chromatography, and the rapid developments in column technology, greatly increased chromatographic resolution can now be attained. The potential of capillary column gas chromatography to the metabolic profiling of steroids has been well recognized for many years[51]; however, its application to the analysis of bile acids has by comparison been slow. Only a limited number of applications have been reported[34,35,52-55], restricted largely to the analysis of serum bile acids in liver disease.

The choice of open-tubular glass capillary column for bile acid analysis is restricted to a limited number of phases. Using a non-selective stationary phase, such as silicone OV-1 or SE-30, the profiling of a wider range of bile acids is possible in a single analysis compared with selective phases, which are unsuitable for the chromatography of bile acids possessing carbonyl functions.

When samples of complex mixtures of components of widely differing polarity and structure require analysis, such as extracts of faecal bile acids, temperature-programmed operation is essential to provide satisfactory peak shapes of those compounds with long retention times.

The separation of methyl ester-trimethylsilyl ether derivatives of a mixture of authentic bile acids by temperature programming using a 25 m capillary column coated with OV-1 is shown in Figure 1.8.

Several methods are available for the introduction of samples to the gas chromatography column[56]; these include split and splitless injection, on-column injection and solid injection. With high-boiling-point compounds such as steroid derivatives, the introduction of the sample by solid injection using an all-glass dropping needle injection device[57] has many advantages over conventional liquid injection. The amount of sample which can be introduced is not restricted to a small volume since the solvent is evaporated from the dropping glass needle and vented to atmosphere before injection. If required the total sample can be loaded thereby enhancing the 'sensitivity' of the analysis and facilitating the identification of minor components. The presence of a solvent front, which occurs when samples are introduced by liquid injection and results in compounds being eluted in the 'tail' of the solvent front, is minimised or eliminated by solid injection and the linear baseline obtained increases the precision and accuracy of the quantification.

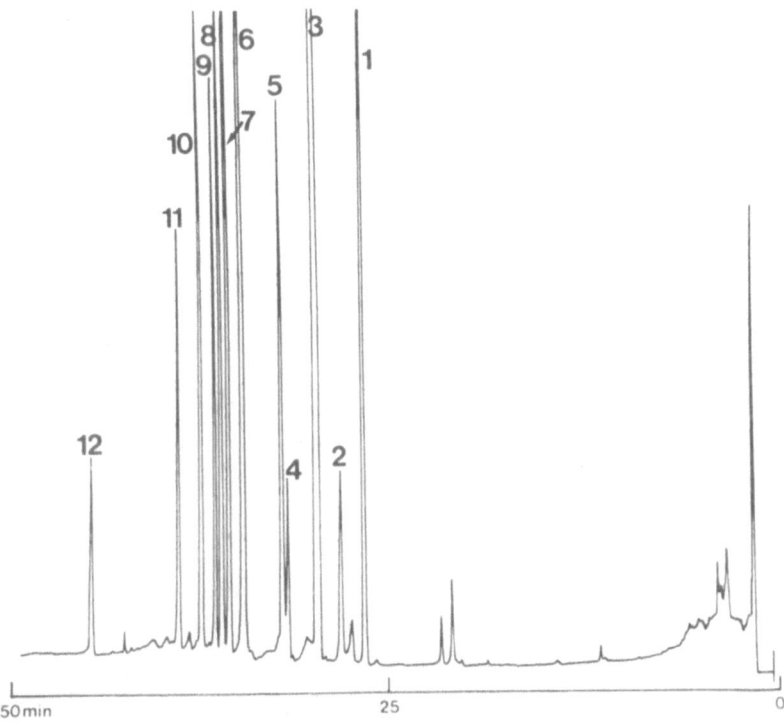

Figure 1.8 Capillary column gas chromatographic recording of the methyl ester-trimethylsilyl ether derivatives of a mixture of approximately equal amounts of bile acids. The bile acid derivatives were separated on a 25 m silicone OV-1 capillary column using helium as the carrier gas and temperature programmed operation from 225 °C to 285 °C in increments of 2 °C/min. Detection was by flame ionization. Bile acids possessing a carbonyl function gave a poor response compared with hydroxylated bile acids. The following acids were indicated: 1, 7α-hydroxy-5β-cholanoic; 2, 12-oxo-5β-cholanoic and 7-oxo-5β-cholanoic (unresolved); 3, coprostanol (internal standard, at a concentration three times greater than the bile acids); 4, 3-oxo-5β-cholanoic; 5, 3α-hydroxy-5β-cholanoic (lithocholic); 6, 3α, 12α-dihydroxy-5β-cholanoic (deoxycholic) and 3β-hydroxy-5-cholenoic (unresolved); 7, 3α, 7α-dihydroxy-5β-cholanoic (chenodeoxycholic); 8, 3α, 7α, 12α-trihydroxy-5β-cholanoic (cholic); 9, 3α, 6α-dihydroxy-5β-cholanoic (hyodeoxycholic); 10, 3α, 7β-dihydroxy-5β cholanoic; 11, 7-oxo-3α-hydroxy-5β-cholanoic; 12, 12-oxo-3α, 7α-5β-cholanoic

Furthermore, non-volatile impurities present in sample extracts are retained on the dropping needle (which can be intermittently removed and cleaned) thereby preventing contamination of the first few coils of the capillary column and increasing its lifetime.

Quantification can be carried out by relating the peak height response of

13

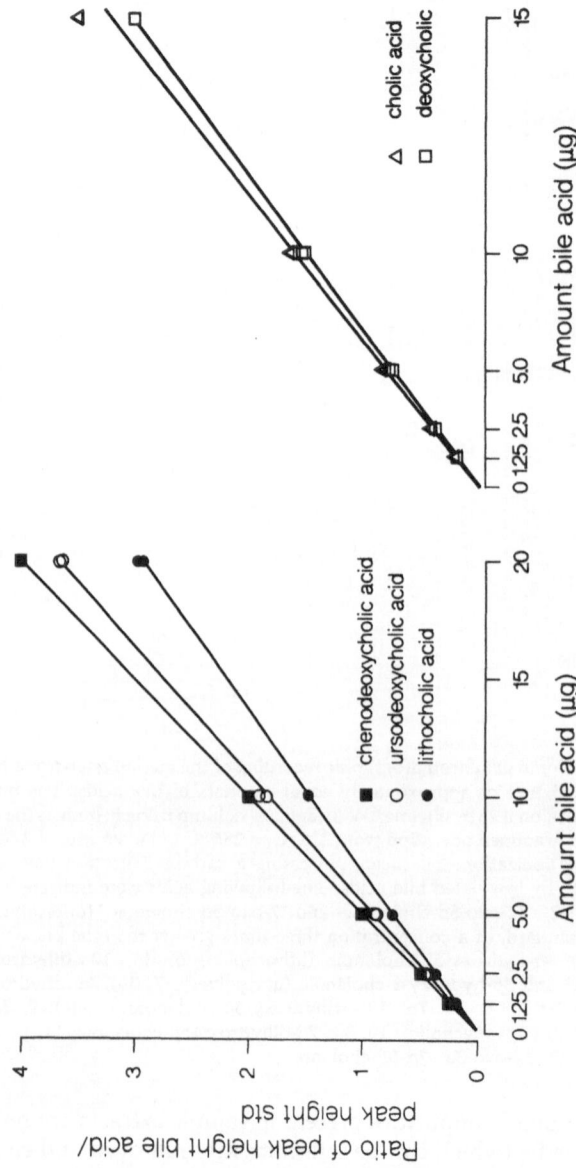

Figure 1.9 Calibration plots for a number of authentic bile acids measured by capillary column gas chromatography with flame ionization detection. Increasing amounts of bile acid (0–20 μg) were added to a constant mass of the internal standard, coprostanol (5 μg). After preparation of the methyl ester-trimethylsilyl ether derivatives the equivalent of about 50 ng (1/25–1/400 sample) was injected on column and the ratio of the peak height of the bile acid to the peak height of the internal standard (std) determined

the bile acid relative to the peak height obtained for a known amount of an internal standard (coprostanol), which is added to the sample prior to derivatization. Calibration curves for the authentic bile acids – cholic, chenodeoxycholic, ursodeoxycholic, deoxycholic and lithocholic acids – are linear over the mass range 0–20 μg and give relative response factors approximating to unity (Figure 1.9). This is not, however, the case for bile acids possessing a free carbonyl group in the nucleus, which in common with trimethylsilyl ethers of steroids[58] give poor responses relative to hydroxylated bile acids (Figure 1.8).

Capillary column gas chromatography offers greatly increased sensitivity compared with gas chromatography using conventional packed columns. A peak in the chromatogram giving a full-scale deflection (FSD) is obtained from approximately 50 ng bile acid (about 0.125 nmol) injected on column. For normal fasting human serum (Figure 1.5) the equivalent of 100 μl of serum is generally injected onto the column (1/20th of total serum sample), so that a bile acid in a concentration of 1.25 μmol/l will give rise to a peak with a FSD (signal:noise ratio of 100:1). Since a much larger proportion of the sample can be loaded using the solid injection device and the amplification of the signal can be further increased if necessary, the limit of detection of a bile acid will correspond to a serum concentration of 0.01–0.02 μmol/l. The sensitivity compares favourably with the sensitivity of most radioimmunoassays for serum bile acids[9–14].

In the limited number of publications which report on the use of capillary column gas chromatography for the estimation of serum bile acids, emphasis has been given to the problem of resolving interfering compounds and sterols, in particular cholesterol, from bile acids during gas chromatography and the use of high resolving capillary columns has been advocated as the solution to these problems. Although capillary column gas chromatography is a powerful analytical tool, to maximise on its high chromatographic resolving power consideration must be given to the purification of samples and as much as possible to the removal of potentially interfering compounds. The most effective means of overcoming the interference due to sterols is to selectively remove them from the sample extract before gas chromatographic analysis. In this way, overloading of the gas chromatography column, which has an adverse effect upon chromatographic efficacy and resolution, is prevented.

With the application of the liquid–gel chromatographic techniques described here and elsewhere[8,34,35,38,42,59,60] for the isolation and purification of bile acids from serum, faeces and other biological samples, maximum benefit can be derived from the use of capillary column gas chromatography for the metabolic profiling of bile acids and related compounds.

References

1. Hofmann, A.F. (1967). Efficient extraction of bile acid conjugates with tetraheptylammonium chloride, a liquid ion exchange. *J. Lipid Res.*, **8**, 55
2. Fransson, B. and Schill, G. (1975). Isolation of acidic conjugates by ion pair extraction, II. Extraction of taurocholic acid derivatives. *Acta Pharm. Soc.*, **12**, 417
3. Sandberg, D.H., Sjövall, J., Sjövall, K. and Turner, D.A. (1965). Measurement of human serum bile acids by gas–liquid chromatography. *J. Lipid Res.*, **6**, 182
4. Makino, I. and Sjövall, J. (1972). A versatile method for analysis of bile acids in plasma. *Anal. Lett.*, **5**, 341
5. Barnes, S. and Chitranukroh, A. (1977). A simplified procedure for the isolation of bile acids from serum based on a batch extraction with non-ionic resin Amberlite XAD-7. *Ann. Clin. Biochem.*, **14**, 235
6. Pageaux, J.F., Duperray, B., Anker, D. and Dubois, M. (1979). Bile acid sulphates in serum bile acid determination. *Steroids*, **34**, 73
7. Axelson, M. and Sahlberg, B-L. (1981). Solid extraction of steroid conjugates from plasma and milk. *Anal. Lett.*, **14**, 771
8. Almé, B., Bremmelgaard, A., Sjövall, J. and Thomassen, P. (1977). Analysis of metabolic profiles of bile acids in urine using a lipophilic anion exchanger and computerised gas–liquid chromatography-mass spectrometry. *J. Lipid Res.*, **18**, 339
9. Simmonds, W.J., Korman, M.G., Go, V.L.W. and Hofmann, A.F. (1973). Radioimmunossay of conjugated cholyl-bile acids in serum. *Gastroenterology*, **65**, 705
10. Murphy, G.M., Edkins, S.M., Williams, J.W. and Catty, D. (1974). The preparation and properties of an anti-serum for the radioimmunoassay of serum conjugated cholic acid. *Clin. Chim. Acta*, **54**, 81
11. Roda, A., Roda, E., Aldini, R., Festi, D., Mazzela, G., Sama, C. and Barbara, L. (1977). Development, validation and application of a single tube radioimmonoassay for cholic and chenodeoxycholic conjugated bile acids in human serum. *Clin. Chem.*, **23**, 2107
12. Spenny, J.G., Johnson, B.J., Hirschowitz, B.I., Mikas, A.A. and Gibson, R. (1977). An ^{125}I radioimmunoassay for primary conjugated bile salts. *Gastroenterology*, **72**, 305
13. Minder, E., Karlaganis, G., Schmied, U., Vitins, P. and Paumgartner, G. (1979). A highly specific ^{125}I-radioimmunoassay for cholic conjugates. *Clin. Chim. Acta*, **92**, 177
14. Schwarz, H.P., Von Bergmann, K. and Paumgartner, G. (1974). A simple method for the estimation of bile acids in serum. *Clin. Chim. Acta*, **50**, 197
15. Murphy, G.M., Billing, B.H. and Baron, D.N. (1970). A fluorimetric and enzymatic method for the estimation of serum total bile acids. *J. Clin. Pathol.*, **23**, 594
16. Mashinge, F., Imai, K. and Osuga, T. (1976). A simple and sensitive assay of bile acids. *Clin. Chim. Acta*, **70**, 79
17. Fauso, O. (1975). Quantitative determination of serum bile acids using a purified 3α-hydroxysteroid dehydrogenase. *Scand. J. Gastroenterol.*, **10**, 747
18. Barnes, S., Gallo, G.A., Trash, D.B. and Morris, J.S. (1975). Diagnostic value of serum bile acid estimation in liver disease. *J. Clin. Pathol.*, **28**, 506
19. Steensland, H. (1978). An automated method for the determination of total bile acids in serum. *Scand. J. Clin. Lab. Invest.*, **38**, 447
20. Siskos, P.A., Cahill, P.T. and Javitt, N.B. (1977). Serum bile acid analysis: A rapid direct enzymatic method using dual-beam spectrophotofluorimetry. *J. Lipid Res.*, **18**, 666
21. Shackleton, C.H.L. and Whitney, J.O. (1980). Use of Sep-pak cartridges for urinary steroid extraction: evaluation of the method for use prior to gas chromatographic analysis. *Clin. Chim. Acta*, **107**, 231
22. Heikkinen, R., Fotsis, T. and Adlercreutz, H. (1981). Reversed-phase C_{18} cartridge for extraction of estrogens from urine and plasma. *Clin. Chem.*, **27**, 1186
23. Whitney, J.O. and Thaler, M.M. (1980). A simple liquid chromatographic method for quantitative extraction of hydrophobic compounds from aqueous solutions. *J. Liquid Chromatogr.*, **3**, 545
24. Setchell, K.D.R. and Worthington, J. (1982). A rapid and quantitative method for the extraction of bile acids from serum using commercially available reverse phase octadecylsilane bonded silica cartridges. *Clin. Chim. Acta*, **125**, 135
25. Ruben, A.T. and Van-Berge-Henegouwen (1982). A simple reverse-phase high pressure

liquid chromatographic determination of conjugated bile acids in serum and bile using a novel radial compression separation system. *Clin. Chim. Acta*, **119**, 41

26. DeMark, B. R., Everson, G. T., Klein, P. D., Showalter, R. B. and Kern, F. Jr. (1982). A method for the accurate measurement of isotope ratios of chenodeoxycholic and cholic acids in serum. *J. Lipid Res.*, **23**, 204

27. Rudman, D. and Kendall, F. E. (1957). Bile acid content of human serum. 1. Serum bile acids in patients with hepatic disease. *J. Clin. Invest.*, **36**, 530

28. Sampson, D. G., Murphy, G. M., Cross, L. M., and Catty, D. (1979). Specificity and cross reactivity in bile acid radioimmunoassays. *Anal. Letters.*, **12**, 927

29. Sjövall, J. and Vihko, R. (1966). Chromatography of conjugated steroids on lipophilic Sephadex. *Acta Chem. Scand.*, **20**, 1419

30. Ellingboe, J., Almé, B. and Sjövall, J. (1970). Introduction of specific groups into poly-saccharide supports for liquid chromatography. *Acta Chem. Scand.*, **24**, 463

31. Almé, B. and Nyström, E. (1971). Preparation of lipophilic anion exchangers from chlorohydroxypropylated Sephadex and cellulose. *J. Chromatogr.*, **59**, 45

32. Setchell, K. D. R., Almé, B., Axelson, M. and Sjövall, J. (1976). The multicomponent analysis of conjugates of neutral steroids in urine by lipophilic ion exchange chromato-graphy and computerized gas chromatography–mass spectrometry. *J. Steroid Biochem.*, **7**, 615

33. Ellingboe, J., Nyström, E. and Sjövall, J. (1970). Liquid-gel chromatography on lipophilic-hydrophobic Sephadex derivatives. *J. Lipid Res.*, **11**, 266

34. Setchell, K. D. R. and Matsui, A. (1982). Serum bile acid analysis – The application of liquid–gel chromatographic techniques and capillary column gas chromatography and mass spectrometry. *Clin. Chim. Acta* (In press)

35. Setchell, K. D. R., Lawson, A. M., Tanida, N. and Sjövall, J. (1982). General methods for the analysis of metabolic profiles of bile acids and related compounds in feces. *J. Lipid Res.* (In press)

36. Smith, S. M., Loria, P., Setchell, K. D. R. and Murphy, G. M. (1982). The measurement of unconjugated bile acids in normal serum. *J. Clin. Pathol.* (In press)

37. Dyfverman, A. and Sjövall, J. (1978). A novel liquid-gel chromatographic method for extraction of unconjugated steroids from aqueous solutions. *Anal. Lett.*, **B11**, 485

38. Dyfverman, A. and Sjövall, J. (1978). Liquid-gel extraction of bile acids. In Paumgartner, G., Stiehl, A. and Gerok, W. (eds.) *Proceedings of 26th Falk Symposium. Biological effects of bile acids*, pp. 281–286. (Lancaster: MTP Press)

39. Nair, P. P. (1969). Enzymatic cleavage of bile acid conjugates. In Schiff, L., Carey, J. B. and Dietschy, J. (eds.) *Bile Salt Metabolism*, pp. 172–183. (Springfield: Il.: C. C. Thomas)

40. Nair, P. P. and Garcia, C. C. (1969). A modified gas liquid chromatographic procedure for the rapid determination of bile acids in biological fluids. *Anal. Biochem.*, **29**, 164

41. Setchell, K. D. R., Lawson, A. M., Blackstock, E. J. and Murphy, G. M. (1981). Meal induced absorption of newly formed secondary bile acids in normal man. *Clin. Sci.*, **60**, 23

42. Setchell, K. D. R., Lawson, A. M., Blackstock, E. J. and Murphy, G. M. (1982). Diurnal changes in serum unconjugated bile acids in normal man. *Gut*, **23**, 353

43. Lewis, B., Panveliwalla, D., Tabaqchali, S. and Wootton, D. P. (1969). Serum bile acids in the stagnant loop syndrome. *Lancet*, **1**, 219

44. Makino, I., Nakagawa, S. and Mashimo, K. (1969). Conjugated and unconjugated serum bile acid levels in patients with hepatobiliary diseases. *Gastroenterology*, **56**, 1033

45. Makita, M. and Wells, W. W. (1963). Quantitative analysis of fecal bile acids by gas-liquid chromatography. *Anal. Biochem.*, **5**, 523

46. Barnes, S., Billing, B. H. and Morris, J. S. (1976). Effect of fasting and ileal resection on the concentration of deoxycholic acid in rat portal blood. *Proc. Soc. Exp. Biol. Med.*, **152**, 292

47. Schlenk, H. and Gellerman, J. L. (1960). Esterification of fatty acids with diazomethane on a small scale. *Anal. Chem.*, **32**, 1412

48. Roovers, R. E., Evrard, E. and Vanderhaeghe, H. (1968). An improved method for measuring human blood bile acids. *Clin. Chim. Acta*, **19**, 449

49. Miyazaki, H., Ishibashi, M. and Yamashita, K. (1978). Use of a new silylating agent for separation of bile acids and cholesterol by selected ion monitoring with the computer

controlled intensity matching technique. *Biomed. Mass Spectrometry*, **5**, 469

50. Barnes, S., Pritchard, D.G., Settine, R.L. and Geckle, M. (1980). Preparation and characterization of permethylated derivatives of bile acids and their application to gas chromatographic analysis. *J. Chromatogr.*, **183**, 269

51. Shackleton, C.H.L., Taylor, N.F. and Honour, J.W. (1980). *An atlas of gas chromatographic profiles of neutral urinary steroids in health and disease.* (Packard–Becker)

52. Laatikainen, T. and Hesso, A. (1975). Determination of serum bile acids by glass capillary gas–liquid chromatography. *Clin. Chim Acta*, **64**, 63

53. Karlaganis, G. and Paumgartner, G. (1978). Analysis of bile acids in serum and bile by capillary column gas–liquid chromatography. *J. Lipid Res.*, **19**, 771

54. Karlaganis, G., Schwarzenbach, R.P. and Paumgartner, G. (1980). Analysis of serum bile acids by capillary gas–liquid chromatography–mass spectrometry. *J. Lipid Res.*, **21**, 377

55. Karlaganis, G. and Paumgartner, G. (1979). Determination of bile acids in serum by capillary column gas–liquid chromatography. *Clin. Chim. Acta*, **92**, 19

56. Jennings, W. (1980). *Gas chromatography with glass capillary columns.* (New York: Academic Press)

57. Van den Berg, P.M.J. and Cox, T.P.H. (1972). All glass solid sampling device for open tubular columns in gas chromatography. *Chromatographia*, **5**, 301

58. Shackleton, C.H.L. and Honour, J.W. (1976). Simultaneous estimation of urinary steroids by semi-automated gas chromatography. Investigation of neonatal infants and children with abnormal steroid synthesis. *Clin. Chim. Acta*, **69**, 267

59. Bremmelgaard, A. and Almé, B. (1980). Analysis of plasma bile acid profiles in patients with liver disease associated with cholestasis. *Scand. J. Gastroenterol.*, **15**, 593

60. Bartholomew, T.C., Summerfield, J.A., Billing, B.H., Lawson, A.M. and Setchell, K.D.R. (1982). Bile acid profiles of human serum and skin interstitial fluid and their relationship to pruritus studied by gas chromatography–mass spectrometry. *Clin. Sci.*, **63**, 65

2
Measurement of the physical–chemical properties of bile salt solutions

MARTIN C. CAREY

INTRODUCTION

This chapter provides a brief critical overview of the techniques employed to probe the physical–chemical properties of bile salt solutions. Since the laws of physics and chemistry are also valid in the biological world, an understanding of the solution properties of bile salts both as simple solutions and when mixed with other macromolecules is central to understanding their physiological functions. It is also clear that an appreciation of the malfunction of bile salts is forthcoming from a knowledge of their physical–chemical properties under pathophysiological conditions.

PHASE EQUILIBRIA AND THE PHASE RULE

The fundamental thermodynamic reference condition of any physical–chemical system is the equilibrium state. A *system* is a defined part of the physical universe, i.e. a substance or mixture of substances isolated in some way from all other substances. At *equilibrium*, a system is at its lowest free energy, that is, is incapable of doing work. Equilibrium involving more than one physically distinct part of a system is called *heterogeneous equilibrium*. For the systematization of heterogeneous equilibria, the US physicist J. Willard Gibbs during 1873–78 theoretically derived the Phase Rule on the basis of *a priori* thermodynamic principles. This Rule represents an important milestone in the history of science, and is valid for all macroscopic systems which are in a state of heterogeneous equilibrium irrespective of whether equilibrium is physical or chemical. Over the past few decades the Rule has found major applications in physics, chemistry, geology, metallurgy, mineralogy and, more recently, in biology. The Phase Rule may be stated as follows:

$$F = C - P + 2$$

19

where F is *Degrees of Freedom, or Variance* of the system, that is the *minimum* number of *variables* of temperature (symbol T), pressure (symbol Π) and concentration that must be fixed in order to define the system, i.e. in order to fix the intensive properties (properties independent of quantity or size, e.g., density, refractive index) of all phases; C is the number of *Components* or *Order* of the system, that is the *smallest* number of *independently variable chemical constituents* required to account for the composition of each and every phase present; and P is the number of *Phases* in the system, that is the number of *homogeneous, mechanically separable*, portions of a system. All parts of a phase are identical in intensive properties. Although a phase must be homogeneous it need not be continuous; crushed ice is an example. Table 2.1 shows some typical systems, with a tabulation of the number of components present and the maximum number of possible phases.

Table 2.1 Examples of systems

System	No. of components	Maximum No. of phases
The water system	1 – H_2O (H_3O^+ and OH^- are not independently variable)	3 – Solid (ice), liquid, vapour (gas)
The air system	⟩ 5 – $O_2/N_2/CO_2/Ar/He$ ...	1 – All gases are miscible
Saturated NaCl solution	2 – $NaCl/H_2O$	4 – Two solids (pure H_2O as ice and the compound $NaCl \cdot 2H_2O$), liquid (NaCl dissolved in H_2O) and vapour (H_2O)
$Hg/CCl_4/H_2O$	3 – $Hg/CCl_4/H_2O$	4 – Three immiscible liquids plus one vapour
$CaCO_3/CO_2/CaO$	2 – CaO/CO_2 ($CaCO_3$ can be described as 50% CaO and 50% CO_2)	3 – Two solids ($CaCO_3$, CaO) and 1 vapour (CO_2)

One of the simplest possible systems is the water system where one component (H_2O) is present throughout all phases. Thus, there are no concentration variables and therefore a plot of pressure versus temperature suffices to determine the state of the system (Figure 2.1). Within the limits of $\Pi \langle 2000$ atm and $T \rangle -40\,^\circ C$ only one solid phase is possible, that is, ordinary ice. Liquid water and its vapour constitute the other possible phases. Within any of the three single-phase regions, ice, liquid or vapour, e.g. A in Figure 2.1, Π and T can be independently varied without a second phase appearing. This can be predicted by the phase rule (Figure 2.1); when for $P=1$ and $C=1$, it follows that $F=2$. Such a system is said to be *bivariant*.

At any point on one of the three linear phase boundaries, i.e. freezing (fusion), sublimation or boiling (vaporization) curves (e.g. B) two phases are in equilibrium. It is obvious from Figure 2.1 that to maintain this relationship a variation in Π or T will automatically fix the other variable, thus Π or T can be varied but *not* independently. As deduced from the phase rule, $P=2$ and $C=1$, therefore $F=1$. Such a system is said to be *univariant*. On curve B, the normal boiling point of water is $T=100\,°C$ at $\Pi=760\,\text{mmHg}$. By extending this curve to $\Pi=218\,\text{atm}$ and $T=374\,°C$, the vapour and liquid become indistinguishable – this is the *critical point* of water. *Supercritical fluids* have properties of both gases *and* liquids.

At point C, solid, liquid and vapour are in equilibrium. To maintain three phases in equilibrium neither Π nor T can be varied, that is at the one temperature, ice and water have the same fixed vapour pressure. As predicted by the phase rule (Figure 2.1), $C=1$ and $P=3$, therefore $F=0$. Such a system is said to be *invariant*. This *triple point* of water at $T=0.0098\,°C$ and $\Pi=4.58\,\text{mmHg}$ is a fundamental constant for the water system and its values cannot be changed in any way. It is so accurately defined $(\pm0.0001\,°C)$ that it is now used as a fixed point on the International Temperature Scale rather than the melting point of ice under atmospheric conditions. The phase diagram also predicts that at Π values below the triple point ($<4.58\,\text{mmHg}$) the liquid phase never appears at any value of T. Hence, with an increase in T across the sublimination curve, there is a direct transition from the solid ice phase to the vapour phase. This phenomenon is put to practical use in freeze-drying.

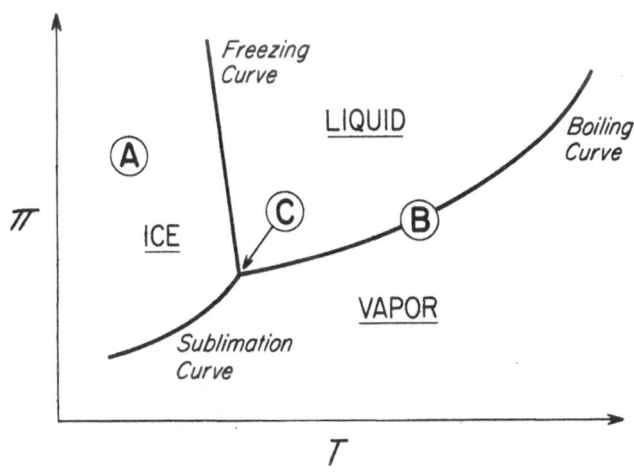

$$F = C - P + 2 \qquad THE\ PHASE\ RULE$$

(A) $F = 1 - 1 + 2$ π and T can be varied independently $(F=2)$

(B) $F = 1 - 2 + 2$ π or T can be varied but <u>not</u> independently $(F=1)$

(C) $F = 1 - 3 + 2$ π and T cannot be varied $(F=0)$

Figure 2.1 Phase equilibria for the solid, liquid and vapour states of a 1-component (water) system and its analysis by the Phase Rule (see text)

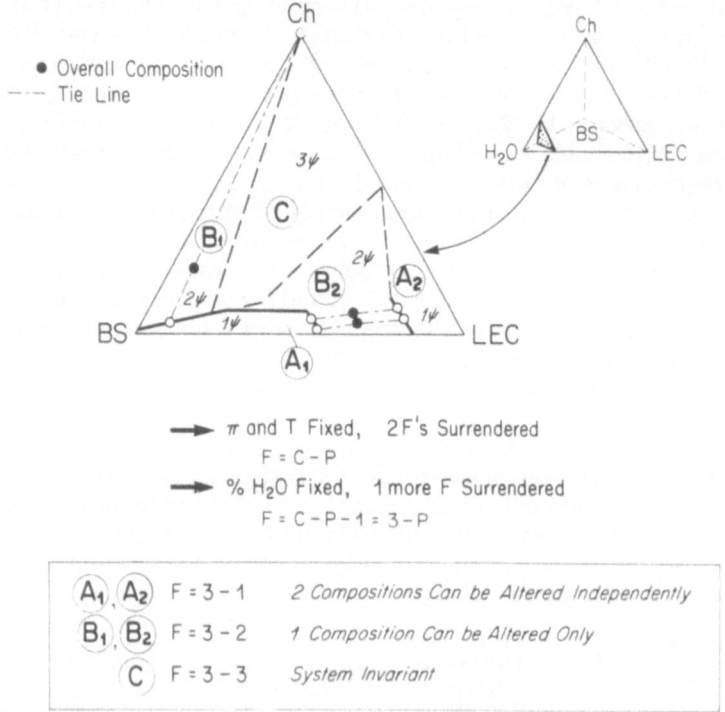

Figure 2.2 Phase equilibria for the solid, liquid (micellar) and liquid–crystalline states of the four-component (bile) system and its analysis by the Phase Rule (see text)

An example of a complex and important biological system is displayed in Figure 2.2, that is, the 'Bile' system. Bile may be simplified to a four-component system containing the independently variable chemical species, H_2O, bile salts, cholesterol and lecithin at 1 atm (isobaric) and 37 °C (isothermal). Thus the variables of temperature and pressure are assigned fixed values from the outset. Such a four-component system is represented in three dimensions as a regular tetrahedron (Figure 2.2, upper right). However, since gallbladder bile contains, on the average, 90% H_2O, this concentration variable is also fixed so that the system reduces to a three-component system of bile salt, lecithin and cholesterol. Thus, a section of the solid model (Figure 2.2) rather than the model itself becomes more convenient for graphic representation. By bringing together various proportions of these substances (in 90% water) and isolating and analysing the phases at equilibrium we can plot the compositions, phases and phase relationships of model 'bile' in two dimensions on an equilateral triangle whose axes represent the solid components only. Because the vapour phase is ignored, the phase diagram is also said to be 'condensed'. Since Π, T and percentage water are fixed for this system, three degrees of freedom are surrendered from the beginning. Hence, the phase rule reduces to:

$$F = C - P$$

where C represents the number of *solid* components, i.e. three. Because percentage H_2O is fixed, an excess water phase cannot be considered as one of the separate coexisting phases on the triangular coordinate plot. As shown in Figure 2.2, this phase diagram defines 2 one-phase (symbol ψ) areas, 2 two-phase areas and 1 three-phase area.

In the one-phase areas, two compositions can be altered independently and the systems remain single phases. In the two-phase areas, only one composition can be altered independently and in the three-phase area the system is invariant, that is, every composition falling within this area is composed of three phases, each with an absolutely *fixed* composition. Within the two-phase areas are shown a series of *tie-lines*. These lines designate compositions of coexisting phases (open circles) which are included in the overall compositions of the phases which they intersect (closed circles). Thus the tie-line in B_1 shows that, at equilibrium, the overall composition described by the closed circle is composed of a saturated micellar phase coexisting with a phase composed of solid cholesterol (monohydrate) crystals. In B_2, the tie-lines show that the compositions represented by the closed circles are composed of coexisting saturated micellar phases (open circles, left) and saturated liposomal (liquid crystalline) phases (open circles, right). The former tie-line is directly applicable to the physical state of cholesterol gallstone containing bile at equilibrium and the latter tie-lines to the equilibrium physical state of bile during established fat digestion.

Historically, the phase rule was used to determine C from experimentally observed values of P and F, and systems were then classified as being 1C, 2C and so forth. With systems containing a small number of components, C is usually known, P can be obtained experimentally and then F can be employed to verify or disprove the numbers of phases. As systems become more complex (three or more C), this application of the Phase Rule increases in value since it can be employed to verify that certain coexisting phases are impossible. Different systems of *identical variance* usually exhibit analogous behaviour no matter how dissimilar the systems may outwardly appear. If the phase rule is apparently 'disobeyed', the reason is that C, P and/or F are identified incorrectly or (more commonly) the system is not at *equilibrium*.

The state of true equilibrium can be tested by a number of well-established criteria: (a) true equilibrium is sensitive to change of external conditions; (b) the equilibrium concentrations are independent of time and (c) are independent of the masses of the phases; (d) identical equilibrium concentrations and states are reached when equilibrium is approached from at least two directions. An example is solubilization in a micellar system where equilibrium can be approached from the supersaturated state and from the unsaturated state.

CRITICAL MICELLAR CONCENTRATION (CMC)

Bile salts are soluble amphiphiles, that is, soluble molecules which are partly hydrophilic (literally, 'water loving') and partly hydrophobic (literally, 'water fearing'). In dilute solution such molecules exhibit a phenomenon known as the CMC, which is the concentration at which the maximum molecular (monomeric) solubility is reached and molecular aggregation begins to occur. These molecular aggregates are termed *micelles*. Micelles are defined as small thermodynamically stable aggregates, whose individual molecules are in constant dynamic equilibrium with neighbouring micelles via a surrounding aqueous medium containing bile salt monomers *at* a concentration equivalent to the CMC. The average number of monomers in a bile salt micelle is called the aggregation number ($Ag\#$ or $\bar{n}$). This number is not fixed but can vary from 2 to over 100, depending on the bile salt species and physical–chemical conditions. The aggregation number multiplied by the molecular weight of the bile salt monomer is termed the micellar molecular weight (M.M.W.).

The importance of the CMC and micellization is central to the physiological function of bile salts, since micelles exhibit the properties of solubilization and detergency. *Solubilization* involves the presence of bile salt micelles that can incorporate, within or upon themselves, otherwise insoluble substances – e.g. insoluble lipids, proteins, polysaccharides, polymers, and so forth. Thermodynamically, *micellization* reflects the desire of the hydrophobic part of a soluble amphiphile to decrease its contact with water. The interaction of bile salts with other hydrophobic surfaces such as receptors, membranes, proteins, polymers, etc. is governed by similar thermodynamic forces. In an aqueous system, bile salt monomers exhibit surface and interfacial activity, whereas micelles and bile salts already bound to surfaces or receptors are not surface active.

Experimental methods for estimating the CMCs of bile salt solutions can be divided into two broad categories: (1) non-invasive methods, which require no physical or chemical additive. These depend purely on the colligative properties of the system, i.e. properties related to the number of particles, measured as a function of bile salt concentration; and (2) invasive methods, which require an additive. An additive is usually an easily measured 'reporter' molecule which changes in some physical–chemical property in the presence of micelles. By definition this adds another component to the bile salt system and this usually alters the monomer–micelle equilibrium. The following methods have been employed to measure the CMC of bile salt solutions:

(A) Non-invasive methods (no additives)
    (1) Surface tension:
        (i) Wilhelmy blade or plate – equilibrium method
        (ii) Maximum bubble pressure
        (iii) Hanging drop   (All non-equilibrium
        (iv) Capillary rise   or dynamic methods)
        (v) Du Noüy ring

(2) Electrical conductivity.
(3) Classical light scattering (turbidimetry).
(4) Micellar spectral change (intrinsic UV spectrum).
(5) Other: (i) osmometry; (ii) calorimetry; (iii) self-diffusion; (iv) ion-specific electrodes; (v) refractive index; (vi) densimetry (molar volumes); (vii) electromotive force; (viii) ultrafiltration; (ix) ultracentrifugation; (x) electron spin resonance; (xi) nuclear magnetic resonance; (xii) sound velocity and absorption.

(B) Invasive methods (with additives)
(1) Spectral change (λ-max, absorbance, fluorescence) of a water-*soluble* dye: methyl orange (cationic), rhodamine 6G (cationic), pinacyanol (cationic), bilirubin IXα (anionic), anilino-naphthalene sulphonate (anionic).
(2) Solubilization of a water-*insoluble* dye or lipid: azobenzene, dansylcadaverine, phenylnaphthalenamine, naphthalene, methylcholanthrene, orange OT, azulene, testosterone (and its derivatives) xylene, griseofulvin, hexestrol, cholesterol, 1-monoolein, fatty acids (including fatty acid nitroxides).
(3) Interfacial tension at liquid–liquid interfaces: toluene–water, vaseline oil–water.
(4) Partition coefficients between aqueous and non-polar phases: 1-octanol-water; 1-octanol/iso-octane-water; iso-octane/chloroform-water.

Ideally, only non-invasive methods should be employed to estimate the CMC of bile salts, but unfortunately, most of these are laborious and technically difficult. The spectral shift of a water-soluble dye (e.g., rhodamine 6G) is fast and technically easy to perform. With the common bile salts, the method gives values within 1–2 mmol/l (on the lower side) of values obtained by most non-invasive methods. Further, in the case of uncommon bile salts, it is extremely useful for defining the possible range of CMC values before the more laborious and rigorous non-invasive methods are attempted. In the author's laboratory the following methods are in use:

(A) Facile; spectral shift (rhodamine 6G, bilirubin at pH ⟩ 9.0).
(B) Intermediate:
(1) Wilhelmy plate – surface tension.
(2) classical light scattering.

(C) Laborious; electrical conductivity.

Since each technique probes a somewhat different colligative property of a bile salt solution, the CMC values derived by two or three techniques are rarely in absolute agreement.

The equilibrium (Wilhelmy) surface tension method gives an accurate estimate of the CMC and, in addition, provides other information on bile salt micellization. A brief account of the physics of surfaces is germane to the understanding of surface tension. Liquids have a surface (interface) between the bulk liquid and another phase, commonly air. A surface occurs when the kinetic energy of molecules is counteracted by strong cohesive forces between molecules. Since a surface is two-dimensional and the bulk liquid three-dimensional, the forces of repulsion and attraction acting on molecules in each state are different (Figure 2.3).

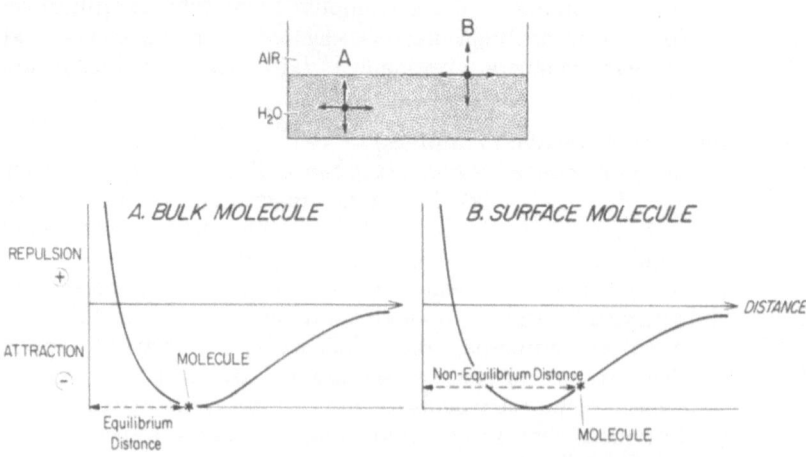

Figure 2.3 Schematic representation of the forces acting on a water molecule at the surface and in the bulk of liquid water. (A) Potential energy–distance diagram for a water molecule in the bulk. (B) Potential energy–distance diagram for a water molecule at the air–water interface

Molecules in the bulk experience the same net forces of attraction and repulsion in all directions. At equilibrium there is no net repulsion, and no net attraction and the potential energy of a molecule in the bulk is shown as a minimum on the curve of potential energy plotted against distance (Figure 2.3(a)). At the surface (Figure 2.3), there are no strong forces attracting from above, so that there is a net inward force acting on the surface molecules. This causes surface molecules to leave the surface and enter the bulk solution. For an infinitesimal amount of time, the spacing between neighbouring molecules in the surface becomes slightly greater. As shown by the potential energy–distance diagram (Figure 2.3(b)), the spacing between nearest neighbour surface molecules is increased and the molecules thereby gain a positive free energy which is expended continually in doing work by *shrinking* the surface. This is loosely equivalent to the existence of a tension in the surface, i.e. surface tension. While surface tension has a physical reality, i.e. the force in dynes acting along the surface of a liquid at right angles to any line 1 cm in length, the tension is really the result of the dissipation of surface free energy with which it is numerically and dimensionally equal ($1 \, erg/cm^2 \equiv 1 \, dyn/cm$). In the Wilhelmy method, surface tension is measured by extending the surface by a known area and actually weighing the surface as shown in Figure 2.4(b)). The numerical value for surface tension is then derived by equating the total area of new surface multiplied by γ (the surface energy or tension) to the weight (mass × the gravitational constant, symbol g) of the surface measured (Figure 2.4(d)).

In estimating the CMC of a bile salt by surface tension, the surface of the solution is employed to report on phenomena occurring in the bulk. By diffusing from the bulk, bile salt molecules align at the surface and decrease the surface cohesion; this results in a fall in surface tension in proportion to the surface concentration of bile salts. If the surface measurements are to report accurately on events in the bulk the surface molecules must be in equilibrium with those in the bulk. Since all methods of measuring surface tension require an expansion of the existing surface, it is obvious that the surface tension must be measured against time until stable equilibrium values are obtained (Figure 2.4(c)). Often, these bulky amphiphilic molecules take a considerable time (e.g., hours) to reach a stable concentration at the surface and hence surface tension–time curves must be obtained. These curves are measured conveniently by the Wilhelmy blade method. However, all other methods are not designed to measure surface tension versus time; as such they are dynamic and non-equilibrium techniques and their use can lead to large errors in the estimation of CMC. Further, in the case of bile salts, it is not possible to employ a fixed time of equilibration, since the rate of surface ageing depends, *inter alia*, on bile salt concentration, hydrophilic–hydro-

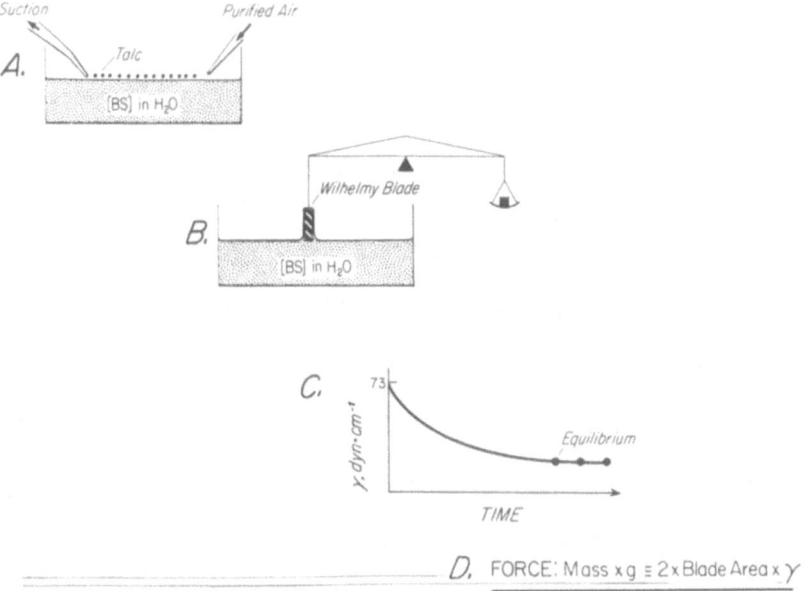

Figure 2.4 Steps in the measurement of equilibrium surface tension of bile salt solutions by means of the Wilhelmy blade method. (A) Sweeping and cleaning the talc-marked surface by means of a fine suction-line and air-jet. (B) Wetting of Wilhelmy blade and 'weighing' the surface. (C) Monitoring changes in surface tension as a function of time to obtain equilibrium values. (D) Calculation of equilibrium surface tension (γ)

phobic balance of bile salts, the critical micellar concentration, ionic strength and experimental temperature. Thus, the practice of using constant equilibrium times which cut across different surface-tension–time curves will lead to non-systematic errors. As shown in Figure 2.4(a) the cleaning of the surface of surface-active contaminants is an important preliminary to the measurement of surface tension.

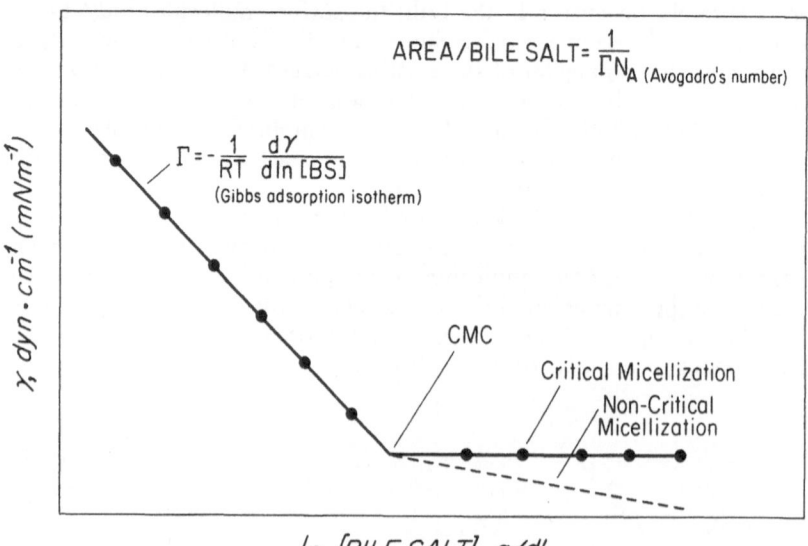

In [BILE SALT], g/dl

Figure 2.5 Mathematical analysis of plots of surface tension versus logarithm of bile salt concentration. Γ represents the surface excess concentration of the bile salt monolayer (g/cm²) (see text)

Figure 2.5 shows a schematic plot of equilibrium surface tension versus logarithm of bile salt concentration. With increasing bile salt concentration, surface tension falls in a linear fashion from a value somewhat less than that for water (about 73 dyn.cm⁻¹) to about 45–55 dyn.cm⁻¹. At the lowest surface tension, a sharp inflection point occurs because the surface is now saturated with bile salt monomers. Further addition of bile salts leads only to a slight depression in surface tension. The bile salt concentration at the intersection of the steep and horizontal curves corresponds approximately to the CMC in the bulk. Examination of the surface using radiotracers suggests that micelle formation can take place in the bulk at a concentration somewhat lower than that corresponding to surface saturation. From the steep slope of the curve, the surface excess concentration can be obtained employing the Gibbs adsorption isotherm. The area per bile salt molecule at the interface can then be derived utilizing the surface excess concentration and Avogadro's number (Figure 2.5). This surface area should correspond to a value which falls between 80 and 95 Å² corresponding to the area of a steroid nucleus lying flat. If a reasonable value is not obtained, the most likely explanation is that the surface molecules were not in equilibrium with the bulk molecules. At concentrations greater than the CMC, the slope of the curve gives a rough indication as to whether critical or non-critical micellization occurs (Figure 2.5). As will be discussed below, there are more precise methods for making this distinction.

Figure 2.6 provides a critical inventory of literature CMC data for four bile salts, unconjugated cholate (C) and deoxycholate (DC) and their corresponding taurine (T) conjugates, grouped as functions of their reported $\bar{n}$ values at the CMC. These data show that when $\bar{n}$ is small, the 'CMC' values by both invasive and non-invasive methods are scattered with the invasive techniques tending, in general, to give higher values. This is presumably due to the fact that when $\bar{n}$ (CMC) is small, continuous self-association continues above this concentration and as a result the initial solubilization of large hydrophobic solubilizates often begins well above the 'true' (non-invasive) CMC. In the case of bile salts with larger $\bar{n}$ (CMC) values, e.g. NaTDC (Figure 2.6), both invasive and non-invasive techniques

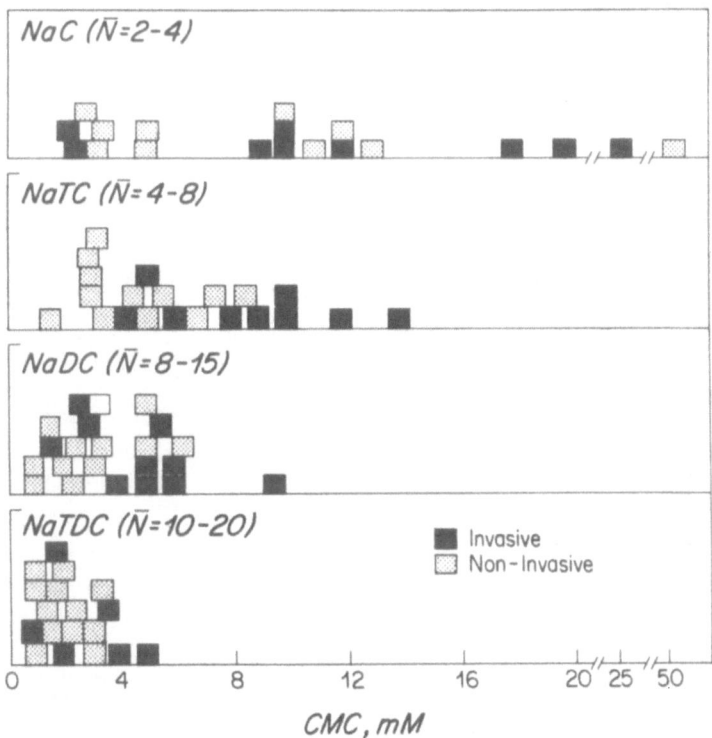

Figure 2.6 Critical inventory of literature critical micellar concentrations (CMCs) by a large variety of methods for sodium cholate (NaC), sodium taurocholate (NaTC), sodium deoxycholate (NaDC) and sodium taurodeoxycholate (NaTDC). Most reported values are for 0.15 mol/l Na$^+$, 25 °C at appropriate pH (see text)

tend to be in agreement. Since the ratio of solubilizate to solubilizer ('saturation ratio') in micellar solutions is often of the order 1:100–1:1500, large insoluble hydrophobic additives do not usually *alter* the intrinsic CMC of a bile salt solution (see below). Further, since $\bar{n}$ (CMC) is apparently not altered by these additives, only a small fraction of micelles can bind the solubilizate at any one time. The major exception to this rule is bile salt solubilization of insoluble swelling amphiphilic lipids, such as phospho- and glycolipids, 'acid soaps', monoglycerides, etc., which is discussed in the next section.

The mixed bile salt micelles of relevance to bile are lecithin/bile salt (L/BS) micelles. The measurement of their CMCs (more correctly, the intermicellar *monomeric* bile salt concentration, IMC) is more difficult since techniques involving dilution alter the L/BS ratio in the mixed micelles and alter the IMC. It has been shown theoretically and experimentally (Figure 2.7) that the IMC lies below the CMC of the pure bile salt and decreases in proportion to the insoluble amphiphile/bile salt ratio. Once the L/BS micellar phase limit is passed, liquid crystalline liposomes form, and the IMC tends to approach a constant value asymptotically (Figure 2.7). General methods for estimating the IMC of mixed bile salt micelles are: (a) equilibrium dialysis and its variants; (b) ultrafiltration; (c) bile salt selective electrodes; (d) ultracentrifugation; (e) preservation of micellar size (by light-scattering)

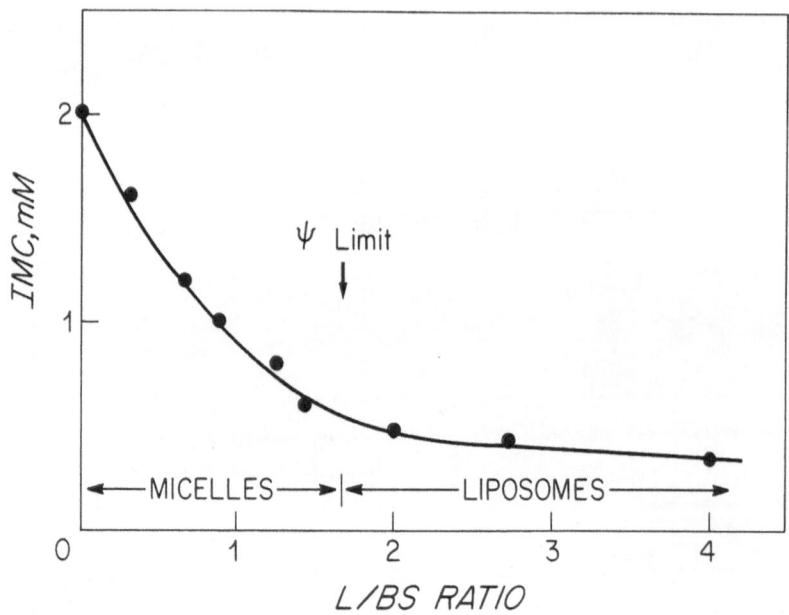

Figure 2.7 Intermicellar (monomeric) bile salt concentration for the TDC-lecithin system as estimated by equilibrium dialysis (Conditions: pH 7, 2 mmol/l Tris-maleate, 1 mmol/l CaCl$_2$, 150 mmol/l NaCl, 0.2% NaN$_3$, 25 °C, starting [TDC] = 12 mmol/l). ψ limit indicates phase limit of the TDC-lecithin micellar phase, L/BS ratio represents the ratio in the particles. (After references 25, 43 and 61.)

when diluted with the IMC; (f) plots of $C_{BS} = \alpha^{-1} C_L + IMC$, where $\alpha = L/BS$ at the macroscopic phase limit and C represents BS and L concentrations. All of these methods perturb the system in some way, hence the development of more accurate methods is required.

Elevation in temperature, and addition of organic solvents such as ethanol, tend to elevate both the CMC and IMC, whereas conjugation with either glycine or taurine, increases in ionic strength, pressure, addition of insoluble swelling amphiphiles (monoolein, 'acid soaps', lecithin, etc.) and a fall in pH, (which protonates bile salts to bile acids) tend to lower the CMC or IMC values. Qualitative and quantitative thermodynamic treatments of some of these effects are given elsewhere (see reading list).

CRITICAL MICELLAR TEMPERATURE (CMT)

As with conventional detergents, bile salts exhibit a typical temperature (CMT) to which a given mixture of bile salt and water must be raised to transform the detergent from a suspension of crystals (or a gel) to a clear micellar phase. For most of the common bile salts, water freezes before the detergent 'freezes', hence the CMT lies below 0 °C. For most of the monohydroxy bile salts including their sulphates (Figure 2.8) and certain uncommon dihydroxy bile salts such as 7α, 12α-dihydroxy-5β-cholanoates and 3α, 6α-dihydroxy-5β-cholanoates (hyodeoxycholates), this temperature may lie above body temperature (Figure 2.8). The Krafft point is not synonymous with the CMT, but should be restricted to the CMT *at* the CMC. Hence, in a two-component system the Krafft point is a triple point where the CMC, CMT and monomeric solubilities intersect. Since at the Krafft point three phases are in equilibrium and since Π is fixed, the phase rule gives an invariant ($F=0$) system, since $F=2-3+1$.

The CMT phenomenon may be explained on the basis of the coupling between the monomer–hydrated solid equilibrium *and* the monomer-micelle equilibrium. This implies that as a suspension of bile salt crystals in water is heated, the monomeric solubility increases along the monomeric solubility curve in Figure 2.8. Once the CMC is reached (dashed curve, Figure 2.8), the system attempts to continue to increase its monomeric solubility, but cannot do so owing to the flow of monomeric bile salts into micelles. Hence, the bile salt solubility curve demonstrates a sharp break at the Krafft point because all monomers leaving the crystals are at concentrations above the CMC. The traditional explanation given for the CMT phenomenon is that the hydrocarbon part of the amphiphile becomes 'melted' at the temperature of the CMT. This is obviously incorrect since the fused steroid skeleton of bile salts is as rigid below the CMT as above it. More correctly stated, the crystals 'melt' at the CMT because the monomers rapidly flow down a concentration gradient from crystals into micelles. In contrast to classic detergents, the CMT of bile salts shows a marked positive slope with increases in bile salt concentration. It can be shown theoretically and experimentally that this is a function of micellar size, i.e. the smaller the micelle at the CMC, the greater the positive slope and this is further evidence

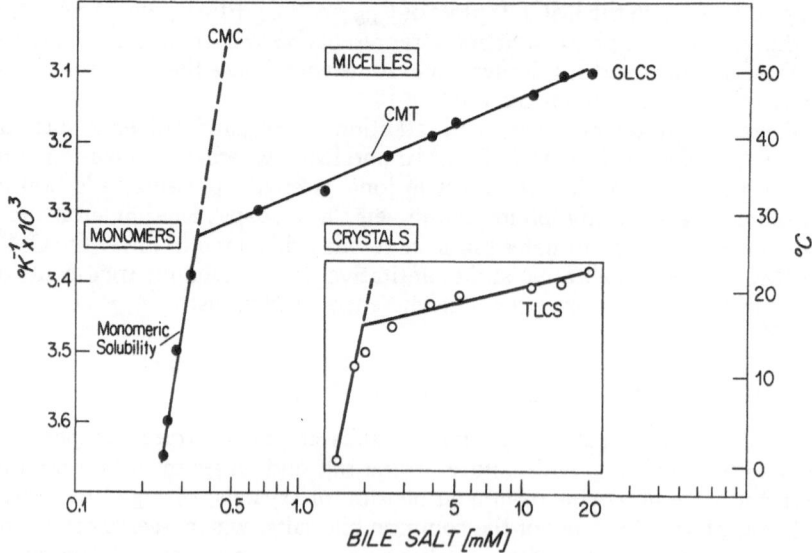

Figure 2.8 Phase equilibria of the disodium salts of sulphated monohydroxy bile salts, glyco-lithocholate sulphate (GLCS at pH 10.0) and taurolithocholate sulphate (TLCS at pH 7.0, inset). The solid solubility curve and the interrupted CMC curve demarcate areas when crystals and monomers, micelles and monomers, and monomers alone are found. The critical micellar temperature (CMT) represents the equilibrium between micelles and hydrated crystals connected via the monomer concentration at the CMC. The Krafft Point is a triple point and only represents the CMT at the CMC (after Carey, Wu and Watkins[51]; see text)

for non-cooperative self-association with certain bile salt species.

The CMT of bile salts is measured by the equilibrium clearing point method. In such an experiment the temperature of clarification of an aqueous suspension of bile salt crystals is monitored by light scattering or other optical methods. In order to obtain equilibrium CMT values it is necessary to buffer the system to an appropriate pH to ensure complete ionization, to have extremely slow rates of temperature elevation (about 1 °C/h) and to agitate constantly. Because of super-cooling in detergent–water systems, the equilibrium CMT of bile salts cannot be obtained by cooling to the CMT no matter how slowly the temperature is reduced.

MICELLAR SIZE AND POLYDISPERSITY

The average size of bile salt micelles and the distribution of micellar sizes around this mean value are important physical–chemical characteristics of a bile salt solution. Traditional methods for characterizing micellar size (listed below) all suffer from some limitations. The most restrictive disadvantage is that most methods require measurement at several finite concentrations, followed by linear extrapolation of these values to the CMC. Micellar sizes so derived are therefore only applicable to just above the CMC, and depend, *inter alia*, on an accurate determination of the CMC. Further, all these methods are insensitive to micellar polydispersity.

Conventional Methods	*Limitations*
Ultracentrifugation (equilibrium, sedimentation)	Buoyancy factor $(1 - \bar{v}\varrho) \cong 1$. Perturbation from charge separation of co-ions and counterions. Electrostatic effects from micelle–micelle interactions. Micellar size is a function of lipid concentration through the sedimentation profile. $\bar{v}$ (partial specific volume) and ϱ (solution density) must be accurately determined.
Conventional light scattering $(\bar{I} \propto \text{M.M.W.} \times C - \text{CMC})$	Micelles and electrolyte concentration must be progressively diluted. Corrections for micelle–micelle and thermodynamic preferential interactions required. (Being highly charged, bile salt micelles do not interact as 'hard spheres' when they collide, they repel one another, thereby increasing $\bar{I}$). Solution clarification is a major problem.
Tracer (free) diffusion to obtain D (diffusion coefficient)	Very long measurement times. Microbial contamination. Major effects from micelle–micelle (non-hard sphere) interactions at low (< 0.4 mol/l) ionic strengths; therefore high ionic strengths required.
Osmometry (vapour pressure, membrane)	Membranes are not impermeable to micelles owing to monomer–micelle equilibrium. True equilibrium cannot be attained. Counterions and added neutral electrolyte contribute significantly to osmotic pressure.
Gel filtration	Large dilution effects on the micellar concentrations. Bile salt monomers adhere to gel bed. Charge effects between micelles and counterions. Equilibration of column with bile salt concentrations $>$ IMC or CMC required.
Small-angle X-ray scattering	Electron charge density between micelles and solvent is small. $\bar{R}_g$ (radius of gyration) obtained by measurements at different detergent concentrations followed by extrapolation to the CMC.
Electron microscopy	Entails dehydration – with ensuing phase changes in the micellar solution.

With the advent of the laser, an important, and highly versatile method, called quasielastic light scattering (QLS), was developed. QLS offers a number of important advantages (see below) for determining micellar size and polydispersity, one of the most crucial being that micellar growth within the micellar phase can be accurately probed for the first time. Hence, QLS can provide information on micellar size and polydispersity at physiologically relevant bile salt concentrations ($< 1-20\,g/dl$).

QLS: Advantages

(1) Permits an accurate measurement of D (diffusion coefficient) at high bile salt concentrations. Therefore dilution and extrapolation to the CMC are not required.

(2) Permits measurements in metastable states.

(3) Provides size and can provide shape of micelles.

(4) Since $\overline{R}_h$ (mean hydrodynamic radius) and $\overline{I}$ (mean intensity of scattered light) can be measured in seconds, nucleation and precipitation phenomena can be studied.

(5) Provides information on micellar polydispersity, and under suitable conditions can distinguish whether polydispersity is unimodal or bimodal.

(6) Dust does not interfere appreciably with the measurement of micellar D.

(7) Native bile and intestinal juice can be examined without sample pre-treatment.

QLS: Disadvantages

(1) Below the hard sphere limit ($< 0.3-0.4\,mol/l\ Na^+$), micellar charge interactions are important (apparent decrease in $\overline{R}_h$). For example, in $0.15\,mol/l\ Na^+$ the error in measurement of $\overline{R}_h$ is about 15%. In addition, micelle–micelle interactions occur with high bile salt concentrations ($> 5\,g/dl$).

(2) At present the 'state of the art' is insensitive to particle sizes of $\overline{R}_h < 10\,\text{Å}$.

(3) Instrumentation sophisticated, expensive and requires considerable maintenance.

The principles of the QLS method for estimating the mean hydrodynamic radii ($\overline{R}_h$) of micelles and the conventional light scattering (CLS) method for estimating micellar weight are shown schematically in Figure 2.9). The QLS method utilizes the temporal fluctuations in the scattered light to derive D (diffusion coefficient) whereas the CLS method utilizes the average intensity of the scattering light to give a complex mathematical function which is proportional to mean micellar weight (MMW). The aggregation number ($\overline{n}$) can be derived directly from MMW by simply dividing this quantity by the anhydrous MW of the bile salt. However, to obtain $\overline{n}$ from $\overline{R}_h$, a calculation

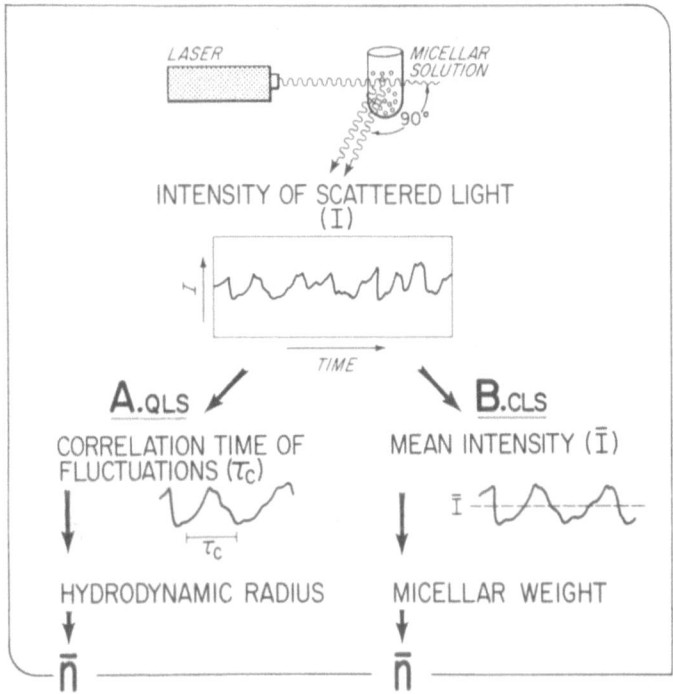

Figure 2.9 Schematic diagram of the two major light-scattering methods (A: QLS, quasielastic light scattering. B: CLS, conventional light scattering.) used to determine mean aggregation number (number of monomers) per micelle ($\bar{n}$). Note that in (A) the correlation time (τ_c) of the fluctuations in the scattered light is measured whereas in (B) the mean intensity of the scattered light is measured (see text)

is required which involves an accurate knowledge of the shape of the micellar particles.

Figure 2.10 displays the $\bar{R}_h$ values derived by QLS measurements of two bile salt–lecithin (BS-L) systems at 10 g/dl as functions of the L to BS ratio and three temperatures. As L/BS ratio is increased, micellar sizes vary markedly. In the taurodeoxycholate (TDC)-L system there is an initial decrease in size and in the taurocholate (TC)-L system an initial increase in size. Beyond the vertical dashed lines in the centre of the plots the micellar sizes are seen to increase strongly to $\bar{R}_h \rangle 80$ Å as the L/BS values reach the phase limit (broad dashed line). It is apparent that these micellar sizes are much larger than the sizes based on the postulated micellar structure proposed by Small and Dervichian (Figure 2.10). This finding led us to propose a new molecular model (the 'mixed-disc' micelle) for these BS-L particles in which bile salts both coat the perimeter and are solubilized within the disc-like fragments of L bilayers. The marked divergence in micellar sizes as the phase limit is approached provides an explanation for the existence of this phase limit since at these lipid ratios the micelles become maximally

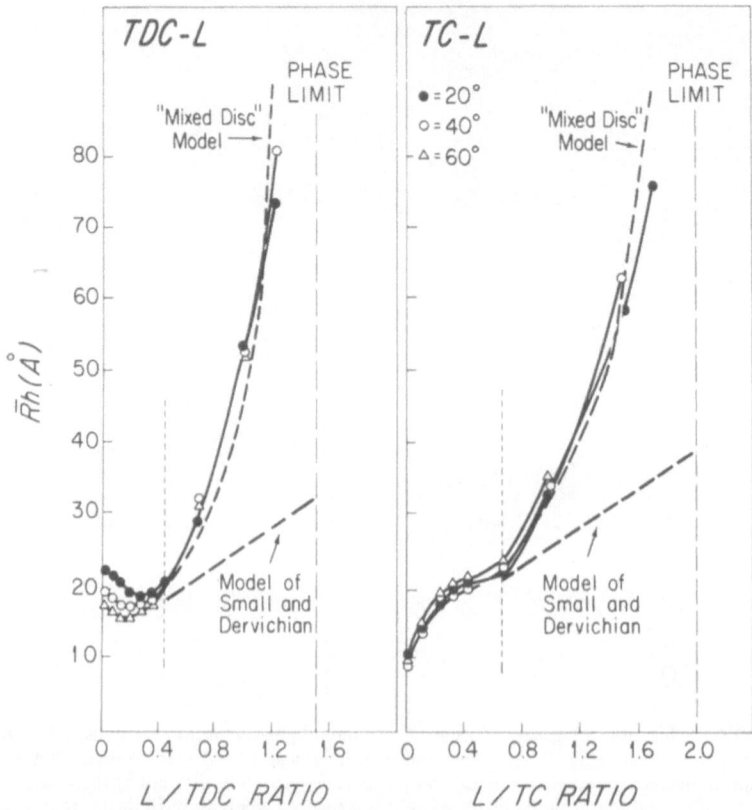

Figure 2.10 Mean hydrodynamic radii ($\overline{R}_h$) in Å of TDC-lecithin (L) micelles (left) and TC-L micelles (right) as functions of L/bile salt ratio and three temperatures (other conditions, 10 g/dl total lipids, 0.15 mol/l NaCl, pH 7.0). To the left of the short vertical hatched lines, the data are consistent with the coexistence of simple bile salt and mixed bile salt-L micelles in varying proportions. To the right of this line the data are consistent with a 'mixed disc' molecular model rather than the 'plain disc' model proposed by Small and Dervichian (From reference 61.)

swollen with L. As the L to BS ratio is increased beyond the phase limit, the excess L plus BS constitute a second lecithin-rich liquid crystalline phase.

The $\overline{R}_h$ values to the left of the narrow-dashed vertical lines show dissimilar behaviour between the two systems, as noted above. In addition there is a pronounced temperature dependence especially in the case of the TDC-L system. A mathematical analysis of these curves, taken together with the *variance* of the data (an index of micellar polydispersity) shows that simple micelles and mixed bile salt–lecithin micelles of fixed composition coexist in varying proportions over these BS-L ratios. Since physiological biliary lipid compositions fall within these BS-L ratios, this hypothesis has relevance to the structure and function of native human and animal biles. The addition of cholesterol, up to the point of saturation of the micellar phase, induces only a small (2–5 Å) increase in micellar size. This suggests that cholesterol incorporation alters neither pre-existing micellar shape nor structure.

MICELLAR SHAPE AND HYDRATION

At low concentrations just above the CMC and at low ionic strengths (< 0.2 mol/l NaCl), nearly all simple bile salt micellar solutions contain spherical or nearly spherical micellar particles. Further, the viscosity of these

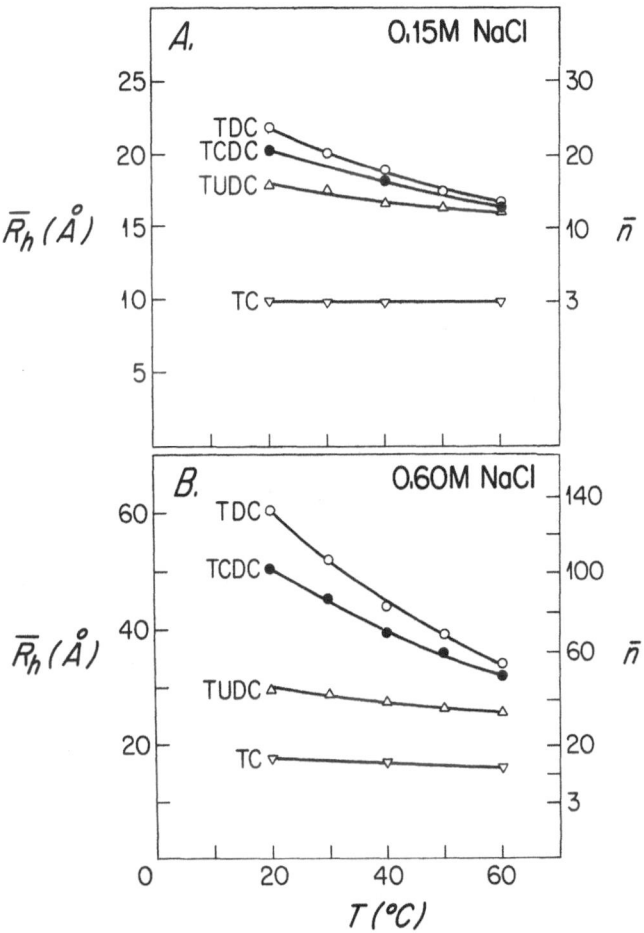

Figure 2.11 Mean hydrodynamic radii ($\bar{R}_h$, in Å) for the taurine (T) conjugates of the four common bile salts (DC, deoxycholate; CDC, chenodeoxycholate; UDC, ursodeoxycholate; C, cholate) in 0.15 mol/l NaCl (A) and 0.6 mol/l NaCl (B) as functions of temperature (From reference 59; see text.)

solutions is consistent with globular and highly hydrated micelles. However, bile salt micelles (like those of other detergents) have been shown by QLS methods to grow markedly under conditions of high detergent concentrations, high ionic strengths and low temperatures. The more hydrophobic bile salts such as deoxycholate and chenodeoxycholate and their conjugates grow more readily under these conditions than the more hydrophilic bile salts, such as ursodeoxycholate and cholate and their conjugates. This growth pattern is shown in Figure 2.11 for the taurine conjugates.

Theoretically, micelles could grow as spheres or as one of the asymmetrical particles (rod, disc, ellipsoid) shown in Figure 2.12. For most practical purposes, the geometry of the prolate ellipsoids is similar to that of rods (Figure 2.12(b)) and the geometry of the oblate ellipsoids is similar to that of discs (Figure 2.12(c)). When the mean scattered light intensity $\bar{I}$ is plotted against each value of $\bar{R}_h$ obtained under the same experimental conditions, the shape of large bile salt micelles can be accurately determined (Figure 2.13(a,b)). When the measured $\bar{R}_h$ and $\bar{I}$ data for TDC (normalized for the scattering of the micellar solution at 60 °C where micellar size is smaller (Figure 2.13(a)), are plotted on the theoretical

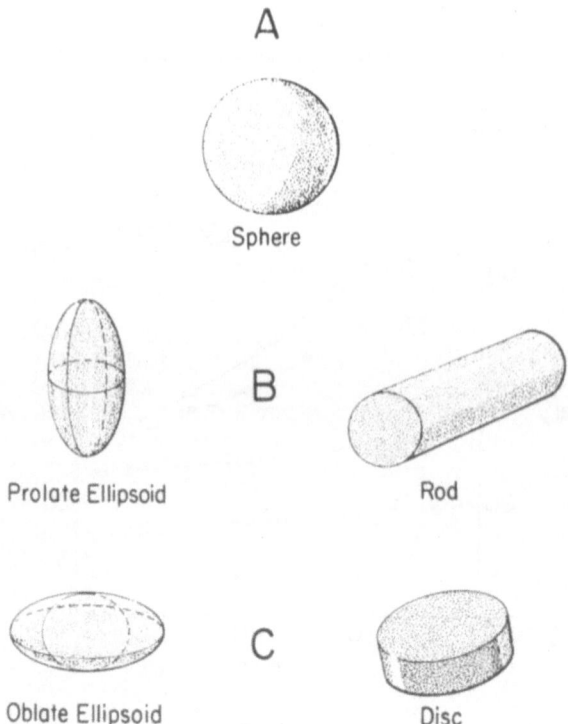

Figure 2.12 Possible growth patterns for enlarging micelles. (A) Spherical; (B) prolate ellipsoid, which is similar to the rod-shape; and (C) oblate ellipsoid, which is similar to the disc-shape (discussed in text)

curves for prolate, oblate and spherical growth (Figure 2.13(b)), all the values fall on the growth curve for the prolate (or rod-like) shape. Thus, we can infer that when spherical bile salt micelles grow, they grow as rod-like or cigar-shaped particles. This implies, by necessity, an interaction between the exterior or hydrophilic surfaces of the primary micelles to form so-called secondary micelles. These polymerization forces have been shown to be hydrophobic in nature (like the thermodynamic forces involved in primary micelle formation), and the aggregates are possibly stabilized by inter-micellar hydrogen bonds. Once the shape of asymmetric bile salt micelles is known, then the hydrodynamic radii ($\overline{R}_h$), i.e. the size of the equivalent spherical particles, can be translated into aggregation numbers ($\overline{n}$) as shown by the non-linear ordinate of Figure 2.11.

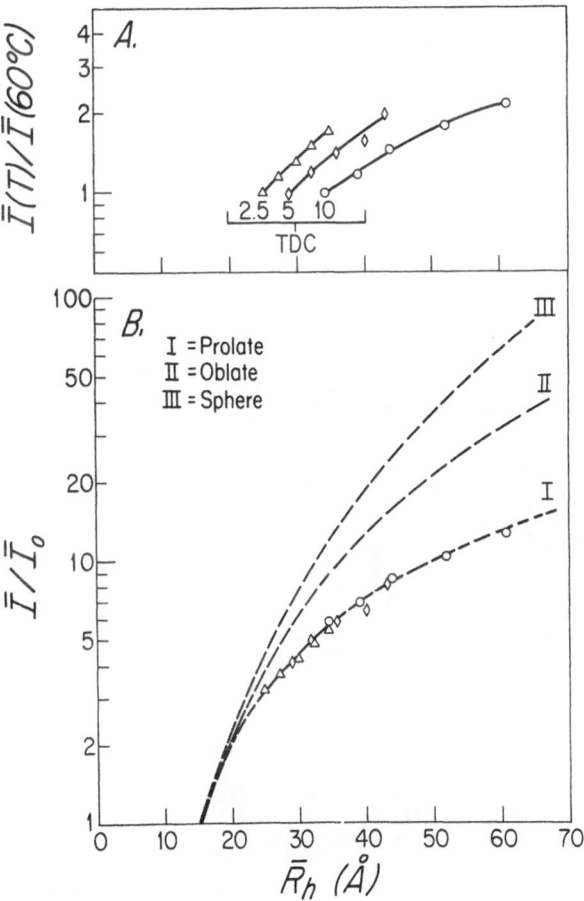

Figure 2.13 The normalized mean intensity of scattered light ($\overline{I}/\overline{I}_{60}$) versus $\overline{R}_h$ (Å). (A) Actual experimental data for TDC. (B) Fitting of experimental data to the theoretical curve for prolate (or rod-like) growth (From reference 59.)

MICELLAR STRUCTURE

Prerequisites for a preliminary determination of bile salt micellar structure are a knowledge of micellar size, shape and the space-filling dimensions of the bile salt monomer. The former are determined by QLS as discussed in the last section, and the molecular structure is determined from crystallographic measurements and space-filling (e.g., Stuart–Briegleb) molecular models of the bile salt. Figure 2.14 shows an accurate scale drawing of the longitudinal and cross-sectional views of such a model for TC showing the bulky steroid hydrocarbon ring structure with α-oriented OH functions (closed ovals) and ionic side chain. In Figure 2.15, the conventional representation of tauro-cholate is shown together with the perspective structure (on the left) and a short-hand representation of the space-filling model (on the right) aligned as the molecule would orient at an air–water interface. Since bile salt molecules have two distinct sides – a hydrophobic side and a hydrophilic side – they are planar amphiphiles and orient on an interface with their hydrophobic surfaces facing upwards and their hydrophilic surfaces projecting into the aqueous phase.

This orientation can be verified by experiment employing a Langmuir–Pockels surface-balance. In operation, a hydrophobic trough is filled with water and a known amount of an insoluble amphiphile is spread from a volatile organic solvent at an air–water interface. By changing the surface area (and hence area per molecule) systematically, the force or surface pressure (in dyn/cm) generated can be measured by a suitable direct-recording device. Since surface pressure is the difference between the surface

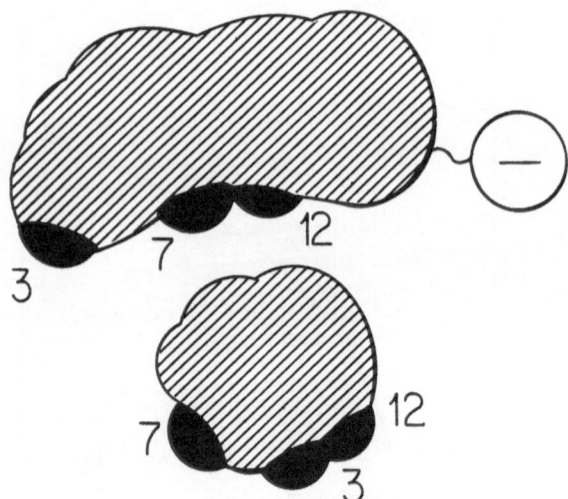

Figure 2.14 Scale-drawing of a Stuart–Briegleb molecular model of taurocholate in longitudinal (top) and cross-sectional (bottom) views. The positions of the 3α, 7α and 12α OH groups are shown as dark ovals. These constitute a hydrophilic side on the steroid nucleus. The charged side chain is represented by a circle with inscribed negative sign (From reference 3.)

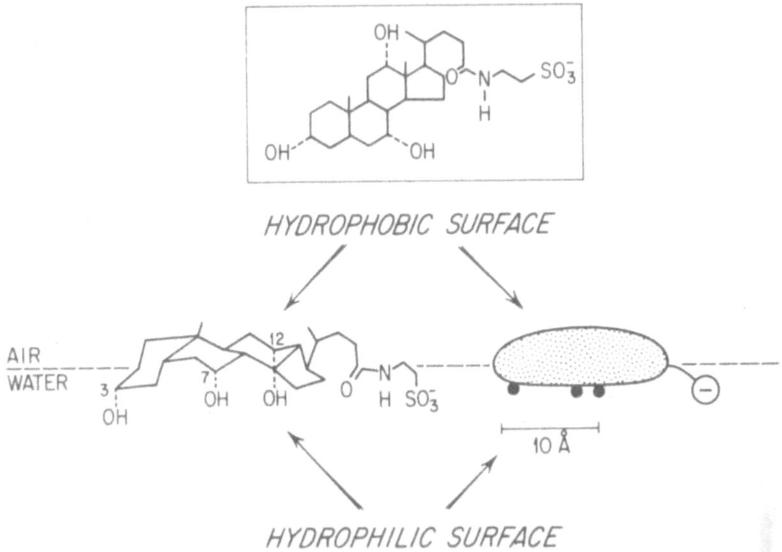

HYDROPHOBIC SURFACE

HYDROPHILIC SURFACE

Figure 2.15 Conventional representation (top) and perspective (left bottom) and space-filling (right bottom) representations of taurocholate as the molecule would lie at an air–water interface. The hydrophilic groups project into the water and the bulky hydrophobic portion lies exposed to air (From reference 59.)

tension of the water minus that of the water with the monomolecular film, surface pressure can also be measured with the Wilhelmy blade technique (see discussion of Figure 2.4). Because bile salts are *soluble* amphiphiles, their surface properties can only be studied after conversion of the salt to the 'insoluble' protonated bile *acid* form. However bile acids are sparingly soluble in water, so that solubility must be further restricted by using a sub-phase of 5–6 mol/l NaCl to salt out OH, N-H, C=O and COOH groups and pH 1–2 to prevent ionization. Because of the appreciable solubility of taurine-conjugated bile salts even at this pH and ionic strength, surface balance experiments cannot be performed with this bile salt. Surface viscosity is estimated from the observed movements of a few grains of talc under an air-jet.

Bile acids appear in general to form gaseous and liquid monolayers, but not condensed or solid films. Pressure–area (Π–A) isotherms typical of those shown for chenodeoxycholate (CDC) and ursodeoxycholate (UDC) (Figure 2.16) are found with most bile acids. Upon comprssion of each surface film, the physical state changes from that of a two-dimensional gas ($A > 8000 \text{ Å}^2$/molecule) to a two-dimensional liquid ($A \approx 90$–150 Å^2/molecule). As the areas are reduced further, the films collapse and usually become three-dimensional with piling of one molecule on top of the other, the first two layers of molecules interacting via their hydrophobic surfaces, the third interacting with the second via their hydrophilic surfaces. This was first discovered by Ekwall, who suggested on the basis of this

41

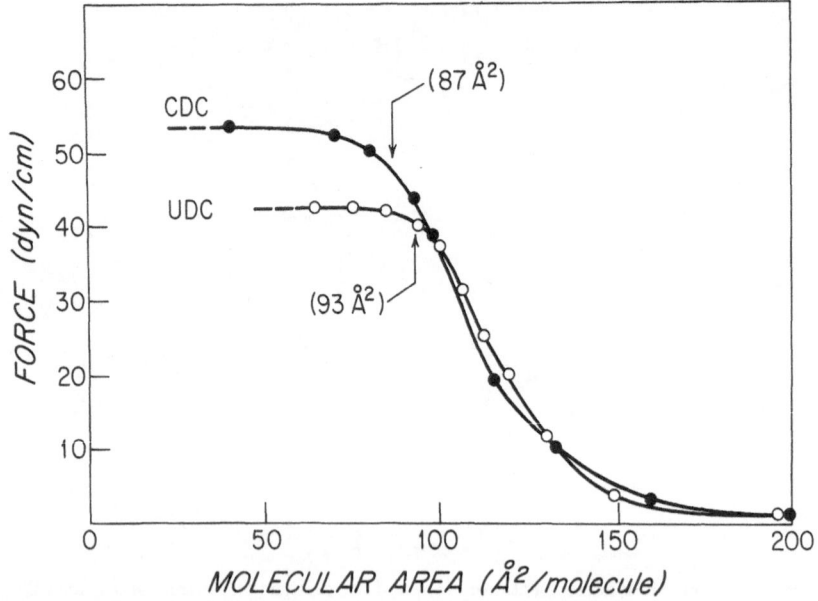

Figure 2.16 Force–Area ($< 200\,\text{Å}^2$) isotherms for the acid form of CDC (chenodeoxycholate) and UDC (ursodeoxycholate) at an air–6 mol/l NaCl, pH 2 aqueous interface (25 °C). The arrowed points represent the areas per molecule at the collapse pressures of the monolayers (40 dyn/cm for UDC and $\approx$ 50 dyn/cm for CDC) (From reference 29; see text.)

interpretation how bile salt molecules might pack to form simple micelles. These principles were extended by Small and our own laboratory to further define the structure of both primary and secondary bile salt micelles.

Crisp derived a two-dimensional phase rule for the analysis of $\Pi\text{-}A$ isotherms:

$$F = C - P_b - (q-1).$$

F and C have the same meanings as before, P_b is the number of bulk phases (which can be one or two) and q is the number of surface phases (which can be one or two). When the area per molecule is very large, say $10\,000\,\text{Å}^2$ ($As > 200\,\text{Å}^2$ are not shown in Figure 2.16), the surface pressure is very low ($<0.1\,\text{dyn/cm}$) but increases slightly with each decrease in area (two-dimensional gas law). Here, q, a gas phase, is $=1$, $P_b=1$, and $F=2-1-(1-1)$ $=1$. The one degree of freedom indicates that Π changes with compression. At a certain range of areas (about $180\,\text{Å} - 8000\,\text{Å}^2$) the isotherm is absolutely flat, i.e. there are zero degrees of freedom ($F=0$) in the surface because $F=2-1-(2-1)=0$: q must be $=2$ to satisfy this equation. This implies the formation of islands of CDC or UDC packed close together floating on the surface in *excess* surface water, i.e. a two-dimensional liquid phase in equilibrium with its two-

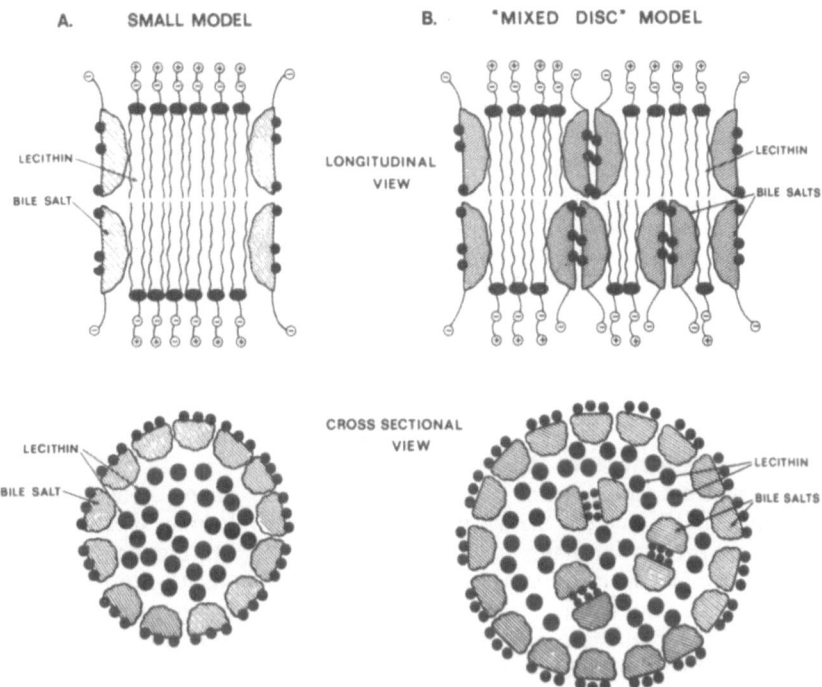

Figure 2.17 Longitudinal and cross-sectional views of the proposed molecular models for the structure of bile salt–lecithin mixed micelles. All recent experimental data are consistent with model B where reversed bile salt aggregates are present in high concentrations within the lecithin disc. Bile salts also coat the perimeter of the disc as a bilayered 'ribbon' (See reference 61.)

dimensional vapour. Between 180 Å² and about 80–90 Å² a degree of freedom is regained (Figure 2.16), i.e. Π rises sharply with compression ($F=1$). We can then write the phase rule as $F=2-1-(1-1)=1$ and conclude that there must be one surface phase as the collapse area is approached, that is a two-dimensional liquid of bile acid molecules packed with increasing tightness. At about 100 Å², there is a rearrangement or a secondary phase transformation in this two-dimensional liquid, as inferred from the change in slope of the isotherms (Figure 2.16). At areas less than 80–90 Å², the isotherms again become flat, meaning that there are zero degrees of freedom ($F=0$). Since there can be only one surface phase, we must conclude that a second *bulk* phase has formed ($P_b=2$) and $F=2-2-(1-1)=0$.

The two-dimensional phase rule does not indicate whether the second bulk phase lies above the surface or is in the subphase. However, if the subphase contains [H⁺] at pH 1–2 and about 6 mol/l NaCl, the second phase must form above the surface. The movement of talc or the rigidity of the Wilhelmy blade in the surface usually suggests the presence of a second surface phase, i.e. multilayer formation.

UDC and CDC give, within experimental error, the same area per molecule at the collapse pressures (arrowed, Figure 2.16). Since this is equivalent to the expected area of the steroid nucleus lying flat (Figure 2.15), it is obvious that both epimers lie horizontal in the interface even when closely packed. However, the UDC film collapses at a $\Pi \approx 10\,\mathrm{dyn/cm}$ lower than CDC, suggesting that UDC more readily forms a second bulk phase. At very small surface areas (not shown in Figure 2.16) there is again an increase in surface pressure ($F=1$), which suggests that no monolayer phase remains and we are dealing with the compression of two bulk phases. Hence, the surface phase rule no longer applies and the formula reverts to its pure Gibbsian form:

$$F = C - P + 1 \quad \text{(since } T \text{ is fixed)}$$
$$= 2 - 2 + 1$$
$$= 1.$$

The fine structure of bile salt and bile salt-mixed micelles can be approached by a number of spectroscopic methods, such as electron spin resonance (ESR), nuclear magnetic resonance (NMR), Raman spectroscopy, fluorescent probes and neutron, electron and X-ray scattering techniques. A rigorous X-ray scattering study of the large bile salt–lecithin micelles has confirmed the mixed disc structure (Figure 2.17) which was originally proposed by our laboratory based on QLS measurements of micellar size and shape. The thermodynamics of simple and mixed bile salt micelles suggest that the enthalpy change for the area of hydrocarbon that loses contact with water when simple micelles form or when cholesterol binds to micelles is $20\,\mathrm{cal\ mol^{-1}\,\mathring{A}^2}$. A comparable value has been found for micellization and cholesterol binding in classic micellar systems.

HYDROPHILIC–HYDROPHOBIC BALANCE OF BILE SALTS

Before the advent of high-performance liquid chromatography (HPLC), it was difficult to quantify the hydrophilic–hydrophobic balance of a homologous series of underivatized bile salts. With the employment of HPLC and reverse-phase columns, a mixture of bile salts elutes in order of decreasing polarity. Figure 2.18 displays the elution profile of a mixture of taurine-conjugated bile salts when the stationary phase is a pure hydro-carbon matrix composed of octadecylsilane chains and the mobile phase is polar, composed of methanol/water. The elution profile is a function of the partition coefficients of bile salt monomers between the polar and non-polar phases; hence, bile salt monomers that spend more time in the polar phase elute first, whereas those that spend more time in the hydrocarbon phase elute last. The order of decreasing hydrophilicity is tauroursocholate (TUC, 3α, 7β, 12α OH), tauroursodeoxycholate (TUDC, 3α, 7β OH), taurohyo-deoxycholate (THDC, 3α, 6α OH), taurocholate (TC, 3α, 7α, 12α OH), taurochenodeoxycholate (TCDC, 3α, 7α OH), taurodeoxycholate (TDC, 3α, 12α OH) and taurolithocholate (TLC, 3α OH). Note that equatorial (7β and 6α) OH functions on the bile salt nucleus are more hydrophilic than α-

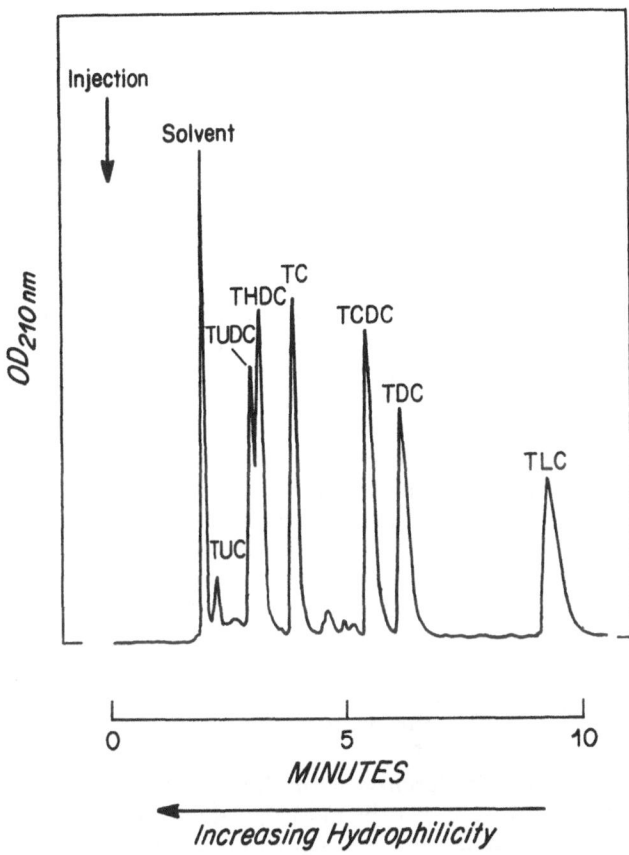

Figure 2.18 The elution pattern of taurine-conjugated bile salts by reverse-phase high-performance liquid chromatography. The stationary phase is octadecylsilane and the mobile phase is MeOH-H$_2$O. The bile salts elute in order of decreasing hydrophilicity with tauroursocholate (TUC 3α, 7β, 12α OH) > TUDC (3α, 7β OH) > taurohyodeoxycholate (THDC, 3α, 6α OH) > TC (3α, 7α, 12α OH) > TCDC (3α, 7α OH) TDC (3α, 12α OH) > tauro-lithocholate (TLC, 3α OH) (After reference 78.)

axial OH functions; therefore, several bile salts are more hydrophilic than TC. This hydrophilic–hydrophobic ordering bears important relationships to lecithin and cholesterol solubilities, dissolution kinetics, to higher order bile salt–lecithin–cholesterol phase diagrams and to other important physical–chemical properties of bile salts such as calcium binding.

We examined quantitatively the interactions of bile salts with cholesterol monohydrate (ChM); (1) by determining the initial dissolution rates of ChM discs in bile salt solutions; (2) by examining the bile salt dissolution rates of ChM incorporated into multilamellar lecithin membranes; (3) by phase equilibria experiments where the maximum capacity of bile salt and BS-lecithin micelles to solubilize ChM was determined; and (4) by constructing

45

condensed phase diagrams of the liquid crystalline and solid phases that coexist with saturated micelles in bile salt–lecithin–cholesterol–water systems. By relating the results of these experiments to the hydrophilic–hydrophobic balance of the bile salts as inferred from their mobility (retention^{-1}), by reverse-phase HPLC, a number of important correlations were derived.

Hydrophilicity of the common free and conjugated bile salts decreases in the order UDC ⟩ C ⟩ CDC ⟩ DC ⟩ LC with T-conjugates ⟩ G-conjugate ⟩ free species. This ordering correlates inversely with micellar dissolution rates of ChM and the equilibrium ChM solubilizing capacities. For each homologous series of conjugated or free bile salts, logarithmic plots of the ChM mole fractions solubilized are linear functions of the HPLC retention factors (mobility^{-1}). It follows that micellar cholesterol-solubilizing capacities of uncommon bile salts can be predicted from their HPLC retention factors. Similarly, in the quaternary phase diagrams, bile salts more hydrophilic than cholate (Figure 2.18) gave a reduced bile salt–lecithin–cholesterol micellar phase and an expanded three-phase region above the micellar zone (where saturated micelles, liquid crystals and solid crystals coexist) (Figure 2.2). Bile salts less hydrophilic than cholate (Figure 2.18) demonstrate a somewhat expanded micellar zone and a reduced three-phase zone (Figure 2.2). By correlation with the respective phase diagram, the HPLC mobility of a bile salt is capable of predicting the predominant molecular mechanism of ChM dissolution. Highly hydrophilic bile salts (most mobile by reversed phase HPLC) dissolve ChM via micellar plus liquid crystalline mechanisms. In contrast, hydrophobic bile salts dissolve ChM via micellar mechanisms only.

Pathophysiological correlations with the hydrophilic–hydrophobic balance of bile salts indicate that the most hydrophilic bile salts have high hepatic secretory maxima, are not cholestatic, have low haemolytic potential, have little, if any, toxicity, and are not secretogenic in the colon. The more hydrophobic bile salts exhibit diametrically opposed characteristics displaying low hepatic secretory maxima, high haemolytic potential and secretogenic effects on colonic epithelia. Since the binding of ChM is but one facet of the hydrophilic–hydrophobic properties of a bile salt, these principles can be extended to systematize the interactions of bile salts with other biological amphiphiles such as lecithin, monoglycerides, 'acid soaps', lipovitamins and phytosterols, and perhaps many receptor-mediated functions. It is likely that these 'Bile Salt Rules' based on the hydrophilic–hydrophobic balance of the molecules will find increasing applicability in predicting pathophysiological function.

MISCELLANEOUS PROPERTIES

Micellar charge and counterion binding

There are a number of indirect methods for determining micellar charge and/or the percentage of counterions bound to bile salt micelles. These include the dependence of CMC and M.M.W. on added ionic strength. However, the most accurate methods involve direct measurements of self-diffusion of radiolabelled counterions and radiolabelled bile salts, ion-specific electrodes sensitive to the activity of the unbound counterion, and nuclear magnetic resonance (NMR) methodologies. At physiological ionic strengths, the association of Na^+ with bile salts is much lower than that observed for classical micellar systems (5–15% vs. $\rangle$ 50%). This implies that approximately 1 Na^+ is bound to a taurine-conjugated bile salt micelle with an average aggregation number ($\bar{n}$) of 10. In contrast, approximately 30 Na^+ counterions are bound to the average sodium dodecyl sulphate micelle of $\bar{n}$=60. Despite its great importance, much less reliable information is available concerning Ca^{2+} binding to bile salt micelles. In equimolar counterion concentrations, divalent metals are bound more tightly and to a greater degree than are Na^+ ions. Recent evidence suggests that Na^+ ions, which are present physiologically in 10–30-fold excess, strongly compete with bound Ca^{2+}. When added to the sodium bile salts, the degree of calcium binding follows the hydrophilic–hydrophobic order (as inferred by reverse-phase HPLC) with UDC $\langle$ C $\langle$ CDC $\langle$ DC $\langle$ LC and T-conjugate $\langle$ G-conjugate $\langle$ free bile salts.

Rates of exchange of intermicellar monomers, counterions and micellar components

Chemical relaxation techniques (Π-jump, T-jump, stopped flow, shock-tube and ultrasonic absorption) and NMR have been used to define the nature and number of relaxation processes in micellar solutions. These include: (1) the counterion association/dissociation to/from micelles (ionization); (2) detergent ion association/dissociation to/from micelles (exchange process); (3) micelle formation/dissolution; and (4) change of micellar shape and/or size. Very few points of agreement have been reached in the literature concerning the origin and characteristics of the relaxation processes. The fastest relaxation process (well below 1 μs) has been attributed to the exchange of detergent ions between solvent and micelles and a slower relaxation process (100–10 μs) has been assigned to micelle formation–dissolution equilibria. The former relaxation process has been measured for sodium deoxycholate at concentrations well above the CMC. The value found (10^9/l/mol^{-1}/s^{-1}) is similar to that for exchange of detergent ions in classic detergent systems.

Techniques for distinguishing *critical* from *non-critical* self-association

Critical self-association implies a strong co-operative interaction of a large number of detergent ions to form micelles over a narrow concentration range, the CMC. *Non-critical* self-association implies that the detergent interactions are non-cooperative and occur usually in a progressive or stepped fashion over a wide concentration range often beginning as dimers. To the purist the latter is not considered micellization but to avoid a complicated nomenclature most cholanologists would also call this initial self-association a micellization initiated at a CMC.

This distinction can be probed physicochemically in a number of ways:

(1) Chemical relaxation methods, especially ultrasonic relaxation spectra: the ultrasonic absorption relaxation spectra of NaC and NaDC show evidence of a distribution of relaxation frequencies rather than a single relaxation frequency as found with classic ionic detergents. Thus these bile salts apparently self-associate over a whole range of concentrations and not at some critical micellar concentration where co-operative interactions occur. Further, since the relaxation frequencies are strongly concentration dependent, the distribution curve of aggregate sizes appears to be wide and shifts upward as bile salt concentration is increased. It must be appreciated, however, that in these studies, the investigators focused on free (un-conjugated) bile salts which have much smaller $\bar{n}$ (CMC) values (see Figure 2.6) than the conjugates, especially in the low ($< 0.2 \, mol/l$) ionic strengths which they employed.

(2) Solubilization of large hydrophobic solubilizates: as illustrated in Figure 2.6, bile salts with non-critical self-association (e.g., NaC) show a broad range of apparent CMC values when micellization is evaluated by both invasive and non-invasive methods. This scatter in the data appears to be a function of the upward shift in mean micellar sizes as the detergent concentration is increased. Bile salts like NaTDC (Figure 2.6) and other taurine-conjugated dihydroxy bile salts do not display this feature (see below) and show true co-operative micellization at a well-defined concentration.

(3) Ratio of slopes of surface tension *versus* concentration above and below the CMC: with most of the taurine conjugates (which form the largest micelles) the semilogarithmic plot of surface tension versus bile salt concentration shows a sharp break point, with little change in slope once the CMC is exceeded (see Figure 2.5). Such data are consistent with a critical (co-operative) phenomenon at the CMC. The plots of NaC or NaDC in low ionic strengths continue to show some fall in surface tension above the CMC consistent with non-cooperative self-association. Curvature of the data around the CMC point is not an indication of non-critical self-association, but usually indicates that the data are non-equilibrium values.

(4) Ratio of slopes of monomer solubility and the CMT as functions of bile salt concentration: The ratio of the changes in bile salt solubility above and below the Krafft point (see Figure 2.8) is a function of cooperativity of self-association at the Krafft point. In general, the greater the ratio of the slope of the CMT-monomer solubility plot, the less critical the CMC. In the case of typical ionic detergents the CMT versus concentration curve has only a slight slope consistent with co-operative self-association at the CMC.

Thus the conclusion as to whether or not a bile salt exhibits a critical or non-critical self-association depends upon the bile salt species and the physical–chemical conditions. For example, NaC in H_2O exhibits continuous non-critical association and $\bar{n}$ at the CMC$=2-4$. In contrast, NaTDC in $0.15 \, mol/l$ Na$^+$ exhibits a true CMC and $\bar{n}$ at the CMC$=20$. If dimers are called micelles (which in my opinion is quite reasonable) then the first concentration at which any self-association is detected can be labelled a micellization with the understanding that it may not be a *critical* phenomenon. It appears counterproductive to suggest a different nomenclature for the micellization patterns of different bile salts or for the same bile salts evaluated under different physical–chemical conditions.

Reversed micelle formation

Probably the most important variety of reversed micelle formation (i.e., initial self-association via the hydrophilic sides of bile salt monomers) is the interaction of bile salts within membranes and with dispersions of membrane lipids, e.g. lecithin. Bile salt–membrane lipid interaction have been studied by phase equilibria, X-ray diffraction, NMR and fluorescent techniques. The bile salt packing is probably similar to that which occurs within the lecithin core of mixed micelles (shown in Figure 2.17). The NMR diffusion coefficients and order parameters suggest that lecithin in mixed micelles or mixed with bile salts in vesicles is much less constrained than that in pure lecithin or pure lecithin–cholesterol vesicles. Further, other studies have shown that bile salts act as 'ionophores' in artificial membranes and also induce rapid flip-flop of lecithin molecules from one side of a vesicle to the other. Whether bile salts themselves diffuse through membranes in reverse di-, tri- or tetramers is not known – nor has the possibility been studied that reversed micelle formation might induce water, macromolecule and electrolyte flow through membranes.

Utilizing the techniques of NMR and Vapour Pressure Osmometry, bile acid methyl esters (MeLC, MeDC, MeC) have been shown to form small reversed micelles to CCl_4, CH_2Cl_2, CS_2 and $CHCl_3$. This type of reversed association may be monomer–dimer, monomer–dimer–trimer, or monomer–dimer–tetramer with the order of affinity for self-association being MeC 〉 MeDC 〉 MeLC. The hydrophilic derivatives are more strongly bound than the hydrophobic ones and self-association in aprotic solvents, e.g. CCl_4, is somewhat greater than in protic solvents, e.g. $CHCl_3$. These findings suggest that hydrogen-bonding is important in stabilizing the complexes. Certain bile salts, e.g. cholate and deoxycholate, have also been shown to form reversed micelles in decanol–water systems at decanol concentrations 〉 70%. Deoxycholate (in the acid form) also self-associates in a monomer–tetramer–hexamer pattern in pure iso-octane–chloroform (80:20 v/v) systems. While of great interest, these micelles have not been rigorously characterized.

Electrochemical properties

Because the properties of bile acids (insoluble amphiphiles) and bile salts (soluble amphiphiles) differ, it is obviously important to know the pK'a of bile acids under a wide variety of physical–chemical states such as those encountered physiologically. To date, potentiometric titrations have been carried out on bile salts as functions of detergent concentration, temperature, ionic strength, added lecithin and mono-olein in aqueous solvents. Because taurine is a much stronger acid than HCl (usually used in such studies), precise $pK'a$ values of *any* taurine conjugates are not yet known. Being sulphonic acids the values probably lie in the pH -1.5 to $+1.5$ range. The following summarizes the apparent dissociation constants of the common bile acids as estimated potentiometrically with HCl. It must be stressed that other methods such as NMR chemical shift and solvent–solvent partition are likely to give somewhat different values.

$$pK'a = pH \text{ at which } \frac{50\% \text{ A}^-(\text{salt})}{50\% \text{ HA (acid)}}$$

pK'a values ($\rangle$ CMC)
    free bile acids $= 5$–6.5
    glycine conjugates $= 3.8$–5.2
    taurine conjugates $=$ not known ($\langle 1.8$ with HCl)
pK'a values of free bile acids: CDCA $\rangle$ DCA $\rangle$ UDCA $\rangle$ CA
pK'a values of glycine conjugates: GDCA $\rangle$ GUDCA $\rangle$ GCDCA $\rangle$ GCA

The pH range over which the corresponding bile acids precipitate (pHppt) from solution represents the maximum solubility of bile acid in bile salt micelles and in the aqueous solvent.

pHppt = pH at which system is saturated with [HA]aq + [HA] micellar
pHppt values ($\rangle$ CMC)

    free bile acids $= 6.4 - 8.1$
    glycine conjugates $= 4.3 - 7.4$
    taurine conjugates $=$ soluble at pH 0

pHppt of free bile acids: UDCA $\rangle$ CDCA $\rangle$ DCA $\rangle$ CA
pHppt of glycine conjugates: GUDCA $\rangle$ GCDCA $=$ GDCA $\rangle$ GCA

Figure 2.19 summarizes these concepts. From the graph, the percentage of free, glycine- and taurine-conjugated bile salts which exist in ionized (A^-) and unionized (HA) form and the physical state of the systems can be estimated at all physiological pH values. It is apparent that when titrated with HCl, protonation of free bile salts begins at pH 9.0, glycine conjugates at pH 8.0 and taurine conjugates possibly at about pH 4.0 though this latter value will probably require a downward adjustment. On account of the high solubility of bile acids in bile salt micelles, precipitation of the HA form (indicated by the two-phase bracket) does not commence until pH 7.25 ± 0.85 (mean $\pm$ range) in the case of free bile salts, and pH 5.85 ± 1.5 in the case of the glycine conjugates. Taurine conjugates remain in micellar solution at pH values as low as 0. No information is available on the ionization (dissociation) constants of bile salts in biliary mixed micelles, intestinal mixed micelles, liposomes, and emulsions or when associated with membranes, receptors, and transport lipoproteins (HDL and albumin).

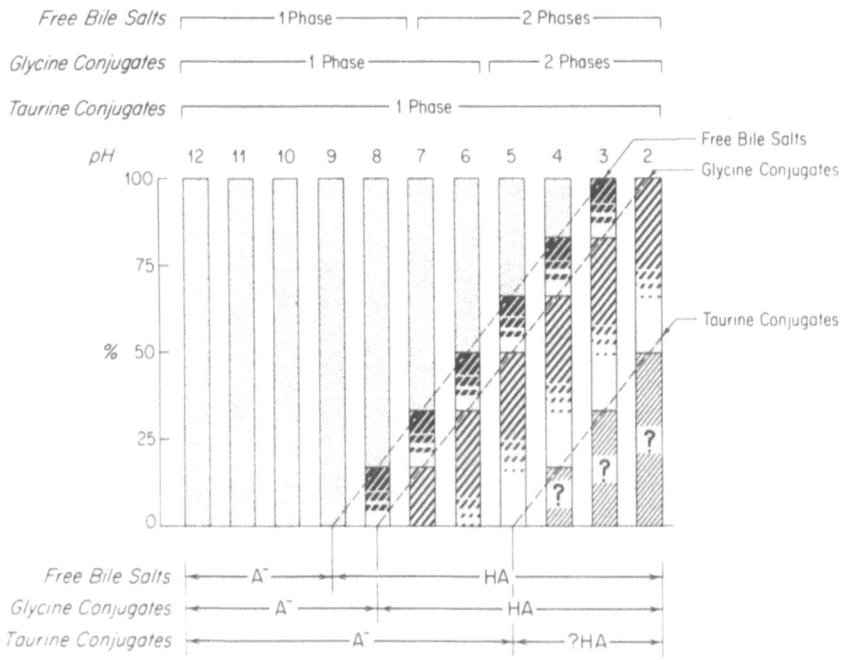

Figure 2.19 Plot of physical state and percentage undissociated acid, (HA) and anion (A⁻) species of pure bile salts as functions of pH (discussed in text) (After references 3, 96, 97, 98.)

Acknowledgements

I wish to recognize the important research contributions toward understanding the physical–chemistry of bile salts from work carried out in my laboratory by N. A. Mazer, A. P. Koretsky, H. Igimi, J. S. Patton, M. J. Armstrong, M. D. Berman, S. P. Lee, Y.-H. Park, R. J. Stafford, G. Salvioli, W. Spivak, R. McCabe, P. J. Missel and C. Y. Young. Ms Rebecca Ankener edited and typed the manuscript.

The author's research is supported in part by NIADDK grant AM 18559 and grants-in-aid from Abbott Laboratories, N. Chicago, IL., Zambon S.p.a., Bresso, Italy and the Cystic Fibrosis Foundation.

Bibliography

This literature classification is arbitrary since there is much overlap in the content of references.

General reviews

1. Carey, M. C. and Small, D. M. (1970). The characteristics of mixed micellar solutions with particular reference to bile. *Am. J. Med.*, **49**, 590
2. Carey, M. C. and Small, D. M. (1972). Micelle formation by bile salts. Physical chemical

51

and thermodynamic considerations. *Arch. Intern. Med.*, **130**, 506

3. Small, D.M. (1971). The physical chemistry of cholanic acids. In Nair, P.P. and Kritchevsky, D. (eds.) *The Bile Acids*, Vol. 1, pp. 249–356 (New York: Plenum Press)

4. Tanford, C. (1979). *The Hydrophobic Effect: Formation of Micelles and Biological Membranes*, 2nd edn. (New York: John Wiley)

5. Shinoda, K. *et al.* (1963). *Colloidal Surfactants: Some Physical–Chemical Properties.* (New York: Academic Press)

6. Shaw, D.J. (1970). *Introduction to Colloid and Surface Chemistry*, 2nd edn. (London: Butterworths)

7. Elworthy, P.H., Florence, A.T. and MacFarlane, C.B. (1968). *Solubilization by Surface Active Agents*, 1st edn. (London: Chapman and Hall)

Phase equilibria and the phase rule

8. Bancroft, W.D. (1897). *The Phase Rule.* (The Journal of Physical Chemistry Publications: Ithaca, New York)

9. Ferguson, F.D. and Jones, T.K. (1966). *The Phase Rule.* (London: Butterworths)

10. Small, D.M. (1968). A classification of biological lipids based upon their interaction in aqueous systems. *J. Am. Oil Chem. Soc.*, **45**, 108

11. Findley, A., Campbell, A.N. and Smith, N.O. (1951). *The Phase Rule and its Applications.* (New York: Dover Publications)

12. Smith, N.O. (1974). *Phase Changes and Equilibria.* The New Encyclopaedia Britannica (Macropaedia), Vol. 14, pp. 204–210. (Chicago: H.H. Benton)

13. Small, D.M., Bourgès, M. and Dervichian, D.G. (1966). The biophysics of lipidic associations I. The ternary systems lecithin–bile salt–water. *Biochim. Biophys. Acta*, **125**, 563

14. Bourgès, M., Small, D.M. and Dervichian, D.G. (1967). Biophysics of lipidic association II. The ternary systems cholesterol–lecithin–water. *Biochim. Biophys. Acta*, **137**, 157

15. Bourgès, M., Small, D.M. and Dervichian, D.G. (1967). Biophysics of lipid association III. The quaternary system lecithin–bile salt–cholesterol–water. *Biochim. Biophys. Acta*, **144**, 189

16. Small, D.M. and Bourgès, M. (1966). Lyotropic paracrystalline phases obtained with ternary and quaternary systems of amphiphilic substances in water: studies on aqueous systems of lecithin, bile salt and cholesterol. *Mol. Cryst.*, **1**, 541

17. Admirand, W.H. and Small, D.M. (1968). The physical–chemical basis of cholesterol gallstone formation in man. *J. Clin. Invest.*, **47**, 1043

18. Carey, M.C. and Small, D.M. (1978). The physical–chemistry of cholesterol solubility in bile. Relationship to gallstone formation and dissolution in man. *J. Clin. Invest.*, **61**, 998

19. Crisp, D.J. (1949). A two-dimensional phase rule I – Derivation of a two dimensional phase rule for plane interfaces. In *Surface Chemistry*, pp. 17–22. (London: Butterworths)

20. Crisp, D.J. (1949). A two-dimensional phase rule II. Some applications of a two-dimensional phase rule for a single interface. In *Surface Chemistry*, pp. 23–35. (London: Butterworths)

21. Ekwall, P., Mandell, L. and Fontell, K. (1969). Solubilization in micelles and mesophases and the transition from normal to reversed structures. *Mol. Cryst. Liq. Cryst.*, **8**, 157

Critical micellar concentration and intermicellar concentration

22. Mukerjee, P. and Mysels, K.J. (1971). *Critical Micelle Concentration of Aqueous Surfactant Systems.* (Washington, D.C.: National Bureau of Standards, US)

23. Mukerjee, P. (1967). The nature of the association equilibria and hydrophobic bonding in aqueous solutions of association colloids. *Adv. Coll. Interface Sci.*, **1**, 241

24. Hartley, G.S. (1936). *Aqueous Solution of Paraffin-Chain Salts.* (Paris: Hermann)

25. Carey, M.C. and Small, D.M. (1969). Micellar properties of dihydroxy and trihydroxy bile salts. Effects of counterion and temperature. *J. Coll. Interface Sci.*, **31**, 382

26. Hofmann, A.F. (1963). The function of bile salts in fat absorption: The solvent properties of dilute micellar solutions of conjugated bile salts. *Biochem. J.*, **89**, 57

27. Kratohvil, J.P. and DelliColli, H.T. (1968). Micellar properties of bile salts. Sodium

taurodeoxycholate and sodium glycodeoxycholate. *Can. J. Biochem.*, **46**, 945
28. Carey, M. C. and Small, D. M. (1978). The apparent critical micellar concentration of bile salt–lecithin micelles: Influence of composition, phospholipid chain length, sodium chloride concentration, and temperature. In Schukin, E. (ed.) *Physical Chemistry of Surface Active Substances*, Vol. 2, pp. 810–827. (Moscow: State Publishing House)
29. Carey, M. C., Montet, J.-C., Phillips, M. C., Armstrong, M. J. and Mazer, N. A. (1981). Thermodynamic and molecular basis for dissimilar cholesterol solubilizing capacities by micellar solutions of bile salts: Cases of sodium chemodeoxycholate and sodium ursodeoxycholate and their glycine and taurine conjugates. *Biochemistry*, **20**, 3637
30. DeVandittis, E., Palumbo, G., Parlato, G. and Bocchini, V. (1981). A fluorimetric method for the estimation of the critical micelle concentration of surfactants. *Anal. Biochem.*, **115**, 278
31. Fisher, L. and Oakenfull, D. (1979). The environment of solubilized molecules in bile salt micelles. *Aust. J. Chem.*, **32**, 31
32. Smith, W. B. and Barnard, G. D. (1981). A study of aqueous sodium cholate by ^{2}H NMR. *Can. J. Chem.*, **59**, 1602
33. Paul, R., Mathew, M. K., Narayanan, R. and Balaram, P. (1979). Fluorescent probe and NMR studies of the aggregation of bile salts in aqueous solution. *Chem. Phys. Lipids*, **25**, 345
34. Thomas, D. C. and Christian, S. D. (1980). Micellar and surface behaviour of sodium deoxycholate characterized by surface tension and ellipsometric methods. *J. Coll. Interface Sci.*, **78**, 466
35. Gupta, P. M., Bahudur, P. and Singh, S. P. (1979). Adsorption characteristics of bile salts at Toluene–water interface. *Ind. J. Biochem. Biophys.*, **16**, 336
36. Vadnere, M., Natarajan, R. and Lindenbaum, S. (1980). Apparent model volumes of bile salts in H_2O and D_2O solution. *J. Phys. Chem.*, **84**, 1900
37. Sugihara, G. and Tanaka, M. (1976). A pH and pNa study of aqueous solution of sodium deoxycholate. *Bull. Chem. Soc. Jpn.*, **49**, 3457
38. Hisadome, T., Nakama, T., Itoh, H. and Furasawa, T. (1980). Physical–chemical properties of chenodeoxycholic and ursodeoxycholic acid. *Gastroenterol. Japon.*, **15**, 257
39 Carey, M. C. and Koretsky, A. P. (1979). Self-association of unconjugated bilirubin 1IXXα in aqueous solution at pH 10.0 and physical-chemical interactions with bile salt monomers and micelles. *Biochem. J.*, **179**, 675
40. Shankland, W. (1970). The equilibrium and structure of lecithin–cholate mixed micelles. *Chem. Phys. Lipids*, **4**, 109
41. Duane, W. C. (1975). The intermicellar bile salt concentration in equilibrium with the mixed micelles of human bile. *Biochim. Biophys. Acta*, **398**, 275
42. Duane, W. C. (1977). Taurocholate- and taurochenodeoxycholate–lecithin micelles: The equilibrium of bile salt between aqueous phase and micelle. *Biochem. Biophys. Res. Comm.*, **74**, 223
43. Borgström, B. (1978). Equilibrium of taurodeoxycholate between mixed micellar and aqueous phases: Effect of amphiphile. *Lipids*, **13**, 187
44. Ulmius, J., Lindblöm, G., Wennerström, H., Johansson, L. B-Å, Fontell, K., Soderman, D. and Arvidson, G. (1982). Molecular organization in the liquid–crystalline phases of lecithin–sodium cholate–water systems studied by nuclear magnetic resonance. *Biochemistry*, **21**, 1553

Critical micellar temperature

45. Krafft, F. and Wiglow, H. (1895). Üeber das Verhalten der Fettsauren Alkalien und der Seifen in Gegenwart von Wasser, III. Die Seifen als Krystalloïde. *Ber. Dtsch. Chem. Gesell.*, **28**, 2566
46. Krafft, F. and Wiglow, H. (1895). Üeber das Verhalten der Fettsauren Alkalien und der Siefen in Gegenwart von Wasser IV. Die Seifen als Colloïde. *Ber. Dtsch. Chem. Gesell.*, **28**, 2573
47. Small, D. M. and Admirand, W. H. (1969). Solubility of bile salts. *Nature (Lond.)*, **221**, 265

48. Démarq, M. and Dervichian, D. G. (1945). Détermination des temperatures de clarification des solutions de savons de Li, Na, K, Rb et Cs. *Bull. Soc. Chim. France*, **12**, 939
49. Murray, R. C. and Hartley, G. S. (1935). Equilibrium between micelles and simple ions, with particular reference to the solubility of long-chain salts. *Trans. Faraday Soc.*, **31**, 183
50. Mazer, N. A., Benedek, G. B. and Carey, M. C. (1976). An investigation of the micellar phase of sodium dodecyl sulfate in aqueous sodium chloride solution using quasielastic light scattering spectroscopy. *J. Phys. Chem.*, **80**, 1075
51. Carey, M. C., Wu, S-F and Watkins, J. B . (1979). Solution properties of sulfated monohydroxy bile salts: Relative insolubility of the disodium salt of glycolithocholate sulfate. *Biochim. Biophys. Acta.*, **575**, 16

Micellar size and polydispersity

52. Small, D. M. (1968). Size and structure of bile salt micelles: Influence of structure, concentration, counterion concentration, pH and temperature. *Ad. Chem. Ser.*, **84**, 31
53. Kratohvil, J. B. and DelliColli, H. T. (1970). Measurement of the size of micelles: The case of sodium taurodeoxycholate. *Fed. Proc.*, **29**, 1335
54. Woodford, F. P. (1969). Enlargement of taurocholate micelles by added cholesterol and mono-olein: self-diffusion measurements. *J. Lipid Res.*, **10**, 539
55. Fung, B. M. and Peden, M. C. (1976). The nature of bile salt micelles as studied by deuterium NMR. *Biochim. Biophys. Acta.*, **437**, 273
56. Gähwiller, C., Von Planta, C., Schmidt, D. and Steffen, H. (1977). Untersuchungen über die Grösse, Struktur und Dynamik von Gallensäure/Lecithin-Mischmicellen. *Z. Naturforsch.*, **32c**, 748
57. Gatt, S., Gazit, B., and Barenholz, Y. (1981). Effect of bile salts on the hydrolysis of gangliosides, glycoprotein and neuraminyl-lactose by the neuraminidase of *Clostridium perfringens*. *Biochem. J.*, **193**, 267
58. Montet, J. C., Lindheimer, M., Reynier, M-O., Crotte, C., Bontemps, R. and Gerolami, A. (1982). Mixed micelle properties and intestinal cholesterol uptake. *Biochimie (Paris)*, **64**, 255
59. Mazer, N. A., Carey, M. C., Kwasnick, R. F. and Benedek, G. B. (1979). Quasielastic light scattering studies of aqueous biliary lipid systems: Size, shape and thermodynamics of bile salt micelles. *Biochemistry*, **18**, 3064
60. Sehlin, R. S., Cussler, E. L. and Evans, D. F. (1975). Bile diffusion and its implications in detergency. *Biochim. Biophys. Acta*, **388**, 385

Micellar shape and hydration

61. Mazer, N. A., Benedek, G. B. and Carey, M. C. (1980). Quasielastic light scattering studies of aqueous biliary lipid systems: Mixed micelle formation in bile salt–lecithin solution. *Biochemistry*, **19**, 601
62. Missel, P. J., Mazer, N. A., Benedek, G. B., Young, C. Y. and Carey, M. C. (1980). Thermodynamic analysis of the growth of sodium dodecyl sulfate micelles. *J. Phys. Chem.*, **84**, 1044
63. Young, C. Y., Missel, P. J., Mazer, N. A., Benedek, G. B. and Carey, M. C. (1978). Deduction of micellar shape from angular dissymmetry measurements of light scattered from aqueous sodium dodecyl sulfate solutions at high NaCl concentrations. *J. Phys. Chem.*, **82**, 1375
64. Schurtenberger, P., Mazer, N. A. and Känzig, W. (1983). Static and dynamic light scattering studies of micellar growth and interactions in bile salt solutions. *J. Phys. Chem.* (in press)
65. Cussler, E. L. and Duncan, C. L. (1972). Activities and viscosities of aqueous bile acid salt–lecithin solutions. *J. Sol. Chem.*, **1**, 269

Micellar structure

66. Müller, K. (1981). Structural dimorphism of bile salt/lecithin mixed micelles: A possible regulatory mechanism for cholesterol solubility in bile? X-ray structural analysis. *Biochemistry*, **30**, 404
67. Menger, F. M. and McCreery, M. J. (1974). Kinetic characterization of bile salt micelles. *J. Am. Chem. Soc.*, **96**, 121
68. Mazer, N. A., Kwasnick, R. F., Carey, M. C. and Benedek, G. B. (1977). Quasielastic light scattering spectroscopic studies of bile salt, bile salt–lecithin, and bile salt–lecithin–cholesterol systems. In Mittal, K. L. (ed.) *Micellization, solubilization and microemulsions*, Vol. I, pp. 383–402. (New York: Plenum)
69. Thomas, D. C. and Christian, S. D. (1981). Mixed solubilization of benzene and cyclohexane in sodium deoxycholate micelles. *J. Colloid Interface Sci.*, **82**, 430
70. Fung, B. M. and Thomas, L., Jr. (1979). The motion of aromatic molecules in bile acid micelles. *Chem. Phys. Lipids*, **25**, 141
71. Upreti, G. C. and Jain, M. K. (1978). Effect of the state of phosphatidylcholine on the rate of its hydrolysis by phospholipase A_2 (Bee venom). *Arch. Biochem. Biophys.*, **188**, 364
72. Olive, J. and Dervichian, D. G. (1968). Action d'une phospholipase sur la lécithine à l'état micellaire. *Bull. Soc. Chim. Biol.*, **50**, 1409
73. Barnes, S. and Geckle, J. M. (1982). High resolution nuclear magnetic resonance spectroscopy of bile salts: Individual proton assignments for sodium cholate in aqueous solution of 400 MHz. *J. Lipid Res.*, **23**, 161
74. Small, D. M., Penkett, S. A. and Chapman, D. (1969). Studies on simple and mixed bile salt micelles by nuclear magnetic resonance spectroscopy. *Biochim. Biophys. Acta*, **176**, 178
75. Martis, L., Hall, N. A. and Thakkar, A. L. (1972). Micelle formation and testosterone solubilization by sodium glycocholate. *J. Pharm. Sci.*, **61**, 1757
76. Leibfritz, D. and Roberts, J. D. (1973). Nuclear magnetic resonance spectroscopy. Carbon-13 spectra of cholic acids and hydrocarbons included in sodium deoxycholate solutions. *J. Am. Chem. Soc.*, **95**, 4996
77. Castellino, F. J. and Violand, B. N. (1979). ^{31}P-nuclear magnetic resonance and $^{31}P[^1H]$ nuclear Overhauser effect analysis of mixed egg phosphatidylcholine–sodium taurocholate vesicles and micelles. *Arch. Biochem. Biophys.*, **193**, 543

Hydrophilic–hydrophobic balance of bile salts

78. Armstrong, M. J. and Carey, M. C. (1982). The hydrophobic–hydrophilic balance of bile salts: inverse correlation between reverse-phase high performance liquid chromatographic motilities and micellar cholesterol solubilizing capacities. *J. Lipid Res.*, **23**, 70

Micellar charge and counterion binding

79. Sesta, B., LaMesa, C., Bonincontro, A., Cametti, C. and DiBiasio, A. (1981). Molecular aggregation of sodium deoxycholate in water and water–urea mixtures. *Ber. Bunsenges. Phys. Chem.*, **85**, 798
80. Lindheimer, M., Montet, J. C., Molenat, J., Bontemps, R. and Brun, B. (1981). Ionic self-diffusion of various bile salts. *J. Chim. Phys. (Paris)*, **78**, 447
81. Lindman, B. and Brun, B. (1973). Translational motion in aqueous sodium n-octanoate solutions. *J. Colloid Interface Sci.*, **42**, 388

Rates of exchange of intermicellar monomers, counterions and micellar components

82. Lang, J., Tondre, C., Zana, R., Bauer, R., Hoffmann, H. and Ulbricht, W. (1975). Chemical relaxation studies of micellar equilibria. *J. Phys. Chem.*, **79**, 276
83. Aniansson, E. A. G., Wall, S. N., Almgren, M., Hoffmann, H., Kielmann, I., Ulbricht, W., Zana, R., Lang, J. and Tondre, C. (1976). Theory of the kinetics of micellar equilibria and quantitative interpretation of chemical relaxation studies of micellar solution of ionic surfactants. *J. Phys. Chem.*, **80**, 905

84. Baumüller, W., Hoffmann, H., Ulbricht, W., Tondre, C. and Zana, R. (1978). Chemical relaxation and equilibrium studies of aqueous solutions of laurylsulfate micelles in the presence of divalent metal ions. *J. Colloid Interface Sci.*, **64**, 418
85. Zana, R. (1975). Brief review of the chemical relaxation studies of micellar equilibria. In Wyn-Jones, E. (ed.) *Chemical and Biological Application of Relaxation Spectroscopy*, pp. 133–38. (Dordrecht, Holland: Reidel Publications)
86. Djavanbakht, A., Kale, K. M. and Zana, R. (1977). Ultrasonic absorption and density studies of the aggregation in aqueous solutions of bile acid salts. *J. Colloid Interface Sci.*, **59**, 139

Techniques for distinguishing critical from non-critical self-association

87. Zana, R., Lang, J., Yiv, S. H., Djavanbakht, A. and Abad, C. (1977). On the use of chemical relaxation methods to distinguish between true micellization and continuous association. In Mittal, K. (ed.) *Micellization, Solubilization and Microemulsion*, Vol. I, pp. 291–304. (New York: Plenum)
88. Mukerjee, P. (1974). Micellar properties of drugs: Micellar and nonmicellar patterns of self-association of hydrophobic solutes of different molecular structures: Monomer fraction availability and misuses of micellar hypothesis. *J. Pharm. Sci.*, **63**, 972
89. Mukerjee, P. (1975). Differing patterns of self-association and micelle formation of hydrophobic solutes. In van Olphen, H. and Mysels, K. J. (eds.) *Physical Chemistry: Enriching Topics from Colloid and Surface Science.* pp. 135–53. (La Jolla, Ca: Theorex)
90. Mukerjee, P. and Cardinal, J. R. (1976). Solubilization as a method for studying self-association: solubility of naphthalene in the bile salt sodium cholate and the complex pattern of aggregation. *J. Pharm. Sci.*, **65**, 882

Reversed Micelle Formation

91. Robeson, J., Foster, B. W., Rosenthal, S. N., Adams, E. T., Jr. and Fendler, E. J. (1981). Vapor pressure, osmometry and nuclear magnetic resonance investigation of some bile acid methyl esters. *J. Phys. Chem.* **85**, 1254
92. Fabre, H., Kamenka, N. and Lindman, B. (1981). Aggregation in three-component surfactant systems from self-diffusion studies: Reversed micelles, microemulsions and transition to normal micelles. *J. Phys. Chem.*, **85**, 3493
93. Fontell, K. (1972). Micellar behavior in solutions of bile-acid salts VI. The solutions of the three-component systems bile-acid salt, n-decanol, and water. *Kolloid Z v. Z. Polymere*, **250**, 825
94. Vadnere, M. and Lindenbaum, S. (1982). Association of deoxycholic acid in organic solvents. *J. Pharm. Sci.*, **71**, 881
95. Vadnere, M. and Lindenbaum, S. (1982). Distribution of bile salts between 1-octanol and aqueous buffer. *J. Pharm. Sci.*, **71**, 875

Electrochemical properties

96. Ekwall, P., Rosendahl, T., Löfman, N. (1957). Studies on bile acid salt solutions I. The dissociation constants of the cholic and desoxycholic acids. *Acta Chem. Scand.*, **11**, 590
97. Ekwall, P., Rosendahl, T. and Sten, A. (1958). Studies on bile acid salt solutions II. The solubility of cholic acid in sodium cholate solutions and that of desoxycholic acid in sodium desoxycholate solutions. *Acta Chem. Scand.*, **12**, 1622
98. Igimi, H. and Carey, M. C. (1980). pH-solubility relations of chenodeoxycholic and urso-deoxycholic acids: Physical–chemical basis for dissimilar solution and membrane phenomena. *J. Lipid Res.*, **21**, 72.

3
Sensitive methods for serum bile acid analysis

ALDO RODA

INTRODUCTION

Although it is well known that the levels of serum bile acid (SBA) increase in liver disease[1-4], the clinical utility of the measurement of SBA levels is not yet established.

The momentary balance between intestinal and hepatic uptake of bile acid (BA) has been identified as the most important physiological determinant of SBA levels[5,6]. Moreover, changes in SBA levels occur in disease: ileal dysfunction decreases SBA (especially after meals) and hepatocyte insufficiency increases SBA.

Because the fractional clearance of BA is very high (80% for chenodeoxy-cholic acid conjugates)[7,8], the peripheral blood contains BA at very low concentration (micromolar levels) compared with that of bile (millimolar levels). In addition, variations in SBA levels related to physiological phenonema (gallbladder emptying, fasting) or to disease are often small[7]. The qualitative pattern of SBA is very complex. We recognize at least 17 different major BA; this derives from the serum bile acids being composed of two primary BA (chenodeoxycholic and cholic acid) and three secondary BA (lithocholic, deoxycholic acid and ursodeoxycholic), each BA occurring in both unconjugated as well as conjugated (glycine/taurine) form. In addition, lithocholyl conjugates are mostly sulphated. Each BA has a slightly different enterohepatic circulation[9,10] so that the qualitative composition of serum BA differs from that of bile.

The peripheral blood compartment is in equilibrium with the entero-hepatic compartment and SBA levels could reflect both liver and intestinal functions; therefore, SBA levels have been proposed as markers for liver and intestinal function[11-16].

In proposing the SBA as a 'test' we have to take into account the following points:

(1) What bile acid or group of bile acids most closely reflects liver or intestinal function?

(2)   What sensitivity is required?

(3)   What other tests are already available?

In developing a new method in clinical chemistry we have to select a BA or a group of BA most involved in a particular disease in order to render the test diagnostically sensitive. In addition, simplicity and rapidity of execution are important factors. From the methodological point of view the sensitivity required is directly related to variations in SBA levels occurring in the mildest or asymptomatic phase of the disease. The earliest methods, such as gas–liquid chromatography or enzymatic assays, lacked sensitivity and consequently the results obtained in patients with liver disease were often contradictory and incomplete. The development of a radioimmunoassay (RIA) for cholyl conjugates was the first step in establishing sensitive (micromolar) and reliable methods for SBA[17]. RIAs for other BA have been introduced and more recently enzyme immunoassays have been reported.

Alternative enzymatic procedures using specific and partially purified steroid dehydrogenase (3α-HSD, 7α-HSD) have been improved using amplified techniques[18,19]. We want to review the more recent methods for measuring SBA with emphasis on immunoassays and enzymatic assays.

The lack of standardization using SBA analyses makes any comparison difficult and limits the diagnostic value of such measurement.

IMMUNOASSAYS

Radioimmunoassays

The first radioimmunoassay (RIA) for bile acids developed by Simmonds et al.[17] represented an enormous improvement in serum bile acid analysis and could be compared with a similar advance followed in developing methods for steroid hormones. Since then, additional RIA methods have been reported[20-38]; their characteristics are summarized in Table 3.1. All the methods reported utilize heterogenous antibodies generally produced in rabbit with a bile acid coupled to a protein (antigen). The carrier protein, usually bovine serum albumin, is covalently linked, by a peptide bond on a C_{24} carboxy group. As a consequence the side chain is completely masked by the protein and the antibodies produced were specific only for the steroid skeletron[39] with rare exceptions. New bile acid–antigen complexes in which the carried protein is bound far from the hydroxy groups and the side chain can be used to produce monoclonal antibodies in vitro. This should result in a more specific and high-affinity antibody and consequently improve the accuracy and sensitivity of the RIA. In addition the production of antibodies specific for unconjugated BA is needed in order to define the physiological role of these BA and their levels in health and disease.

Despite slight differences in the bile acids measured by individual RIAs we found[39] an acceptable agreement when different commercial methods were compared. Table 3.1 reports also the normal values obtained using different methods for SBA. The sensitivity of the RIA method is relatively high (micromolar levels) and appears suitable for measuring variation in SBA

Table 3.1 Characteristics of the RIA methods

Reference	BA measured	Acts direct on serum	Labelled antigen	Separation of B/F	Sensitivity (pmol/tube)	Normal values (μmol/l)
17	CCA	Yes	3H	PEG	5	0.54±0.04
20	CCA	No	3H	$(NH_4)_2SO_4$		0.55±1.8
21	CCA	Yes	3H	$(NH_4)_2SO_4$	10	0.27±0.03
21	CCDCA	Yes	3H	$(NH_4)_2SO_4$	10	0.70±0.03
21	SLCA	Yes	3H	$(NH_4)_2SO_4$	10	0.06±0.01
21	DCA	Yes	3H	$(NH_4)_2SO_4$	10	0.06±0.01
23	CCA	Yes	3H	Solid phase		1.4 ±0.3
24	CCA	Yes	3H	$(NH_4)_2SO_4$	5	0.45±0.12
24	CCDCA	Yes	3H	$(NH_4)_2SO_4$	5	1.05±0.35
25	CCDCA	Yes	3H	$(NH_4)_2SO_4$	2	0.3 +3.8
26	CCA+CCDCA	Yes	125I	Charcoal	0.5	3.47±2.16
27	CCA	Yes	3H	PEG		0.62±0.4
28	DCA	Yes	3H	PEG	7.5	0.18÷0.92
29	LCA	Yes	3H	PEG	20	0.25±0.016
30	SLCA	Yes	3H	$(NH_4)_2SO_4$	10	1.56±0.11
31	CLCA	Yes	3H	$(NH_4)_2SO_4$	5	0.085±0.04
32	UDCA	Yes	3H	PEG	10	0.15±0.11
33	CCA+Free	No	125I	PEG	2	0.43±0.17
33	CCDCA+Free	No	125I	PEG	0.5	0.47±0.23
33	DCA+Free	No	125I	Charcoal	2	0.33±0.11
34	CCA	Yes	125I	Charcoal	9.5	0.4 ÷1.9
35	CCA	Yes	125I	Charcoal		—
36	3 choleic	No	125I	$(NH_4)_2SO_4$	0.6	0.08÷0.45
37	CCA	Yes	3H	$(NH_4)_2SO_4$	5	0.49÷1.32
37	CCDCA	Yes	3H	$(NH_4)_2SO_4$	2	0.55+2.02
38	CCDCA	Yes	125I		1	1.0 ±0.6

CCA=Conjugated cholic acid; CCDCA=conjugated chenodeoxycholic acid; DCA = deoxycholic acid; CLCA=conjugated lithocholic acid; SLCA=sulpholithocholic acid; UDCA = ursodeoxycholic acid.

occurring both in physiological condition (after meals) and pathological ones. With these methods it is also possible to detect ileal dysfunction which is signalled by lower postprandial levels of cholyl conjugates. As far as the method is concerned no major problem exists. Serum bile acids are usually albumin bound (50–60% for cholyl conjugates and 90–96% for chenodeoxycholic conjugates) with an affinity constant ranging from 0.26×10^4 to 4.9×10^4 mol/l[40].

A higher affinity constant of the antibody *vs.* the bile acids (100–1000 times) compared with that of the BA–albumin complex allows us to measure the bile acids direct on serum without any preliminary extraction of bile acids or protein denaturation. The kinetics of the reaction bile acid–antibody association is very fast, and a few minutes of incubation are sufficient to reach the equilibrium. The use of 125I-labelled bile acid instead of 3H-labelled bile acids avoids the use of liquid scintillation equipment but presents the disadvantage of a limited half-life (approximately 30 days) of the 125I-labelled BA. The separation of the antigen-antibody complex from the free antigen is carried out using different methods: $(NH_4)_2 SO_4$, polyethylene glycol (PEG), charcoal, and a solid-phase method (Becton-Dickinson Kit;

antibody immobilized on a solid matrix) has been reported more recently. Despite high sensitivity and simplicity the RIA methods are still expensive (radioactive counting, licence and disposal) and consequently limited to a few specialized laboratories.

Enzyme immunoassay

Enzyme immunoassay (EIA) has become an established tool in clinical chemistry. The assay fulfills the requirements of simplicity and sensitivity previously shown only by RIA. In contrast to RIA the EIA employs stable reagents, requires less expensive equipment, and is more suitable for automation.

Recently, EIAs have been developed for SBA analysis[41-44]. The principle of most EIA (heterogeneous) is similar to that of RIA: the 'tracer' is a BA covalently linked with an enzyme (peroxidase, β galactosidase) instead of a radioisotope. Matern[41] and Makino[32,42] developed EIA methods for cholic acid conjugates and ursodeoxycholic acid respectively based on a 'competitive principle'. The enzyme-labelled BA competes with the BA in the sample for a limited number of binding sites on the antibody. Once equilibrium is reached the antibody-bound antigen is separated (usually by solid-phase techniques or with a second antibody) and the enzymatic activity is recorded spectrophotometrically by measuring specific colour-producing substrates. The absorbance is inversely proportional to the amount of BA present in the sample.

Baquir et al.[43] developed another EIA called 'homogeneous enzyme immunoassay' for chenodeoxycholic acid conjugates not based on the same principles as the common competitive or not-competitive immunoassay. This assay is called 'homogeneous' because no separation steps are required. It is based on the principle that when a BA-enzyme interacts with the specific BA-antibody the enzymatic activity is drastically reduced. An increased proportion of a BA standard or sample in respect to a fixed amount of BA-enzyme will result in a release of the enzymatic activity which is directly proportional to the concentration of BA. No separation of 'bound' and 'free' antigen is required but a kinetic measurement (2 point) of the enzymatic activity is needed. The homogeneous method is in principle less sensitive than the 'heterogeneous' enzyme immunoassay, but enough for SBA analysis. The only disadvantage is that a kinetic measurement of the enzymatic activity is required. The characteristic of the EIA published methods are reported in Table 3.2.

The production of monoclonal antibodies in combination with a more sensitive substrate for the enzyme activity measurement should further improve these methods.

ENZYMATIC ASSAYS

The enzymatic method using a specific hydroxysteroid dehydrogenase (HSD) from pseudomonas testosterone was the first bioassay for BA.

Table 3.2 Characteristics of the enzymatic immunoassays for serum bile acids

Reference	Specificity	Acts direct on serum	label	Principle of the method	Sensitivity	Precision (CV%)	Normal values (μmol/l)
41	chl-gly/ chl-tau	Yes	Peroxidase	Competitive	0.05 μmol/l	18–22	(Not reported)
43	chn-gly/ chn-tau	Yes	Peroxidase	Homogeneous	50 pmol	8.6	(Not reported)
42	urs	Yes	Galactosidase	Competitive	0.08 pmol		(Rabbit)
44	chl-gly/ chl-tau	Yes	Alkaline phosphatase	Competitive	0/2 μg/ml	6–12.8	(Not reported)
45	urs	Yes	Alkaline phosphatase	ELISA	20 pmol	3.22 ± 1.28	0.27 ± 0.12

chl-gly = Cholylglycine; chl-tau = cholyltaurine; chn-gly = chenodeoxycholylglycine; chn-tau = chenodeoxycholyltaurine; urs = ursodeoxycholic acid; CV = coefficient of variation.

61

The 3α-HSD catalyse the oxidation of the 3α-OH group of all BA to a 3-oxo group in presence of NAD as a co-factor. The NADH formed is then measured with different techniques. Iwata *et al.*[46] first applied this assay in 1964 to serum BA. The absorbance of NADH was measured spectrophotometrically at 340 nm. According to the molar coefficient of NADH (6.1 mol/l) it is clear that this method is extremely insensitive and large amounts of serum (3–5 ml) are needed for the analysis, introducing a high background and clinical impracticability. The sensitivity was increased several times by measuring NADH fluorimetrically[47-51]. Despite increased sensitivity, a preliminary extraction of BA from serum was still required.

The first direct enzymatic method with a significant improvement in sensitivity and clinical usefulness was reported by Mashige *et al.*[18] in 1976, now commercialized by Nygaard company (Oslo, Norway). The method includes the use of two enzymes: the 3α-HSD in combination with an NADH-dependent diaphorase (lipoamide reductase, EC 1.6.4.3). This enzyme used NADH as a co-factor in the catalysis of resazurin to resorfin. The fluorescence is measured at 580 nm with excitation at 560 nm. This method may be carried out directly on serum, and a sensitivity of 0.5 μmol/l has been reported. More recently[52] the same group reported a further improvement of the method using spectrophotometry detection instead of fluorimetry. Using the same couple of enzymes they used a coloured dye: the hydrogen of generated NADH is transferred with diaphorase catalysis in nitrotetrazolium blue to yield diformazan which is measured spectrophotometrically at 540 nm. The lowest point of the standard curve was 5 μmol/l (200 ml serum sample).

More recently Nicolas *et al.*[19] developed an extremely sensitive enzyme 'cycling' method (Table 3.3). BA are oxidized by 3α-HSD and after selective destruction of NAD excess the NADH is determined by an enzymatic cycling reaction. The amplifying steps uses 3β- or 17β-HSD to reduce dehydroepiandrosterone to 5-testosterone; then a 3-ketosteroid-5-isomerase enzyme catalyzes the formation of testosterone which is measured spectrophotometrically at 248 μm. This method is very sensitive (0.3 pmol/tube) but requires long incubation, two determinations of absorbance and a UV spectrophotometer (quartz tube).

The use of a 3α-HSD presents some disadvantage: there are other 3α-OH steroids in serum (androsterone, testosterone, etc.). Partially purified HSD such as commercial preparations could contain other dehydrogenase.

The steroid dehydrogenase 7α-HSD has been developed for serum BA[51]. The advantage of a 7α-HSD is that no steroids other than BA contains a 7α-hydroxy group; in addition, with this enzyme it is possible to measure only the primary bile acid, which might be more useful than total bile acid in liver disease diagnosis[4,11].

Using this 7α-HSD, we recently developed an extremely sensitive method for SBA based on bioluminescence measurement[54]. We immobilized three enzymes on Sepharose 4B beads: 7α-HSD, NADH-FMN oxidoreductase and bacterial luciferase. The principle is: the 7α-HSD catalyzes the conversion of the bile acid 7α-hydroxyl group to a keto group. NADH is produced in the reaction and in the presence of NAD:FMN oxidoreductase, it converts FMN

Table 3.3 Characteristics of the more recent enzymatic methods for serum bile acids

Reference	Enzyme	Volume of serum required (ml)	Act direct	NADH detection	Sensitivity (pmol/tube)	Normal values (μmol/l)
47	3α-HSD	3	No	F	1500	0–8.2
48	3α-HSD	2	No	F	1	0.3–9.3
49	3α-HSD	1–3	No	F	630	0.9–6.3
50	3α-HSD	0.8	Yes	F	±1	3–6
51	7α-HSD	1–5	No	F	1000	1.2–6.3
18	3α-HSD	0.1	Yes	S	0.5	6.3±2.9
53	3α-HSD	0.2	Yes	S	2000	1–7
19	3α-HSD	0.05	Yes	S	0.3	3.03+1.13
53	3α-HSD	0.2	Yes	S	2.5	3.2 ±1.3
54	7α-HSD	0.01	Yes	B	2	—

F=fluorimetry; S=spectrophotometry; B=bioluminescence.

63

to its reduced form. This, in the presence of bacterial luciferase, reacts with decanal and oxygen to produce FMN, decanoic acid, and light.

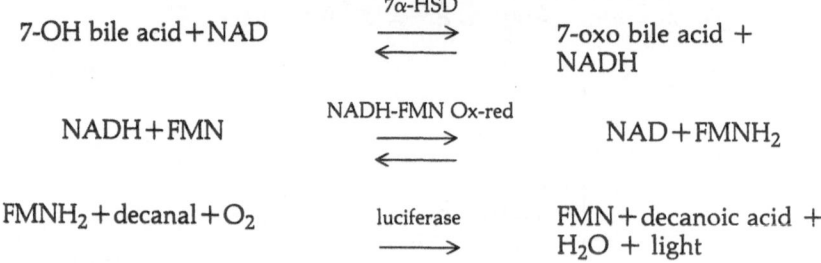

$$7\text{-OH bile acid} + NAD \xrightleftharpoons{7\alpha\text{-HSD}} 7\text{-oxo bile acid} + NADH$$

$$NADH + FMN \xrightleftharpoons{NADH\text{-}FMN\ Ox\text{-}red} NAD + FMNH_2$$

$$FMNH_2 + decanal + O_2 \xrightarrow{luciferase} FMN + decanoic\ acid + H_2O + light$$

The light emission is proportional to the amount of BA present in the test tube. This method is extremely sensitive (2 pmol/tube), precise and rapid. No incubation time is required (1 minute after the addition of reagent) and the enzyme preparation is very stable. It is carried out direct on serum sample and the volume required is very small (5–10 μl).

The method could be used to measure the concentration of the other major serum bile acids by performing a second assay with immobilized 12α-HSD and 3α-HSD.

In addition using this technique it is possible to set up an automated system based on the use of a flow cell inside in the luminometer, containing the three immobilized enzymes.

COMPARISONS OF A SINGLE METHOD

The normal values using RIA techniques for individual classes of BA, as reported by different authors, are listed in Table 3.1. Data are often contra-dictory. For example, the mean normal values for conjugated cholic acid ranged from 0.18 to 1.4 μmol/l, and for conjugated chenodeoxycholic acid from 0.2 to 1.05 μmol/l. Even greater differences exist for deoxycholic acid (0.06–0.33 μmol/l) and for sulpholithocholic acid (0.06–1.56 μmol/l). It appears clear that the data on SBA levels in health and disease depend to some extent on the methodology, and that contradictory results obtained for patients with liver disease can be explained in part by methodology differences. Unfortunately, not all methods have been validated using an independent well-established method such as gas–liquid chromatography. In addition, important factors such as antibody titer and specificity, protein effect, and differences in 'tracer' may play an important role in the reliability of the RIA results. In a previous study we compared six different RIA methods for primary BA which were commercially available[39]. An acceptable agreement of values for BA was observed when measured in a series of 25 serum samples using the six different kits. In addition the normal values using these kits were quite similar. We concluded that for the analysis of the two primary BA the current commercially available methods offer reliable results and despite differences in antibody specificity, results obtained can be compared. For other BA such as deoxycholate, lithocholate, and sulpholithocholate, the methods proposed require further improvement and needed to be validated using independent methods.

As far as the enzymatic method is concerned the normal values reported by different authors ranged from 0.1 to 9.3 μmol/l. Only one kit is commercially available and no comparisons were reported.

COMPARISONS BETWEEN METHODS

We compared values obtained with RIA with those obtained using an enzymatic method (3α Sterognost), an EIA method and with a GLC method – Table 3.4 shows the results obtained: a good agreement at high levels was observed and a poor one below 5 μmol/l, at which the enzymatic and GLC methods lack sensitivity. In the last 2 years the emerging interest in SBA as a candidate for liver function tests encouraged us to organize a national quality control in order to verify the reliability of results and unify normal values.

Table 3.4 Comparison of different methods for serum bile acid analysis

Sample (μmol/l)	GLC	3α-HSD	RIA ^{3}H	EIA
		Glychocholic acid		
0.1	Traces	0.25	0.14	0.20
1	0.90	1.45	1.08	1.5
10	9.25	11.05	10.70	12.0
100	102	100.5	98.5	107
		Glycochenodeoxycholic acid		
0.1	0.25	0.35	0.18	0.26
1	1.21	1.82	1.11	1.35
10	11.0	13.2	9.61	10.7
100	96	98	113	96

Sample = Charcoal extracted human serum and increased amount of bile acids.

To this study 11 different laboratories located in different parts of Italy have been admitted[55]. The protocol included the blind measurements of SBA of different serum specimens for a period of 1 year. The sample[50] included normal serum, pathological sera, BA added to a bile acid free serum, and serum with disproportionated amount of BAs. Some samples were sent differently labelled. The methods used included: RIA (all the commercially available kits, Abbott, Becton and Dickinson, Nordic Lab, Sorin, and that produced in our laboratory)[24,3], enzymatic method (3α Sterognost) and two gas–liquid chromatography techniques. The data were computerized. The preliminary results obtained (to be published elsewhere) can be here summarized.

(1) The analysis of a normal serum using the RIA presented the lower 'intralab' coefficient of variation (15–20%) compared with the

enzymatic method (25–30%) and gas–liquid chromatography (40–60%); when pathological sera were analyzed a similar intralab coefficient of variation was found for all methods (25–40%).

(2) A high coefficient of variation was observed when independent methods were compared (greater than 50%).

(3) Interlab accuracy using the same technique is lower even if unacceptable values are obtained (coefficient of variation ⟩ 20%).

These results suggest that at the present time the analysis of serum bile acid requires further standardization mainly when independent methods are compared; this derives from different analytical informations obtained using different techniques (conjugated BA by RIA, total BA by enzymatic method, unconjugated BA by GLC etc.). Among the intercompared methods the RIA seems to be the more sensitive one.

CONCLUSION

The immunological methods for SBA seem to be the more sensitive. Several kits both from Europe and USA are commercially available but for 'unknown' reasons none of them measure the same bile acid. It appears clear that even if normal values are quite similar, levels related to disease can greatly differ. The sensitivity of this method is adequate to measure not only increases in SBA which occur in liver disease but also reduction in SBA (mainly after meals) occurring in patients with bile acid malabsorption. The enzymatic method, on the other hand, measures total bile acid with low sensitivity. These methods are still sensitive enough to be applied in monitoring patients with liver disease but not in patients with ileal dysfunction. More recently 'amplified' methods including both 3α-HSD and more recently 7α-HSD[54] have improved the sensitivity of the latest technique. The sensitivity is similar or greater than RIA. This technique may be used in both liver and intestinal disease. The enzymatic method with elevated sensitivity offers a series of advantages compared with RIA in terms of automation and cost.

In conclusion, analytical biochemistry can offer the specialist physicians a series of good methods for SBA. The problem of its usefulness in diagnosis is still unsolved and a large-scale prospective study on SBA related to disease is needed. However, documentation of the clinical utility is extremely difficult, as one must show that a new test offers information which correctly influenced physician or patient behaviour and that such information is not available at an identical cost from existing tests.

References

1. Sherlock, S. and Walshe, V. (1948). Blood cholates in normal subjects and in liver disease. *Clin. Sci.*, 6, 223
2. Rudman, D. and Kendall, F. E. (1957). Bile acid content of human serum. I. Serum bile acids in patients with hepatic disease. *J. Clin. Invest.*, 36, 530
3. Skrede, S. *et al.* (1978). Bile acids measured in serum during fasting as a test for liver

disease. *Clin. Chem.*, **24**, 1095

4. Barbara, L. *et al.* (1976). Diurnal variations of serum primary bile acids in healthy subjects and hepatobiliary disease patients. *Rendic. Gastroenterol.*, **8**, 194

5. Hofmann, A. F. *et al.* (1977). Serum bile acid levels: a compartmental model for the dynamics of the enterohepatic circulation. In Paumgartner, G. and Stiehl, A. (eds.) *Bile Acid Metabolism in Health and Disease*, p. 151. (Lancaster: MTP Press)

6. La Russo, N. F. *et al.* (1974). Intestinal absorption. The major determinant of serum bile acids in patients with normal liver function (abstract). *Gastroenterology,* **67**, 806

7. Glasinovic, J. O. *et al.* (1975). Hepatocellular uptake of taurocholate in the dog. *J. Clin. Invest.*, **55**, 419

8. Reichen, H. and Paumgartner, G. (1968). Uptake of bile acids by perfused rat liver. *Am. J. Physiol.*, **231**, 734

9. Dietshy, J. M. (1968). Mechanism for the intestinal absorption of bile acids. *J. Lipid. Res.*, **91**, 297

10. Schiff, E. R. *et al.* (1972). Characterization of the kinetics of the passive and active transport mechanisms for bile acid absorption in the small intestine and colon of the rat. *J. Clin. Invest.*, **51**, 1351

11. Korman, M. G. *et al.* (1976). Assessment of activity in chronic active liver disease. *N. Engl. J. Med.*, **290**, 1399

12. Neale, G. *et al.* (1971). Serum bile acids in liver disease. *Gut*, **12**, 145

13. Roda, A. *et al.* (1978). Le dosage radio-immunologique des acids biliaires: sa signification diagnostique et prognostique. *Acta Gastro-Ent. Belg.*, **41**, 653

14. Barbara, L. (1978). Bile acids as markers of liver disease. *Ital. J. Gastroenterol.*, **10** (Suppl. 1), 8

15. Fausa, O. and Gjone, E. (1976). Serum bile acid concentrations in patients with liver disease. *Scand. J. Gastroenterol.*, **11**, 537

16. Bouchier, I. A. D. and Pennington, C. R. (1978). Serum bile acids in hepatobiliary disease. *Gut*, **19**, 492

17. Simmonds, W. J. *et al.* (1973). Radioimmunoassay of conjugated cholyl bile acids in serum. *Gastroenterology*, **65**, 705

18. Mashige, F. *et al.* (1976). A simple and sensitive assay of total serum bile acids. *Clin. Chim. Acta*, **70**, 79

19. Nicolas, J. C. *et al.* (1980). Enzymatic microassay of serum bile acids: increased sensitivity with an enzyme amplification technique. *Anal. Biochem.*, **103**, 170

20. Murphy, G. M. *et al.* (1974). The preparations and properties of an antiserum for the radioimmunoassay of serum conjugated cholic acid. *Clin. Chim. Acta*, **54**, 81

21. Demers, L. M. and Hepner, G. W. (1976). Radioimmunoassay of bile acids in serum. *Clin. Chem.*, **22**, 602

22. Matern, S. *et al.* (1976). Radioimmunoassay of serum conjugated cholic acid. *Clin. Chim. Acta*, **72**, 39

23. van der Berg, J. W. O. *et al.* (1976). Solid phase radioimmunoassay for determination of conjugated cholic acid in serum. *Clin. Chim. Acta*, **73**, 277

24. Roda, A. *et al.* (1977). Development, validation, and application of a single tube radioimmunoassay for cholic and chenodeoxycholic acid conjugated bile acids in human serum. *Clin. Chem.*, **23**, 2107

25. Schalm, S. W. *et al.* (1977). Radioimmunoassay of bile acids: development, validation and preliminary application of an assay for conjugates of chenodeoxycholic acid. *Gastroenterology*, **73**, 285

26. Spenney, J. G. *et al.* (1977). An ^{125}I-radioimmunoassay for primary conjugated bile salts. *Gastroenterology*, **72**, 305

27. Mihas, A. A. *et al.* (1977). A critical evaluation of a procedure for measurement of serum bile acids by radioimmunoassay. *Clin. Chim. Acta*, **76**, 389

28. Matern, S. *et al.* (1977). Radioimmunoassay of serum-conjugated deoxycholic acid. *Scand. J. Gastroenterol.*, **12**, 641

29. Cowen, A. E. *et al.* (1977). Radioimmunoassay of unsulfated lithocholates. *J. Lipid Res.*, **18**, 692

30. Cowen, A. E. *et al.* (1977). Radioimmunoassay of sulphated lithocholates. *J. Lipid Res.*, **18**, 698

31. Roda, A. *et al.* (1978). A radioimmunoassay for lithocholic acid conjugates in human serum and liver tissue. *Steroid,* **32,** 13
32. Makino, I. *et al.* (1978). Radioimmunoassay of ursodeoxycholic acid in serum. *J. Lipid Res.,* **19,** 443
33. Mentausta, O. and Janne, O. (1979). Radioimmunoassay of conjugated cholic acid, chenodeoxycholic acid and deoxycholic acid from human serum, with use of ^{125}I-labelled ligands. *Clin. Chem.,* **25,** 264
34. Minder, E. *et al.* (1979). A highly specific ^{125}I-radioimmunoassay for cholic acid conjugates. *Clin. Chim. Acta,* **92,** 177
35. Miller, P. *et al.* (1981). Specific ^{125}I-radioimmunoassay for cholylglycine, a bile acid, in serum. *Clin. Chem.,* **27,** 1698
36. Minder, E.I. *et al.* (1978). Radioimmunoassay determination of serum 3β-hydroxy-5-cholenoic acid in normal subjects and patients with liver disease. *J. Lipid Res.,* **20,** 986
37. Baqir, Y.A. *et al.* (1979). Radioimmunoassay of primary bile salts in serum. *J. Clin. Pathol.,* **32,** 560
38. Beckett, G.J. *et al.* (1979). The preparation of ^{125}I-labelled bile acid for use in the radioimmunoassay of bile acids. *Clin. Chim. Acta.,* **93,** 145
39. Roda, A. *et al.* (1980). Results with six 'kit' radioimmunoassays for primary bile acids in human serum intercompared. *Clin Chem.,* **26,** 1647
40. Roda, A. *et al.* (1982). Quantitative aspects of the interaction of bile acids with human serum albumin. *J. Lipid Res.,* **23,** 490
41. Matern, S. *et al.* (1978). Enzyme labelled immunoassay for a bile acid in human serum. In Pal-Walter de Gruyter, S.B. (ed.) *European Labelled Immunoassays of Hormones and Drugs,* pp. 457–467
42. Maeda. Y. *et al.* (1979). Development of a solid-phase enzyme immunoassay for ursodeoxycholic acid: application to plasma disappearance of injected ursodeoxycholic acid in the rabbit. *J. Lipid Res.,* **20,** 960
43 Baqir, Y.A. *et al.* (1979). Homogeneous enzyme immunoassay of chenodeoxycholic acid conjugates in serum. *Anal. Biochem.,* **93,** 361
44. Immunotechnical Corporation Cambridge, Ma,; *Endab cholylglycine EIA Kit.*
45. Ozaki, A. *et al.* (1979). Enzyme linked immunoassay of ursodeoxycholic acid in serum. *J. Lipid Res.,* **20,** 2340
46. Iawata, T. and Yamasaki, K. (1969). Enzymatic determination and thin layer chromatography of bile acid in blood. *J. Biochem.,* **56,** 424
47. Murphy, G.M. *et al.* (1970). A fluorimetric and enzymatic method for the estimation of serum total bile acids. *J. Clin. Path.,* **23,** 594
48. Schwartz, H.P. *et al.* (1974). A simple method for the estimation of bile acids in serum. *Clin. Chem. Acta,* **50,** 197
49. Fausa, O. (1975). Quantitative determination of serum bile acids using a purified 3-alpha hydrosteroid dehydrogenase. *Scand. J. Gastroenterol.* **10,** 747
50. Siskos, P.A. *et al.* (1977). Serum bile acids analysis: a rapid direct enzymatic method using dual beam spectrophotometry. *J. Lipid Res.,* **18,** 666
51. Fausa, O. and Skalhegg, B.A. (1977). Quantitative determination of serum bile acid using a 7-alpha-hydroxysteroid dehydrogenase. *Scand. J. Gastroenterol.,* **12,** 44
52. Mashige, F. *et al.* (1981). Direct spectrophotometry of total bile acids in serum. *Clin. Chem.,* **27,** 1352
53. Steensland, H. (1978). An automated method for the determination of total bile acid in serum. *Scand. J. Clin. Lab. Invest.,* **38,** 447
54. Roda, A. *et al.* (1982). Bioluminescent measurement of bile acids using immobilized 7-alpha-hydrosteroid dehydrogenase: application to serum bile acids. *J. Lipid. Res.* (in press)
55. Attili. A. (Roma), Baccini, C. (Ravenna), Cenciotti, L. (Cesena), Galeazzi, R. (Ancona), Fiaccadovi, F. (Parma), Morselli, A., Capelli, M., Roda, A. (Bologna), Narducci, F. (Perugia), Sanguineti, M. (Genova), Ruggeri, R. (Forli), Salvioli, C. (Modena), Spaccesi, E. (Macerata): Controllo di qualità del dosaggio degli acidi biliari sierici (dati in corso di pubblicazione)

4
Evaluation of hepatic cholesterol synthesis in man: results with the HMG-CoA reductase activity assay

NICOLA CARULLI, MAURIZIO PONZ DE LEON AND
FRANCA ZIRONI

INTRODUCTION

The liver plays a key role in the metabolism and disposition of cholesterol. Input of the sterol to the liver derives from three sources: circulating lipoprotein cholesterol, absorption of dietary cholesterol and local neosynthesis. The liver disposes of its cholesterol by exporting it as lipoprotein into the circulation or secreting it into the bile, either as intact molecule or after its degradation to bile acids. All these processes are somewhat interlocked so that, in physiological conditions, cholesterol balance is kept in equilibrium. One of the factors responsible for this homeostasis is the capacity of the liver to adapt its own cholesterol synthesis.

The pathway leading to cholesterol is rather complex, starting with a simple two-carbon molecule, such as acetate, and ending with a cyclic compound which is the steroid nucleus of cholesterol. The speed of this synthetic process is regulated by many effectors which act on some critical steps of the pathway. Of these steps the transformation of 3-hydroxy-3-methylglutaryl Coenzyme A (HMG-CoA) into mevalonate appears to be of primary importance, although subsequent steps of the pathway could also play a role [1-3].

The rate of hepatic synthesis of cholesterol can be estimated *in vitro* by means of the isotope incorporation principle, using labelled substrates and suitable liver preparations. All the employed procedures have advantages and disadvantages and give only relative estimates of cholesterol synthesis rate. Recently it has been demonstrated that the use of tritiated water, under appropriate conditions and given some assumptions, allows the calculation of values close to the absolute rates of synthesis [4].

Unfortunately, reliable techniques to measure hepatic cholesterol synthesis are not suitable for studies in man. So far the only approach used has been the assay of HMG-CoA reductase activity on liver biopsies not-withstanding the many limitations due both to the physiology of this enzyme and to the methodology of its assay.

Recently it has been shown that HMG-CoA reductase could exist in two forms: a phosphorylated one which is inactive and a dephosphorylated one which is active[5]. We do not know as yet the physiological relevance of the two forms but it may be that the mechanism of phospho-dephosphorylation is responsible for the rapid changes in the reductase activity[6] as has been reported to occur *in vivo* following glucagon administration[7].

The other way by which the activity of HMG-CoA reductase is regulated involves changes of the synthesis or degradation of the enzymic protein. Most likely this latter mechanism accounts for the changes of the reductase activity related to the light–dark cycle, fasting and feeding, the administration of cholesterol and other sterols or hormones, but this problem is not yet well defined[2,8].

The assay of HMG-CoA reductase activity is based on the irreversible transformation of HMG-CoA into mevalonic acid and CoA in the presence of microsomes and an NADPH-generating system. Of the formed products of the reaction mevalonate appears to be the most suitable to measure. This can be accomplished by different procedures, the most common being chloroform extraction, separation of mevalonate on TLC and quantitation of its recovery by means of synthetic tritiated mevalonate added as internal standard[9]. The measured HMG-CoA reductase activity depends on critical conditions such as preparation of microsomes, buffer, pH and quantitation of biosynthetic mevalonate. In conclusion the estimation of the reductase activity could be influenced by many variables; however, in different experimental conditions the enzyme activity has proved to be correlated to the cholesterol synthetic rate as measured by other procedures[10].

Additional limitations should be considered when extrapolating HMG-CoA reductase values obtained in human liver specimen to hepatic cholesterol synthesis. Usually the groups of patients compared when studying the effect of whatever treatment are different and, mainly for ethical reasons, rarely does a subject act as his or her own control[11]. Sometimes the liver specimen is obtained by needle aspiration, but more often it is taken at surgery and in this case the effect of anaesthetic should be taken into account. Most important of all the liver specimen is usually obtained after a prolonged fast and in the morning, when the HMG-CoA reductase is at its nadir. These two latter factors greatly reduce the sensitivity of the measured enzyme activity as index of hepatic cholesterol synthesis rate. Finally, methodological settings for the assay differ from laboratory to laboratory.

HMG-CoA REDUCTASE ACTIVITY IN DIFFERENT CONDITIONS IN MAN

From all the above considerations a wide scattering of reductase activity values in human liver specimen could be expected. Indeed this seems to be the case as shown in Figure 4.1 which illustrates the 'normal' values of

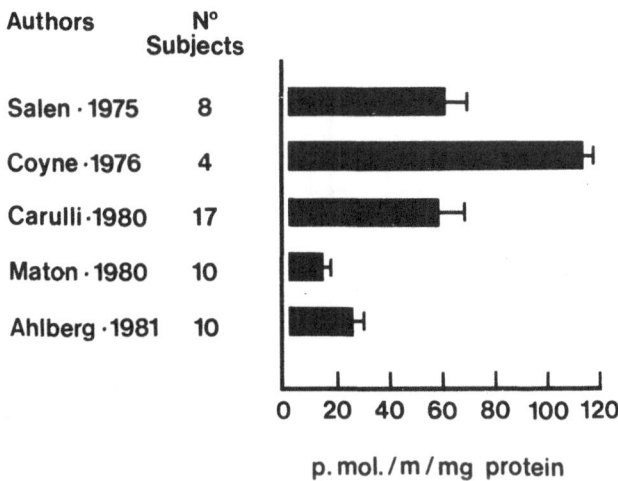

Figure 4.1 HMG-CoA reductase activity in man. 'Normal' values have been obtained on liver specimen taken by needle aspiration or, in the majority of the cases, at surgery for duodenal ulcer, gallbladder adenomyoma, Hodgkin's staging and other unexplained pathology. In all cases light microscopy of the specimen did not reveal morphological alterations.

reductase activity reported by different investigators [12-16]. It can be noted that the range of reductase activity spans over a nearly ten-fold difference from less than 15 to about 120 pmol min^{-1} (mg protein)$^{-1}$.

However, regardless of the absolute figures, once the operative conditions have been standardized, it could be presumed that the estimation of HMG-CoA reductase activity could be used at least for comparative purposes in the same laboratory; that is, for studying the effect of a disease or of a treatment on hepatic cholesterol synthesis rate.

This seems to be true for some conditions known to be associated with alterations of sterol synthesis such as cirrhosis, type IV hyperlipidaemia (HPL), obesity and cerebrotendinous xanthomatosis (CTX). In fact, in patients with these diseases, hepatic HMG-CoA reductase activity has been shown to change accordingly: reduced in cirrhosis[17], and increased in type IV HPL[18], obesity[19] and CTX[20].

The same seems to hold true for treatments with drugs known, from animal studies, to produce an increased reductase activity. It is what we have observed in two patients treated with cholestyramine who showed a twofold increase of HMG—CoA reductase activity (unpublished observations) and Coyne *et al.* have reported similar results in subjects treated with phenobarbital[13].

However, when we do evaluate HMG-CoA reductase activity in those conditions in which there are not consistent changes of hepatic cholesterol synthesis, then equivocal results could be observed. This appears to be the case of cholesterol cholelithiasis. Figure 4.2 illustrates the results on HMG—CoA reductase reported by different investigators. It is evident that

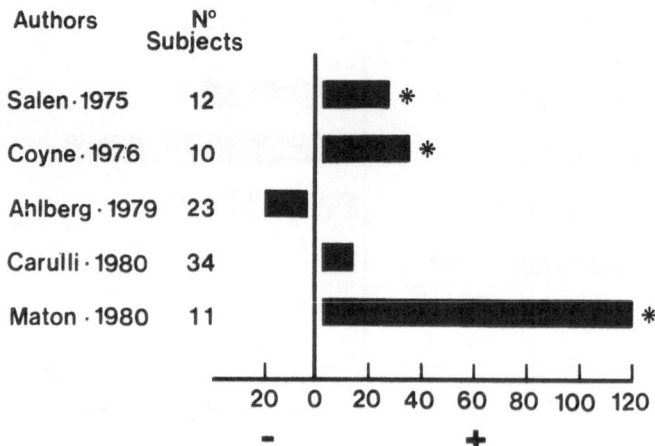

Figure 4.2 HMG-CoA reductase activity in subjects with cholesterol gallstones. The results are expressed as percentage variation (−or+) from the 'normal' values of each laboratory.

whereas some authors have found a striking[15] or, at least, a significant[12,13] increase of the reductase activity, others could not find any difference between controls and patients with gallstones[14,16].

Another controversial issue is the one concerning the effect of bile acid administration on cholesterol synthesis in man, as judged by hepatic HMG-CoA reductase activity. Table 4.1 summarizes the results on the reductase activity reported by different authors in gallstone subjects treated with individual bile acids. While there seems to be no doubt on the capacity of

Table 4.1 Effect of individual bile acid administration on HMG-CoA reductase activity in subjects with cholesterol gallstones

Administered bile acid	No. of subjects	HMG-CoA reductase activity; % variation from control	Reference
CDCA	2	−50	21
	4	−40	13
	9	−60	22
	8	−55	14
	6	−51	15
	9	−40	16
UDCA	2	−65	11
	8	+100	14
	9	−40	15
	?	Unchanged	Angelin*
CA	12	Unchanged	16
DCA	9	−45	23

*Data by Angelin are quoted in reference 24.

chenodeoxycholic acid (CDCA) administration to decrease HMG-CoA reductase to less than 50% of the untreated value[13-16,21,22], the results on the effect of ursodeoxycholic acid (UDCA) are rather controversial. In our hands the administration of UDCA, on a short-term basis, led to a two-fold increase in HMG-CoA reductase activity[14]. Other investigators have found either no change[24] or a significant decrease of the reductase activity[11,15]. In addition the administration of cholic acid (CA) has been reported to be ineffective in changing the specific activity of HMG-CoA reductase[16] whereas the administration of deoxycholic acid (DCA), in our laboratory, did produce a decrease of the reductase activity similar to that observed with CDCA[23].

From this rapid review it could be concluded that: (1) the evaluation of HMG-CoA reductase activity gives, at the best, relative values of the rate of hepatic cholesterol synthesis; (2) methodological limitations reduce its sensitivity in predicting changes of hepatic cholesterol synthesis in man; (3) the results obtained so far are too preliminary to establish the assay of HMG-CoA reductase as a useful and practical means to study hepatic cholesterol synthesis in man.

REFERENCES

1. Dietschy, J. M. and Wilson, J. D. (1970). Regulation of cholesterol metabolism. *N. Engl. J. Med.*, **282**, 1179
2. Rodwell, V. W., Nordstrom, J. L. and Mitschelen, J. J. (1976). Regulation of HMG-CoA reductase. *Adv. Lip Res.*, **14**, 1
3. Brown, M. S. and Goldstein, J. L. (1980). Multivalent feedback regulation of HMG-CoA reductase, a control mechanism coordinating isoprenoid synthesis and cell growth. *J. Lipid Res.*, **21**, 505
4. Andersen. J. M. and Dietschy, J. M. (1979). Absolute rates of cholesterol synthesis in extrahepatic tissues measured with ^{3}H-labelled water and ^{14}C-labelled substrates. *J. Lipid Res.*, **20**, 740
5. Beg, Z. H., Stonik, J. A. and Brewer, H. B. Jr. (1978). 3-Hydroxy-3-methylglutaryl coenzyme A reductase: regulation of enzymatic activity by phosphorylation and dephosphorylation. *Proc. Natl. Acad. Sci. USA*, **75**, 3678
6. Brewer, H. B. and Beg, Z. H. (1981). Short-term regulation of cholesterol biosynthesis. In Paumgartner, G., Stiehl, A. and Gerok. W. (eds.) *Bile Acids and Lipids*, pp. 23–29. (Lancaster: MTP Press)
7. Beg, Z. H., Stonik, J. A. and Brewer, H. B. (1980). *In vitro* and *in vivo* phosphorylation of rat liver 3-hydroxy-3-methylglutaryl coenzyme A reductase and its modulation by glucagon. *J. Biol. Chem.*, **255**, 8541
8. Arebalo, R. E., Tormanen, C. D., Hardgrave, J. E., Noland, B. J. and Scallen, T. J. (1982). *In vivo* regulation of rat liver 3-hydroxy-3-methylglutaryl-coenzyme A reductase: immunotitration of the enzyme after short-term mevalonate or cholesterol feeding. *Proc. Nat. Acad. Sci. USA*, **79**, 51
9. Goldfarb, S. and Pitot, H. C. (1971). Improved assay of 3-hydroxy-3-methylglutaryl coenzyme A reductase. *J. Lipid Res.*, **12**, 512
10. Brown, M. S., Goldstein, J. L. and Dietschy, J. M. (1979). Active and inactive forms of 3-Hydroxy-3-methylglutaryl coenzyme A reductase in the liver of the rat. Comparison with the rate of cholesterol synthesis in different physiological states. *J. Biol. Chem.*, **254**,5144
11. Salen, G., Colalillo, A., Verga, D., Bagan, E., Tint, G. S. and Shefer S. (1980). Effect of high and low doses of ursodeoxycholic acid on gallstone dissolution in humans. *Gastroenterology*, **78**, 1412

12. Salen, G., Nicolau, G., Shefer, S. and Mosbach, E. H. (1975). Hepatic cholesterol metabolism in patients with gallstones. *Gastroenterology*, **69**, 676
13. Coyne, M. J., Bonorris, G. G., Goldstein, L. I. and Schoenfield, L. J. (1976). Effect of chenodeoxycholic acid and phenobarbital on the rate-limiting enzymes of hepatic cholesterol and bile acid synthesis in patients with gallstones. *J. Lab. Clin. Med.*, **87**, 281
14. Carulli, N., Ponz de Leon, M., Zironi, F., Pinetti, A., Smerieri, A., Iori, R. and Loria, P. (1980). Hepatic cholesterol and bile acid metabolism in subjects with gallstones: comparative effects of short term feeding of chenodeoxycholic and ursodeoxycholic acid. *J. Lipid Res.*, **21**, 35
15. Maton, P. N., Ellis, H. J., Higgins, M. J. P. and Dowling, R. H. (1980). Hepatic HMG-CoA reductase in human cholelithiasis: effects of chenodeoxycholic and ursodeoxycholic acids. *Eur. J. Clin. Invest.*, **10**, 325
16. Ahlberg, J., Angelin, B. and Einarsson, K. (1981). Hepatic 3-hydroxy-3-methylglutaryl coenzyme A reductase activity and biliary lipid composition in man: relation to cholesterol gallstone disease and effects of cholic and chenodeoxycholic acid treatment. *J. Lipid Res.*, **22**, 410
17. Carulli, N. Zironi, F., Bosco, F. and Zambarda, E. (1977). Relationship between rate-limiting enzymes of hepatic cholesterol and bile acid metabolism and bile lipid composition (abstract). *Arch. Hell. Med. Soc.*, **3**, Suppl. 8
18. Ahlberg, J., Angelin, B., Bjorkhem, I., Einarsson, K. and Leijd, B. (1979). Hepatic cholesterol metabolism in normo- and hyperlipidemic patients with cholesterol gallstones. *J. Lipid Res.*, **20**, 107
19. Reuben, A., Maton, P. N., Murphy, G. M. and Dowling, R. H. (1981). Cholesterol synthesis and biliary cholesterol secretion in obesity. In Paumgartner, G., Stiehl, A. and Gerok, W. (eds.) *Bile Acids and Lipids*. pp. 203–209. (Lancaster: MTP Press)
20. Nicolau, G., Shefer, S., Salen, G. and Mosbach, E. H. (1974). Determination of hepatic 3-hydroxy-3-methylglutaryl CoA reductase activity in man. *J. Lipid Res.*, **15**, 94
21. Salen, G., Nicolau, G. and Shefer, S. (1973). Chenodeoxycholic acid inhibits elevated HMG-CoA reductase activity in subjects with gallstones (abstract). *Clin. Res.*, **21**,523
22. Key, P. H., Bonorris, G. G., Marks, J. W. and Schoenfield, L. J. (1978). Mechanism of cholesterol desaturation of bile by chenodeoxycholic acid in gallstone patients (abstract). *Gastroenterology*, **74**, 1161
23. Carulli, N., Ponz de Leon, M., Zironi, F., Iori, R. and Loria P. (1980). Bile acid feeding and hepatic sterol metabolism: effect of deoxycholic acid. *Gastroenterology*, **79**, 637
24. Einarsson, K., Ahlberg, J., Angelin, B. and Ewerth, S. (1981). Bile acids and hepatic HMG-CoA reductase in man. In Paumgartner, G., Stiehl, A. and Gerok, W. (eds.) *Bile Acids and Lipids*. pp. 67–71. (Lancaster: MTP Press)

5

Measurement of bile acid and cholesterol kinetics in man by isotope dilution: principles and applications

ALAN F. HOFMANN AND SUSAN A. CUMMINGS

INTRODUCTION

In man, the cholesterol molecule is a major constituent of cell membranes, and most body tissues synthesize cholesterol continuously. Excessive cholesterol retention is associated with elevated serum cholesterol levels and arterial disease. Thus, it is necessary for the adult organism to have a means of eliminating cholesterol. This has been achieved chemically by converting cholesterol to water-soluble derivatives, the bile acids, which are secreted into bile, and physically by excreting cholesterol as such in the mixed micelle present in bile.

In the physical sciences it is useful to distinguish intensity qualities from capacity qualities. For example, temperature is an intensity factor, whereas heat content is a capacity factor. Similarly, pH is an intensity measurement, whereas buffering power is a capacity measurement. This reasoning may be considered to apply, by analogy, to bile acids and cholesterol. The serum level of bile acids may be considered an intensity factor, whereas the exchangeable bile acid pool may be considered a capacity factor. The same is also true for cholesterol: the serum cholesterol may be considered an intensity factor and the exchangeable pools a capacity factor.

The technique of isotope dilution is the only non-invasive method which permits quantitation of the exchangeable pools of bile acids and cholesterol. In this brief article, I will review current concepts of isotope dilution measurements of cholesterol and bile acids – their principles, practical aspects of methodology, and applications in health and disease. A previous review[1] has dealt with selected aspects of isotope dilution techniques for characterizing bile acid metabolism. A book by Sodhi, Kudchodkar and Mason[2] offers a readable introduction to cholesterol and bile acid metabolism and discusses experimental methodology in considerable detail.

OVERALL VIEW OF CHOLESTEROL AND BILE ACID METABOLISM

The simplest schematic view of cholesterol and bile acid metabolism is shown in Figure 5.1. An exchangeable 'pool' of cholesterol has two inputs: synthesis of cholesterol and absorption of dietary cholesterol. Cholesterol is eliminated by excretion as such or by conversion to bile acids. The conversion of cholesterol to bile acids generates an 'input' of bile acids into the exchangeable bile acid pools, from which bile acids are excreted. There is no input into the bile acid pool by absorption of dietary bile acids, as usually the diet contains no bile acids.

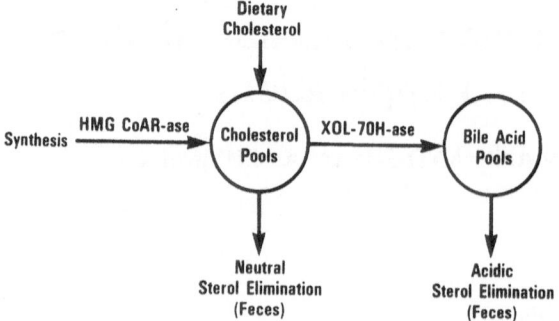

Figure 5.1 Simplified compartmental model of cholesterol and bile acid metabolism. The rate-limiting enzymes are indicated. The term 'dietary cholesterol' refers to the new dietary cholesterol which enters the exchangeable pools of cholesterol. In the sterol balance technique, acidic and neutral sterols are measured. To calculate cholesterol synthesis, the amount of dietary cholesterol which is absorbed must be known. HMG-CoAR-ase = hydroxy-methyl-glutaryl-coenzyme A reductase; XOL-ase = cholesterol 7α-hydroxylase

The exchangeable cholesterol pools may be divided into additional pools – a rapidly exchangeable pool and one or more slowly exchangeable pools[3], as will be discussed. Similarly, the bile acid pool may be divided into two primary bile acid pools, since cholesterol is converted to the two primary bile acids – cholic acid and chenodeoxycholic acid. Thus, with four exchangeable pools, one can in principle represent the major exchangeable pools of body cholesterol and the primary bile acids in man[4]. However, two pools are insufficient to describe bile acid metabolism in man, since the secondary bile acid, deoxycholic acid, which is formed from cholic acid by bacterial 7-dehydroxylation, is a major biliary bile acid, also. After deoxycholic acid is formed, it is absorbed in part from the distal intestine and enters the enterohepatic circulation. Accordingly, one must add a third bile acid pool, i.e. a deoxycholic acid pool, for a more complete description of bile acid metabolism in man[4].

The two primary bile acids and the secondary bile acid, deoxycholic acid, constitute more than 95% of the bile acid pool in most healthy individuals. The two remaining bile acids in man, ursodeoxycholic and lithocholic, are present in only trace amounts (< 5% of biliary bile acids), so it is not necessary to consider them for an approximate description of the enterohepatic circulation of bile acids in man. Both ursodeoxycholic and lithocholic are formed from chenodeoxycholic acid. Their metabolism is more complex than that of the major biliary bile acids, as will be discussed.

DIFFERENCES BETWEEN BILE ACID AND CHOLESTEROL METABOLISM

Virtually all of the bile acids secreted in bile are reabsorbed from the intestine, so that bile acids undergo an enterohepatic circulation which is conveniently depicted by a loop (Figure 5.2). The left arm represents spillover of bile acids into the general circulation. The right arm reflects secretion of bile acids into the intestine, and their subsequent absorption. In principle, each bile acid has its own loop so that the exchangeable bile acid pool shown in Figure 5.1 is in fact composed of at least five loops.

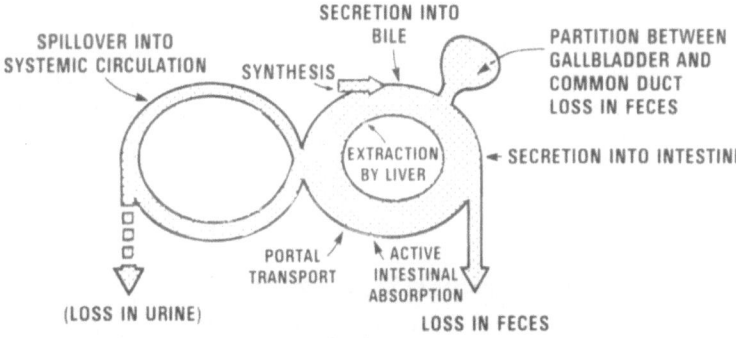

Figure 5.2 Schematic depiction of the enterohepatic circulation of primary bile acids in man. The liver is present at the junction of the two rings. There is no urinary loss in healthy individuals

Cholesterol does not undergo an enterohepatic circulation, in that the molecules which are absorbed from the intestine in the physical form of chylomicrons exchange rapidly with cholesterol molecules at many sites in the body and are not promptly re-excreted into bile, as occurs with the bile acids. In addition, cholesterol also differs from bile acids in being ubiquitous in its tissue distribution, whereas bile acids are localized to the liver, bilary tract, intestinal tract, and plasma compartment. Cholesterol also differs from bile acids in another key respect: cholesterol is synthesized by many body tissues, whereas bile acids are synthesized exclusively in the liver[5]. Thus, there is no simple way to depict cholesterol metabolism in a semi-schematic way as has been done for bile acids. Finally, the rate of exchange of injected tracer varies strikingly between bile acids and cholesterol, as will be detailed. Bile acids exchange completely and relatively rapidly – within a few hours. In contrast, equilibration of injected cholesterol with exchangeable pools requires weeks or months. For all of these reasons, bile acid metabolism is far simpler to characterize than cholesterol metabolism.

There is also an additional fundamental problem of great importance.

Cholesterol is transported in blood in various classes of lipoproteins, and these have different clinical significance. Thus, low-density lipoprotein is considered a form of cholesterol designed for transport to peripheral tissues. The low-density lipoprotein function is considered atherogenic and dangerous. In contrast, high-density lipoprotein cholesterol is considered to represent cholesterol returning from peripheral tissues designed for export in bile, either as bile acids or cholesterol[6]. High-density lipoprotein cholesterol is considered anti-atherogenic and health-promoting. Cholesterol exchanges between these two classes which are considered to have opposing physiological significance. Accordingly, characterization of cholesterol metabolism by isotope dilution provides no direct information on the cholesterol content of these two lipoprotein classes and is unlikely to be of prognostic significance, unless there is a correlation between the mass of the exchangeable pool and the level of either low-density lipoprotein or high-density lipoprotein cholesterol. Thus, the determination of cholesterol kinetics is time consuming and of uncertain physiological meaning, whereas the determination of bile acid kinetics is rapid and simple, and provides some very unambiguous physiological information about bile acid metabolism. For this reason, there are many more measurements of bile acid kinetics than cholesterol kinetics.

In this brief review, bile acid kinetics will be considered before cholesterol kinetics.

ISOTOPE DILUTION METHOD OF BILE ACID KINETICS

History

The history of the development and application of isotope dilution measurements of bile acids was summarized some years ago by Hoffmann and Hofman[1]. In brief, Bergstrom et al. in 1953 prepared 24 ^{14}C-labelled bile acids[7] which were used by Lindstedt, who gave [24 14C]cholic acid to healthy volunteers[8]. Bile was collected daily from the duodenum, after cholecysto-kinin had been given intravenously to contract the gallbladder. Cholic acid was isolated from hydrolysed bile by the methods of reversed-phase partition chromatography that Sjovall and Norman had developed. The specific activity of the cholic acid decreased exponentially with time, and Lindstedt concluded that the bile acid pool behaved as a single well-mixed compartment in a steady state. Using the paper chromatographic methods of Sjovall[9], Lindstedt determined biliary bile acid composition and used those data to calculate total bile acid pool size.

By 1959, Bergstrom's group had developed combustion techniques for measuring ^{3}H and had used ^{3}H-labelled bile acids for metabolic experiments in animals; in the early 1960s [^{14}C]cholic acid and [^{3}H]chenodeoxycholic acid were given to two human volunteers[10]. This important study showed that deoxycholic acid was derived solely from cholic acid and that lithocholic acid was derived solely from chenodeoxycholic acid, indicating that the primary bile acids have separate metabolic pathways. In addition, the data suggested different turnover rates of chenodeoxycholic acid and cholic acid, implying that any complete description of bile acid metabolism would require characterization of the metabolism of both primary bile acids.

Lindstedt et al.[11] used the isotope dilution technique to test whether unsaturated fats increased bile acid excretion when they decreased serum cholesterol levels. In the meantime, several groups reported values for faecal excretion of bile acids[12,13], but none of these groups attempted to compare synthesis rates obtained in this manner with those obtained by isotope dilution. When Lack and Weiner[14] showed that the terminal ileum actively transported bile acids and that ileal resection caused profound bile acid malabsorption in the dog, bile acid metabolism became a subject of interest to the gastroenterologist. Heaton et al., in 1968[15], used a modification of the Lindstedt procedure to establish the diagnosis of bile acid malabsorption in patients with ileal dysfunction. At the same time, Wollenweber and Kottke[16] used the technique to define bile acid metabolism in patients with hyperlipidaemia.

In 1970, Vlahcevic et al., in a classical study, carried out isotope dilution measurements of bile acids for both primary bile acids – cholic and chenodeoxycholic acid[17]. A similar study was carried out a few years later by Danzinger et al.[18] and since then several additional studies have been carried out in which the kinetics of the two primary bile acids were defined in healthy individuals. Subsequently, isotope dilution measurements of bile acid kinetics were carried out for deoxycholic[19] and lithocholic[20,21], so that by 1975 the kinetics of each of the major primary and secondary bile acids had been defined. A series of studies from the Mayo Clinic defined the simultaneous turnover of not only the steroid, but also the amino acid moiety[22-24]. The amino acid moiety was shown to turn over more rapidly than the steroid moiety and to be lost from its exchangeable pool after release by bacterial deconjugation. The slower turnover of the steroid moiety reflects intestinal deconjugation and hepatic reconjugation (with unlabelled amino acid moiety) during enterohepatic cycling. In the last decade, the technique of isotope dilution has been widely accepted and applied to patients with a variety of diseases affecting the enterohepatic circulation. A series of excellent studies from the Stockholm group led by Einarsson and Hellstrom has detailed bile acid metabolism in the hyperlipidaemias, and the relationship of bile acid metabolism to triglyceride metabolism (reviewed in reference 25).

As noted, each primary bile acid is converted into a secondary bile acid. The exact intermediates in this conversion have not been defined. A reasonable hypothesis is that a Δ^7 compound is involved[26], as shown in Figure 5.3. A certain fraction of the secondary bile acid which is formed is absorbed. The subsequent fate of the two secondary bile acids, deoxycholic and lithocholic, is not identical, and the metabolism of each bile acid must be discussed individually.

For deoxycholic, about one-third to one-half of that which is formed in the large intestine is absorbed and passes to the liver where it is conjugated with glycine or taurine and secreted into bile[23]. It then mixes with its exchangeable pool, so that input of newly formed deoxycholic acid from the intestine is exactly analogous to de novo synthesis of bile acid in the liver from

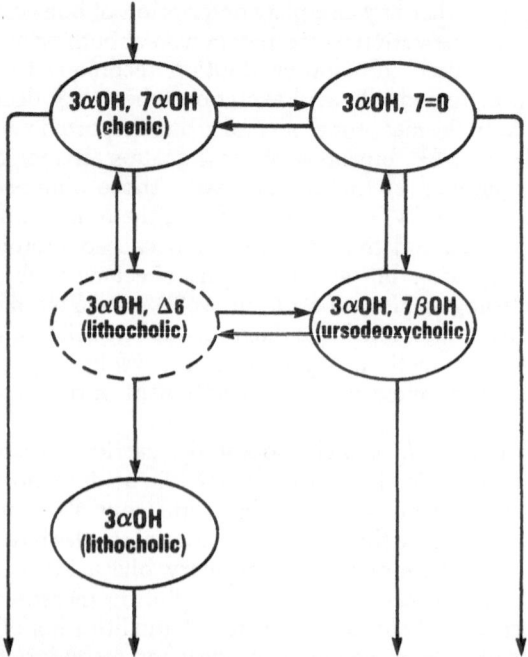

Figure 5.3 Probable biotransformations of chenodeoxycholic acid (here termed chenic) during enterohepatic cycling. The Δ^6 intermediate is likely, but has never been isolated. The 7-oxo compound may be converted to ursodeoxycholic or chenodeoxycholic acid by either hepatic or bacterial enzymes

cholesterol. It is now quite clear that if deoxycholic acid is injected as a tracer dose, its specific activity decay curve manifests first-order kinetics; the input reflects absorption of newly formed deoxycholic acid from the large intestine and the pool size is the exchangeable pool size.

Since the kinetics of the two primary bile acids, cholic and chenodeoxycholic, and that of the secondary bile acid, deoxycholic, may all be described

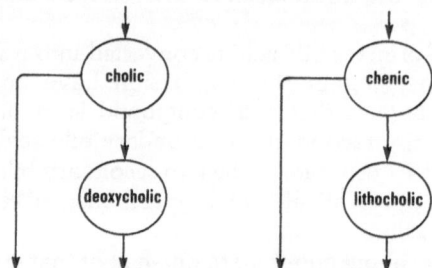

Figure 5.4 Compartmental model for bile acid metabolism in man. The metabolism of each of the bile acids is represented by a single compartment, although it is now known that the metabolism of lithocholic acid in contrast to that of the other bile acids cannot be described by a single compartment

by a single compartmental model, it is convenient to discuss the isotope dilution methods of these three bile acids together (Figure 5.4). The more complex problems of lithocholic and ursodeoxycholic kinetics will be discussed subsequently.

Method

Principle

When a tracer dose of radioactive bile acid is administered, it mixes with the bile acid pool – the pool being defined as that mass of bile acid that dilutes an injected dose of tracer. The pool may then be sampled from the duodenum after time has been allowed for adequate mixing. The following two assumptions have generally been made about the bile acid pool: (1) it behaves as a single compartment; and (2) it is in steady state (pool size is constant).

From conventional analysis of a one-compartment system in a steady state, it can be shown that:

$$SA_{(t)} = SA_{(0)}e^{-kt}$$

in which $SA_{(t)}$ and $SA_{(0)}$ are specific activities (disintegrations per minute per mass) at time t and time 0, respectively, and k is the fractional turnover rate (time^{-1}).

From this equation it is clear that a plot of the natural logarithm of specific activity against time would have a slope of $-k$ and an intercept of $\ln (SA_0)$. From $SA_{(0)}$ and size of the injected dose, pool size can be calculated (pool size = dose injected/$SA_{(0)}$). Because the enterohepatic circulation is in the steady state:

Daily synthesis rate = Pool size × Fractional turnover rate

Inherent in the assumption of steady state is an averaging of the events over many enterohepatic cycles. Fractional turnover rate has the unit of (days^{-1}) and usually is measured over a period of 5–7 days. During each day there are 6–12 enterohepatic cycles. In this technique of isotope dilution, the influence of cycle-to-cycle variation is avoided by averaging over many cycles. This appears to be justifiable in health but may not be so in disease states such as severe bile acid malabsorption.

Recently, van Trappen et al.[27] have described a novel approach to the measurement of bile acid kinetics by isotope dilution in man. In this technique, the bile acid pool is labelled sequentially with two isotopes, e.g. ^{14}C and ^{3}H. The two tracers are given intravenously; the first isotope is given 24 hours before the second. A single bile sample is obtained a day later, and its isotope ratio is defined. From its isotope ratio, the pool size and turnover rate can be calculated. The method is quite correct in principle, and should be satisfactory. However, the ratio of the two isotopes must be measured with high accuracy and one must be certain that both labels are stable during enterohepatic cycling. Further validation and application of this method is desirable.

Route of administration

Accurate calculation of pool size depends on exact knowledge of the amount of radioactivity administered. Accordingly, the labelled bile acid should be given by intravenous injection, which avoids the uncertain absorption via the oral route.

Time of administration

It seems rational and convenient to give the label before a meal. During digestion, the label is well mixed with the bile acid pool, so that sampling of the bile acid pool some time later (⟩6h) gives a valid point on the specific activity decay curve. It often is convenient to administer bile acids before the evening meal and to begin bile collections the following day.

Sampling the bile acid pool

For an estimate of the average specific activity of the bile acid pool, one must sample a well-mixed portion of the pool. This is done by recovering as much of the gallbladder contents as possible after an overnight fast. A duodenal tube containing a perforated metal olive on its end is passed and vigorous gallbladder contraction is induced. This can be achieved by the intravenous administration of cholecystokinin–pancreozymin or its terminal octapeptide, by intraduodenal administration of divalent cations (such as Mg^{2+} or Ca^{2+}) or a mixture of essential amino acids[28], or by ingestion of a glass of milk. As much concentrated bile as possible is collected and mixed well. A sample (usually 1–2 ml), which should contain less than 50 mg of bile acids, is saved for analysis, and the remainder is returned to the duodenum. The duodenal tube may be inserted each day or left in place for the duration of the study. Bile samples may also be obtained by using a paediatric endoscope, a Dreiling tube, or a steerable catheter.

In our opinion, at least five samples are necessary to establish a valid specific activity decay curve, and they usually are obtained over a period of 5–7 days. When the specific activity is decreasing rapidly, the samples may be obtained at shorter intervals over a 3-day period. Some workers have attempted to estimate pool size by injecting tracer during continuous bile acid secretion induced by continuous infusion of a meal or an amino acid mixture into the duodenum[29]. It has been claimed[30], however, that this technique may give an erroneously small estimate of the bile acid pool because the gallbladder may not contract completely. A fairly precise measurement of the bile acid pool size may also be obtained by determining a single early point on the specific activity decay curve and taking an arbitrary value for the fractional turnover rate (the slope of the curve)[31]. This method gives a slight (about 10%) overestimate of the bile acid pool, since the intercept of the extrapolated specific activity curve cannot be known precisely.

The bile acid pool also may be sampled by using a capsule of dialysis tubing containing cholestyramine[32]. For 5–7 days a marked capsule is given each day with a meal; the capsule traps conjugated bile acids during intestinal passage. The capsule is recovered from the faeces, the bile acids are eluted and isolated chromatographically, and the specific activity of the appropriate steroid moiety is determined. The technique appears to yield data identical with those obtained by duodenal sampling but with much less precision. However, it does offer a means of determining bile acid kinetics in children or in population studies when intubation is difficult. Its major advantage is that the capsules may be taken and the faecal samples collected at home, so that the patient merely mails the stool specimens to the laboratory, using a convenient 'faecal field kit'[33].

The single-compartment model for bile acid kinetics assumes that bile acid metabolism can be described by a single, well-mixed compartment. If the compartment were completely well mixed, every group of bile acid molecules would have the identical specific activity. This is, of course, an over-simplification, since the specific activity decay curve falls because of the input of newly synthesized unlabelled bile acids from the liver. The Lindstedt treatment assumes that newly synthesized bile acid mixes completely with the exchangeable bile acid pool before the pool is sampled in the duodenum. The linearity of the specific activity decay curve and the close agreement between values for bile acid synthesis obtained by the isotope dilution technique with those obtained by direct chemical measurement of faecal bile acids (see below) suggests that this assumption is generally correct.

The bile acids present in serum originate from the spillover of bile acids absorbed from the intestine. Newly synthesized primary bile acids are added to the bile acid pool in the liver. Accordingly, the specific activity of the serum primary bile acids should be identical with that in duodenal bile. In principle, the isotope dilution technique should give identical results if serum samples are used in place of duodenal bile samples as a source of bile acids. In practice, however, serum samples cannot be used, since the specific activity of serum bile acids is too low to permit an accurate and precise measurement, when the usual amounts of tracer are administered. For example, if a 10 mmol bile acid pool was labelled with 10μCi, the specific activity, even if there were instant equilibration, would be only 1μCi/mmol. Thus, since the average bile acid concentration is about 1μmol/l, there is 1 nmol/ml. Hence, 1 ml of plasma would contain 2 dpm of bile acid radioactivity.

A solution to this problem is to enrich the serum bile acids greatly in an isotopically tagged bile acid. Such is easily achieved by administering bile acids tagged with the stable isotopes such as deuterium (^{2}H) or ^{13}C. One may give a sufficient amount of tagged bile acid that every tenth bile acid molecule is labelled. Mass spectrometry is sufficiently accurate to determine the atoms percent excess, i.e. enrichment in the stable isotope.

This technique has recently been developed in the laboratory of Peter Klein[34] and applied and validated in a collaborative study between his group and that of Fred Kern[35]. It has also been reported from a Japanese laboratory[36]. The method has been applied to show that bile acid kinetics can be determined with acceptable accuracy and precision in man using serum samples after the bile acid pool has been labelled with ^{13}C-labelled bile acids.

This method may not be valid for secondary bile acids. These enter the exchangeable pool from the intestine and there is the possibility that serum bile acids might have a momentarily lower specific activity if intestinal input of newly formed secondary bile acids exceeded disproportionately intestinal absorption of secondary bile acids already in the exchangeable bile acid pool.

The careful study of Whiting and Watts[37] has shown that the profile of serum bile acids is closely correlated with that of biliary bile acids, the difference of course reflecting the differing first-pass clearance values for individual bile acids. These data provide additional indirect evidence that isotope dilution techniques should be valid if based on serum samples.

Choice of tracer

The three major human bile acids – cholic, chenodeoxycholic, and deoxycholic – are commercially available labelled with ^{14}C in the carboxyl moiety. This is a satisfactory label in every respect. Bile acids with ^{14}C in other positions have not been synthesized, but would offer no advantage over 24-^{14}C bile acids unless one were concerned with a reaction involving bile acid decarboxylation.

Bile acids labelled with ^{3}H in a variety of locations have been described and used. As noted, Lindstedt prepared bile acids by Wilzbach tritiation, and other authors have also used bile acids randomly labelled with tritium. The problem for any investigator using a ^{3}H-labelled bile acid is the biological and chemical stability of the label, and whenever a new tritiated compound is used, it is mandatory to define the biological stability of the tritium label. This is done most easily by carrying out isotope dilution measurements of bile acid kinetics using ^{14}C and the ^{3}H bile acid in question and showing that the specific activity decay curves of the two radioisotopes are identical, i.e. that the ^{3}H/^{14}C ratio of bile acids remains constant[38,39].

Bile acids, randomly labelled with tritium, were used in the earliest isotope dilution methods by Lindstedt, and Kallner has continued to use such bile acids for studies in man. This group showed that the label was acceptably stable *in vivo*, if the isotope was purified extensively before use[40]. Similar conclusions were reached in a careful study by Panvelliwalla *et al.*[41]

Bile acids labelled with ^{3}H in the 2,2',4,4' positions are readily prepared by enolic exchange[42] and such bile acids are now available commercially. The biological and chemical stability of this label has been documented in a careful study by LaRusso *et al.*[38]. However, it must be stressed that this label is lost during the conversion of cholic acid to deoxycholic acid. The simplest explanation is that there is simultaneous desaturation and resaturation of the A ring.

Chenodeoxycholic acid labelled in the 11,12 position has been prepared by Cowen *et al.* by reductive tritiation of the 11,12 compound which, in turn, had been prepared by dehydration of the 12-hydroxy group of cholic acid[43]. This label possesses both biological and chemical stability; however, it is lost as chenodeoxycholic acid is converted to lithocholic acid, suggesting bacterial desaturation of the C ring.

Recently, our laboratory has prepared bile acids with a double bond at the 22,23 position and prepared [22,23-³H] bile acids by reductive tritiation (R. DiPietro, personal communication). The biological and chemical stability of this label is unknown at this time.

Bile acids labelled with a tritium atom at the 3-beta or 7-beta position are steadily obtained by oxidation to the keto group followed by reduction with borotritide[44]. The reduction favours the alpha configuration, but labile tritium may be moved in alkali. However, this is in principle a risky site for tritium as reversible oxidation at both the 3 and 7 positions is now considered to occur during enterohepatic cycling. Indeed, such bile acids could be used to quantitate the degree of this oxidation and reduction; they should not be used for isotope dilution measurements of bile acids until there is convincing evidence of the biological stability of trace in this position.

Chemical form of tracer

The labelled bile acid should be injected in the chemical form of the un-conjugated bile acid only. Estimates of the total bile acid pool derived from the specific activity decay curve obtained after the injection of a conjugated bile acid may be quite erroneous, based on our calculations from a compart-mental model of the enterohepatic circulation[45].

Measurement of specific activity

In conventional isotope dilution measurements of bile acid kinetics, the mixture of bile acids in bile is hydrolysed either by an enzymatic procedure or by strong alkali to generate the unconjugated bile acids. They are then separated chromatographically, and the specific activity of the isolated unconjugated bile acid is determined by measuring the amount of mass and its radioactivity. The mass of the isolated bile acid may be measured by an enzymatic procedure or by gas–liquid chromatography. Generally, bile acids are chromatographed as trifluoroacetates on QF-1 columns or as acetates on QF-1 on AN-600 columns; trimethylsilyl ethers are well separated on HiEff8B columns. Good quantification of underivatized methyl esters has proved difficult to achieve for most workers. Hydroxy keto hyodeoxycholic, nordeoxycholic, and hyocholic acids have been used as internal standards, but the last may be difficult to derivatize completely.

In principal, one can measure the specific activity of the individual conjugates, i.e. the glycine conjugate and the taurine conjugate, and add these, i.e. the sum of the radioactivities divided by the sum of the masses, to obtain the identical figure that one would obtain if the specific activity of the unconjugated bile acid obtained by hydrolysis is determined. The precision of such an approach should be less.

Expressions of data

The primary data derived from regression analysis of the specific activity decay curve are pool size and daily fractional turnover rate. The product of these two is the daily synthesis rate. The half-life of label $(t_{1/2})$ is commonly reported in place of k, the fractional turnover rate. There is no point in reporting both since $t_{1/2} = \ln 2/k$. For a pool that remains constant in size, we prefer to use k.

Some authors report pool size and daily synthesis in units of mass; others report molar units. As we wrote some years ago[1], we think the latter is preferable, particularly if free and conjugated bile acids are to be compared.

One further problem is the normalization of data. Should data be expressed in terms of actual body weight, ideal body weight, body surface area, or some other variable? Because the purpose of normalization is to decrease the variance within groups believed not to vary with respect to the factor under investigation, the correct method of normalization must be arrived at experimentally. As we wrote some years ago, insufficient data are available to allow a clear choice. We recommend that authors publish bile acid kinetics in comparable terms, including data in micromoles per kilogram of body weight or micromoles per square metre of body surface area. Recommendations for calculating body surface area from height and weight have been published[46]. Reports should include – or archive – full patient data (age, sex, weight and height); this practice will permit the appropriate method of normalization to become apparent in time.

Meaning of the single compartment model

For both cholic and chenodeoxycholic, the exponential decay of the specific activity decay curve reflects synthesis from cholesterol.

For deoxycholic acid, the decay in the specific activity decay curve is caused by the input of newly formed deoxycholic acid molecules which are formed in the distal intestine by bacterial dehydroxylation of cholic. If labelled cholic acid is given, the label appears in deoxycholic acid in a conventional product–precursor relationship (Figure 5.5). The input reflects the amount of newly formed deoxycholic acid which is absorbed which must be less than that formed from cholic. In principle, the maximal amount of deoxycholic acid that could be formed is equal to cholic acid synthesis; the maximal amount which could be absorbed is the amount which is formed. It is useful to define the fraction f_{abs} which reflects deoxycholic acid input divided by the maximum amount of deoxycholic acid which could be formed. Since in most individuals virtually all of the cholic which enters the large intestine is converted to deoxycholic, it is reasonable to equate the maximal amount of deoxycholic acid which could be formed to the amount of cholic acid synthesis[45].

To determine f_{abs} one must carry out simultaneous measurements of cholic and deoxycholic acid kinetics, as has recently been reported by van Berge Henegouwen and his colleagues[47]. The input of deoxycholic divided by the input (or synthesis) of cholic is equal to f_{abs}. However, it is always desirable to validate the assumption that cholic acid is fully converted to deoxycholic; this can only be done by determination of the faecal bile acid pattern.

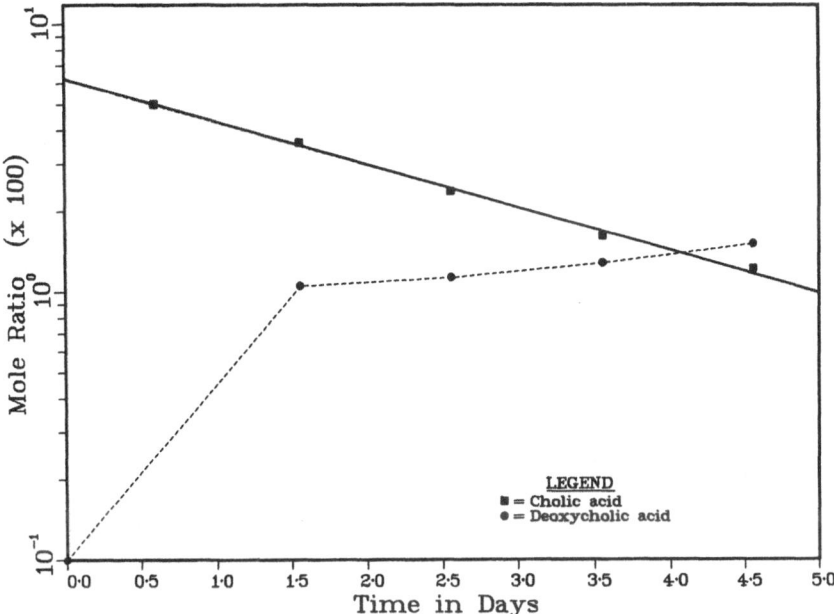

Figure 5.5 Semi-logarithmic plot of 'specific activity' decay curve of cholic acid in a healthy subject. (The term 'mole ratio' is used, as the experiment was carried out with ^{13}C-carbon, a stable isotope, and the unit of stable isotope enrichment is mole ratio (or atoms % excess).) The curve shows the exponential loss of isotopic carbon from the cholic acid pool and its appearance in the deoxycholic acid pool. The relationship of the curves is that of precursor and product. (From reference 124.)

Single compartment versus multiple compartments

As noted, Lindstedt reported that the specific activity decay curve of cholic acid suggested that the metabolism of this bile acid could be described by a single well mixed compartment. It is clear now that the metabolism of chenodeoxycholic acid and deoxycholic acid can also be described by a single-compartment model.

The 'lumping' procedure of Lindstedt has had considerable utility, but it is self-apparent that such a treatment of bile acid metabolism neglects the amino acid moiety, as well as the lower specific activity in the hepatocyte. It also neglects bile acid secretion – a key parameter of bile acid metabolism.

To solve this problem, we expanded the Lindstedt model some years ago and developed a model with separate compartments for the three chemical species of a given bile acid – the glycine conjugate, the taurine conjugate, and the unconjugate[45]. This model allowed one to simulate quite satisfactorily the behaviour of tracer when injected in any chemical form into the bile acid pool. Since that time, in collaboration with Molino, Milanese, and Belforte, the model has been further expanded to include time-dependent aspects, i.e. the increase in bile acid secretion that occurs during digestion[48]. As yet this complete multicompartmental model has only been described for cholic acid; extension to chenodeoxycholic and deoxycholic acids is in progress.

Exceptions to the Lindstedt model

Lithocholic acid

The specific activity decay curve of lithocholic is bi-exponential and the metabolism of lithocholic is thus unique among the bile acids (Figure 5.6)[21]. The bi-exponential form of the SADC of lithocholic is probably explained by its unique hepatic metabolism: lithocholic is not only amidated with glycine or taurine, but in addition, it is sulphated at the 3 position to form two novel bile acid conjugates – sulpholithocholylglycine and sulpholithocholyltaurine[49]. This sulphation is not complete – only about 60% – so that bile contains lithocholic in two forms: the majority as sulphated amidates, and the minority as unsulphated amidates.

The subsequent behaviour of these two classes of conjugates has been studied to only a very limited extent. In all probability, the sulphated amidates pass through the small intestine with little absorption[50]. In the colon, there is desulphation and deconjugation so that some unconjugated lithocholic returns to the exchangeable bile acid pool. In contrast, the unsulphated amidates are probably well absorbed from the small intestine.

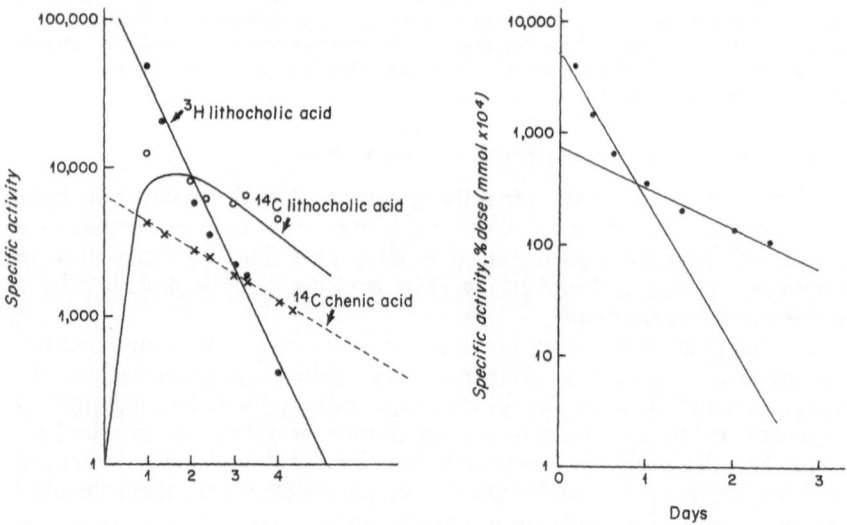

Figure 5.6 (a) Early study of Cowen *et al.*[20] showing specific activity decay curve of chenodeoxycholic (chenic) acid; the precursor–product specific activity decay curve of [14C]lithocholic acid; and the (apparently) linear specific activity decay curve of [3H]lithocholic acid, when the data are plotted on semi-logarithmic coordinates. (b) Bi-exponential specific activity decay curve of lithocholic acid in a patient ingesting chenodeoxycholic acid[21]. The early part of the curve was not detected in the study of Cowen *et al.*[20] because samples were not collected early enough after the administration of tracer

They return to the liver and again are sulphated (60–80%) during hepatic transport. The minority of lithocholylglycine and lithocholyltaurine is again secreted in bile, reabsorbed from the intestine, and again mostly sulphated during hepatic passage. If 70% of lithocholyl amidates are sulphated during hepatic passage, then it can be calculated after four hepatic passes; more than 99% of lithocholic will be sulphated (Figure 5.7).

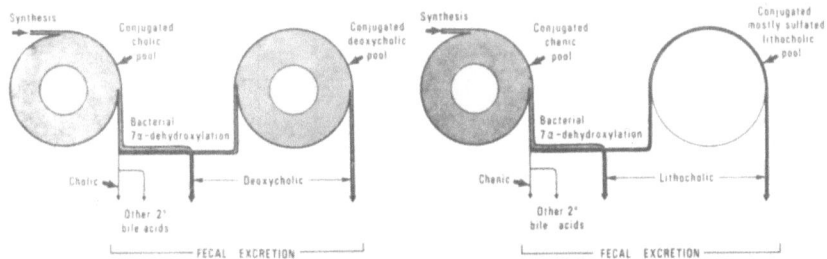

Figure 5.7 Schematic depiction of the intestinal part of the enterohepatic circulation of the four major bile acids in man. The ring corresponds to the right part of the loop shown in Figure 5.2. Note that the enterohepatic cycling of deoxycholates is much greater than that of lithocholates because the latter is sulphated and the sulpholithocholates are poorly absorbed from the intestine. The loop corresponds to the exchangeable pools indicated as compartments in Figure 5.4. Each loop in Figure 5.7 and each compartment in Figure 5.4 contains three chemical species – the glycine conjugate, the taurine conjugate and the unconjugated species. As noted above, the lithochocolate compartment contains not only the glycine and taurine amidates, but also their sulphates

The complex kinetics of lithocholic have received little investigation to date. Allan et al.[21] calculated the input of newly formed lithocholate using the input–output method described by Samuel and Lieberman[51] for cholesterol metabolism. (This is based on the indicator dilution equations of Stewart[52] and Hamilton et al.[53].) These workers found that about one-fifth of newly formed lithocholate was reabsorbed. However, much more investigation of lithocholic kinetics is needed, especially in patients receiving chenodeoxycholic or ursodeoxycholic for gallstone dissolution.

Ursodeoxycholic, the 7β-epimer of chenodeoxycholic, is present in biliary bile acids in trace amounts (2–5%) in most individuals. Ursodeoxycholic acid is not formed directly from cholesterol in man, but is derived from chenodeoxycholic acid (Figure 5.8). Two routes of formation are likely. Probably the majority of ursodeoxycholic acid is formed in the intestine from chenodeoxycholic; the intermediate is either the Δ^7 or the 7-keto compound[54,55]. In addition, ursodeoxycholic may also be formed in the liver by hepatic reduction of its 7-keto derivative which is formed in the intestine by bacterial 7-dehydrogenation of either ursodeoxycholic or chenodeoxycholic[56,57]. However, hepatic reduction is stereospecific, greatly favouring the 7-OH epimer; none the less, small amounts of ursodeoxycholic are also formed.

The very limited isotope dilution measurements of bile acid kinetic studies on ursodeoxycholic acid suggest that its metabolism resembles that of the primary bile acids in having a single well-mixed pool[58]. It may well be,

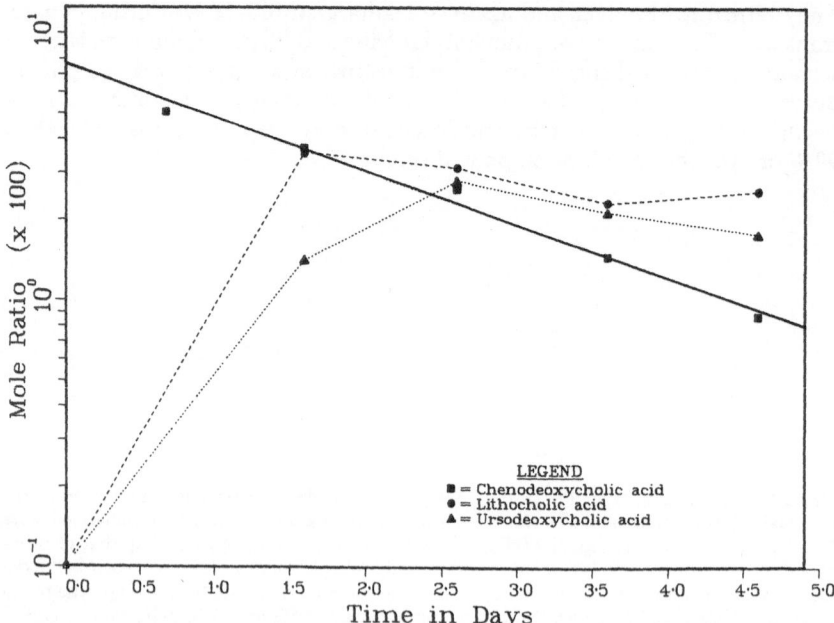

Figure 5.8 Time course of change in molar ratio of [^{13}C]chenodeoxycholic acid in a healthy subject showing subsequent appearance in lithocholic and ursodeoxycholic acid, indicating that these two bile acids were derived from chenodeoxycholic acid (From reference 124.)

however, that the specific activity decay curve of ursodeoxycholic acid is pseudo-first order, in that current concepts of ursodeoxycholic acid metabolism suggest that ursodeoxycholic acid is converted in part to chenodeoxycholic acid which in turn is partly reconverted to ursodeoxycholic acid. The steps could involve bacterial dehydrogenation to form the 7-keto derivative followed by either bacterial or hepatic reduction to form chenodeoxycholic acid. If the biotransformation of ursodeoxycholic to chenodeoxycholic is relatively slow, it should not influence the estimate of the pool size, which as noted above is obtained by extrapolation of the specific activity decay curve to zero time. However, the validity of calculating 'input' of ursodeoxycholic acid by multiplying the slope of the specific activity curve times the pool size is unclear.

Validation of isotope dilution measurements

The pool of bile acid was operationally defined as that mass of bile acids that dilutes a tracer. This should be equal approximately to the mass of bile acids drained by an acute biliary fistula (minus the bile acids synthesized during the time of drainage). Experimental confirmation of this prediction is scarce. In the rat, Mok et al.[59] found that the pool measured by biliary drainage was considerably larger than that estimated by isotope dilution, and similar observations have been made for the rhesus monkey (cited in reference 60).

On the other hand, there is good agreement between the bile acid pattern estimated by gas–liquid chromatography and that estimated by summing the individual bile acid pools estimated by isotope dilution[61].

Bile acid synthesis can be estimated by direct chemical measurement of faecal bile acids[29]. This is not a simple technique for two major reasons: it is difficult to get a complete faecal collection in man and it is difficult to measure faecal bile acids accurately. The reasons for the latter are multiple: difficulty of quantitative hydrolysis and extraction, contamination of the final extract by non-bile acid substances which gives peaks on the GLC, etc. One problem interfering with complete extraction is the presence of sulphated bile acids in faeces, such as sulphated lithocholyl species. If enzymatic deconjugation is carried out, these are hydrolyzed extremely slowly; if alkaline hydrolysis is carried out, sulpholithocholate may be destroyed. The consensus of current opinion is that less than 20% of faecal bile acids are sulphated[62] (and A. Roda, personal communication), despite a claim to the contrary[63]. It is most likely that lithocholic acid is the major sulphated faecal bile acid.

Despite all these problems, there is fair agreement between estimates of bile acid synthesis obtained by isotope dilution and by direct chemical measurement[64].

APPLICATION

Primary bile acids

Measurement of pool size and synthesis has been carried out in health, and has shown that in general, cholic acid synthesis is about twice that of chenodeoxycholic acid. In Table 5.1, we have tabulated all published data in which isotope dilution measurements of bile acid kinetics were carried out according to the recommendations made above. In Table 5.2, calculations of total pool size are collated. The fractional turnover rate of chenodeoxycholic acid is considerably below that of cholic acid, and as a consequence pool sizes are nearly identical. Primary bile acid synthesis and pool size has also been measured in patients with cholesterol cholelithiasis. In general, but not invariably, pool sizes are smaller and synthesis rates tend to be lower (Table 5.1, Part V).

Primary bile acid synthesis has also been measured in the different types of hyperlipidaemia (Table 5.1; Part VII). In general, bile acid synthesis is lower in type II hyperlipidaemia (familial hypercholesterolaemia, heterozygous), and in this condition, cholic acid synthesis is disproportionately decreased. In type IV hyperlipidaemia, bile acid synthesis tends to be increased, with a normal ratio of cholic to chenodeoxycholic acid synthesis.

Decreased primary bile acid synthesis has also been induced by feeding bile acids. Specifically, the synthesis of chenodeoxycholic acid was decreased during cholic acid feeding[65]; the synthesis of cholic acid was decreased during chenodeoxycholic acid feeding[18]; and the synthesis of both cholic and chenodeoxycholic acid was decreased during deoxycholic acid feeding[66]. Decreased bile acid synthesis, especially that of cholic acid, has

Table 5.1 Isotope dilution measurements of bile acid kinetics*
I. HEALTHY SUBJECTS

Reference	Patient description	Age (years)	Weight (kg)	Tracer	Pool (μmol/kg)	Cholic Pool (g)	FTR (day^{-1})	Synthesis (μmol kg^{-1}day^{-1})	Synthesis (mg/day)
8	8 M	20-25	—	po 24-^{14}C	—	1.376±.569	0.24±0.08	—	364±137
10	2	—	—	po r^{3}H	—	1.19, 0.54	0.17, 0.35	—	200, 190
101	3 F	20-22	60-66	po 24-^{14}C	—	1.597	0.21	—	355
102	6F, 3M	19-40 (26)	55-70 (63)	po 24-^{14}C	45.23±14.47	1.120±.282	0.22±0.10	11.57±4.37	295±84
103	9 M	32-76	—	po 24-^{14}C	—	1.18±.36	0.33±0.15	—	358±149
17	10M	41-72 (54)	—	po 24-^{14}C	—	1.04±.21	0.32±0.13	—	333±149
104	2	—	—	—	—	—	—	—	—
105†	7 F	32	—	po 24-^{14}C	—	0.70±.21	0.28±0.14	—	180±68
18	6 F	54	74	iv 24-^{14}C	23.8±7.6	0.595±.228	0.37±0.12	9.0±5.4	222±142
76	2F, 5M	48-67	—	po 24-^{14}C	—	0.779±.209	0.39±0.13	—	308±95
111	11	54	71	po 24-^{14}C	28.4±14.8	0.821±.428	0.38±0.27	8.76±4.8	253±139
106	2F, 4M	30	77	po 24-^{14}C	25.5±3.8	0.79±.120	0.36±0.15	8.80±2.3	276±73
107	3F, 6M	45	73	—	—	—	—	—	—
81	4F, 3M	55	66	—	19.5±11.9	0.523±320	—	—	—
66	7 M	23-34	78	iv 24-^{14}C	47.7±16.4	1.514±.520	0.22±0.08	9.3±2.9	289±85
108	10	—	—	iv 24-^{14}C	—	0.85±.45	0.28±0.05	—	239±136
109	9 M	22-61	—	po 24-^{14}C	—	0.69±.27	0.54±0.27	—	316±117
75	5F, 1M	39-60	—	po 24-^{14}C	—	0.834±.409	0.44±0.15	—	330±130
47	7 M	18-25	70	iv 2,4-^{3}H	50±28	1.425±.798	0.25	12.5±4.8	356±137
72	5 M	53-64	—	iv 24-^{14}C	—	0.860±.400	0.44±0.13	—	328±103
71	7F, 1M	21-58	—	iv 24-^{14}C	51.7±20.9	—	0.31	16±9.1	—
27	4F, 6M	45	—	iv 24-^{14}C / iv 24-^{14}C 2,4-^{3}H	—	1.336±.687 / 1.344±.598	0.29±0.18 / 0.28±0.18	—	387 / 376
73	4F, 6M	23-55 (34)	—	iv 24-^{14}C	—	1.168±.439	0.35±0.19	—	409±153
110	5	—	—	po 24-^{14}C	—	—	—	—	—

BILE ACID AND CHOLESTEROL KINETICS

	Chenodeoxycholic					Total		
Tracer	Pool (μmol/kg)	Pool (g)	FTR (day^{-1})	Synthesis ($\mu mol\,kg^{-1}\,day^{-1}$)	Synthesis (mg/day)	Synthesis ($\mu mol\,kg^{-1}\,day^{-1}$)	Synthesis (mg/day)	% Cholic
—	—	1.45±.40	—	—	—	—	—	—
po 24-^{14}C	—	2.52,2.42	0.12, 0.16	—	290, 390	—	490, 580	36
—	—	0.849	—	—	—	—	—	—
—	48.23	1.19	—	—	—	—	—	—
—	—	0.83±0.17	—	—	—	—	—	—
po 24-^{14}C	—	0.81±0.17	0.23±0.10	—	162±56	—	495±159	67
iv ^{2}H & ^{3}H	—	1.05, 1.15	0.07, 0.19	—	75, 215	—	—	—
po 24-^{14}C	—	0.64±0.14	0.21±0.09	—	129±41	—	311±79	58
iv 2,4-^{3}H	26.5±7.1	0.626±0.228	0.19±0.07	4.7±2.0	106±34	13.7±5.8	328±146	68
po r^{3}H	—	0.672±0.247	0.27±0.08	—	194±109	—	502±144	61
po r^{3}H	20.7±9.3	0.575±0.259	0.27±0.17	4.72±4.75	131±132	—	384±192	66
po 2,4-^{3}H	17.6±3.2	0.526±0.096	0.27±0.12	4.55±1.44	137±44	—	413±85	67
iv 24-^{14}C	23.7±8.3	0.677±0.237	0.23±0.06	5.43±2.14	155±61	—	—	—
iv 2,4-^{3}H	27.9±12.2	0.720±0.315	0.32±0.13	7.9±2.8	—	—	—	—
iv 11,12-^{3}H	46.9±15.3	—	0.18±0.05	8±2.4	239±68	17.3±3.76	528±109	55
—	—	0.98±0.55	—	—	—	—	—	—
po 24-^{14}C	—	0.66±0.17	0.35±0.14	—	213±57	—	529±130	60
po 24-^{14}C	—	0.768±0.257	0.32±0.10	—	226±39	—	556±136	59
—	30±27	—	—	—	—	—	—	—
iv 24-^{14}C	—	0.643±0.256	0.40±0.14	—	249±123	—	577±160	57
—	—	—	—	—	—	—	—	—
—	—	—	—	—	—	—	—	—
iv 11,12-^{3}H	—	1.322±0.347	0.20±0.09	—	264±69	—	673±168	61
po 24-^{14}C	—	—	—	—	—	—	390±67	—

*In this and subsequent tables, values are expressed as mean ± standard deviation. In this and subsequent tables, data shown were either published as such or calculated from the primary data given in the cited reference. Calculations involved conversion of ratios to absolute values, conversion of moles to mg or g, dividing absolute values by body weight to obtain relative values, conversion of $t_{1/2}$ values to fractional turnover rates (FTR), or determination of synthesis rate by multiplying pool size by the fractional turnover rate.
†Southwestern American Indians.
iv=Intravenous; po=by mouth

Table 5.1 *continued*

II. HEALTHY SUBJECTS INGESTING SYNTHETIC DIETS

Reference	Patient description	Age (years)	Weight (kg)	Tracer	Cholic				
					Pool (μmol/kg)	Pool (g)	FTR (day^{-1})	Synthesis (μmol kg^{-1} day^{-1})	Synthesis (mg/day)
11*	2 M[1]	20	—	po 24-[14]C	—	0.71, 1.0	0.41, 0.20	—	140, 410
	3 M[2]	20-28	—	po 24-[14]C	—	1.0, 1.64	0.07-0.26	—	110-260
	2F, 2M[3]	19-21	—	po 24-[14]C	—	0.83-1.76	0.12-0.26	—	130-240
	2F, 2M[4]	19-21	—	po 24-[14]C	—	0.53-0.99	0.14-0.28	—	110-210
102†	6F, 3M	26 (19-40)	54-68	po 24-[14]C	—	1.29±0.45	0.22±0.09	—	314±111

*1=formula - 60% fat (corn oil); 2=formula - 60% fat (coconut oil); 3=solid - 35% cal (corn oil); 4=solid - 35% cal (coconut oil)
†40% fat - corn oil. Chenodeoxycholic acid pool:1.187g.

III. VEGETARIANS - CHOLIC ACID*

Reference	Patient description	Age (years)	Weight (kg)	Tracer	Cholic				
					Pool (μmol/kg)	Pool (g)	FTR (day^{-1})	Synthesis (μmol kg^{-1} day^{-1})	Synthesis (mg/day)
47	7M	20-26	70	2, 4[3]H	45±23	1.29±0.66	0.21	8.2±2.6	234±74

*Chenodeoxycholic acid pool: 37±30 μmol/kg.

Table 5.1 continued

IV. ALTERATIONS WITH DRUGS

Reference	Patient description	Age (years)	Weight (kg)	Cholic Tracer	Cholic Pool (µmol/kg)	Cholic Pool (g)	Cholic FTR (day⁻¹)	Cholic Synthesis (µmol kg⁻¹ day⁻¹)	Cholic Synthesis (mg/day)
76*	2F, 3M	48–67	—	po 24-¹⁴C	—	0.779±0.209	0.39±0.13	—	308±95
74†	5 F	52–61	45–74	po ¹⁴C	—	1.072±0.230	0.58±0.10	—	737±474
74‡	5 M	45–61	73–92	po ¹⁴C	—	0.906±0.496	0.99±0.14	—	987±577
75*	5F, 1M	39–60	—	po 24-¹⁴C	—	1.404±0.679	0.96±0.42	—	1131±747
112†	6F, 4M	41–62	47–96	po 24-¹⁴C	—	0.918±0.607	0.33±0.32	—	216±82
112‡	5 M	43–53	67–82	po 24-¹⁴C	—	0.968±0.324	0.34±0.22	—	274±58
35*	8 F	21	55	po 24-¹³C	40.0±12.4	0.895±0.277	0.36±0.20	13.9±6.5	311±144

Chenodeoxycholic Tracer	Pool (µmol/kg)	Pool (g)	FTR (day⁻¹)	Synthesis (µmol kg⁻¹ day⁻¹)	Synthesis (mg/day)	Total Synthesis (µmol kg⁻¹ day⁻¹)	Total Synthesis (mg/day)	% Cholic
po r³H	—	0.672±0.247	0.27±0.08	—	194±109	—	502±204	61
po r³H	—	0.317±0.134	1.16±0.19	—	379±130	—	1116±492	66
po r³H	—	0.630±0.371	0.99±0.28	—	650±228	—	1637±620	60
po 24-¹⁴C	—	0.312±0.152	1.72±0.34	—	503±171	—	1634±919	69
—	—	0.702±0.357	0.23	—	138±54	—	354±130	61
—	—	0.667±0.186	0.28±0.22	—	157±45	—	431±201	64
po 24-¹³C	37.1±13.0	0.798±0.280	0.26±0.14	9.2±4.5	198±96	23.1±7.9	508±175	61

1=Cholic acid, 0.5 g/day ×1 week and 1 g/day ×1 week; 2=cholestyramine, 10–12 g/day ×approximately 4 weeks; 3=cholestyramine, 12 g/day ×2 weeks; 4=nicotinic acid, 3–6 g/day ×3–12 months; 5=contraceptive steroids.
*Normals; †hyperlipoproteinaemia, type IIa; ‡hyperlipoproteinaemia, type IV.

Table 5.1 continued

V. BILIARY DISEASE
(a) Radiolucent Gallstone Patients

Reference	Patient description	Age (years)	Weight (kg)	Tracer	Cholic				
					Pool (μmol/kg)	Pool (g)	FTR (day^{-1})	Synthesis (μmol kg^{-1}day^{-1})	Synthesis (mg/day)
113	8 M	32–76	—	po 24-^{14}C	—	0.56±0.24	0.36±0.15	—	206±64
78	10 M	35–75	—	po 24-^{14}C	—	0.42±0.13	0.66±0.20	—	277±86
67	11 F*	35 (27–60)	—	po 24-^{14}C	—	0.12–0.88 (0.43±0.22)	0.28–0.74 (0.56±0.15)	—	75–353 (222±98)
114	1F, 9M	48–60	—	po 24-^{14}C	5.27–25.27 (12.99±6.67)	—	0.39–1.18 (0.63±0.25)	5.12±13.48 (7.3±3.05)	—
18	7F	53	74	iv 24-^{14}C	4.4–34.7 (18.7±11.1)	0.111–0.903 (0.531±0.273)	0.12–0.71 (0.42±0.08)	3.1–8.2 (5.8±0.21)	79–289 (173±69)
111	4†	—	—	po 24-^{14}C	—	0.427±0.330	0.65±0.24	—	231±130
81	4F, 3M	55 (42–69)	68 (47–88)	—	10.5–21.9 (14.4±4.6)	0.399±0.128	—	—	—
65	2F, 4M	57 (40–69)	86 (59–112)	—	9.9–23.5 (17.4±5.4)	0.430–0.565	—	—	—
107	6F, 1M	63 (46–75)	73 (60–82)	—	—	—	—	—	—
108	10	—	—	iv 24-^{14}C	—	0.52±0.20	0.38±0.27	—	117±118

Tracer	Chenodeoxycholic					Total		
	Pool (μmol/kg)	Pool (g)	FTR (day^{-1})	Synthesis (μmol kg^{-1}day^{-1})	Synthesis (mg/day)	Synthesis (μmol kg^{-1}day^{-1})	Synthesis (mg/day)	% Cholic
—	—	0.51±0.11	—	—	—	—	—	—
po 24-^{14}C	—	0.23–0.61 (0.44±0.14)	0.24–0.62 (0.40±0.13)	—	90–368 (170±76)	—	206–721 (391±124)	57

96

Tracer	Pool (µmol/kg)	Pool (g)	FTR (day⁻¹)	Synthesis (µmol kg⁻¹ day⁻¹)	Synthesis (mg/day)	Synthesis (µmol kg⁻¹ day⁻¹)	Synthesis (mg/day)	%
po 24-¹⁴C	8.79-22.34 (14.29±4.03)	—	0.28-0.67 (0.39±0.13)	3.70-6.96 (5.24±1.06)	—	8.82-20.44 (12.54±3.23)	—	58
iv 2,4-³H	5.1-23.9 (13.1±7.7)	0.142-0.598 (0.357±0.190)	0.11-0.39 (0.27±0.13)	1.48-4.88 (2.78±1.03)	55-117 (77±22)	5.4-13.08 (8.58±1.05)	134-322 (250±72)	68
po r³H	—	0.380-0.150	0.38±0.12	—	136±42	—	367±198	63
iv 2,4-³H	13.0-28.9 (19.7±6.8)	0.525±0.181	0.13-0.54 (0.34±0.15)	3.3-14.0 (6.4±3.6)	171±96	—	—	—
iv 2,4³H	14.7-29.8 (23.2±6.6)	0.401-0.687	0.13-0.67 (0.38±0.20)	3.8-14.0 (8.2±4.2)	112-547 (374±213)	—	—	—
iv 24-¹⁴C	—	0.510±0.166	0.21±0.10	—	120±36	—	—	—
	—	0.47±0.10	—	—	—	—	—	—

*Eight patients with stones, three with lithogenic bile.
†Gallbladder disease.

(b) Post-cholecystectomy Patients

Reference	Patient description	Age (years)	Weight (kg)	Tracer	Chenodeoxycholic Pool (µmol/kg)	FTR (day⁻¹)	Synthesis (µmol kg⁻¹ day⁻¹)	Pool (g)	Synthesis (mg/day)	Cholic Pool (µmol/kg)	Pool (g)	FTR (day⁻¹)	Synthesis (µmol kg⁻¹ day⁻¹)	Synthesis (mg/day)	Total Synthesis (µmol kg⁻¹ day⁻¹)	Synthesis (mg/day)	% Cholic
114	1F, 9M	48-60	—	po 24-¹⁴C	5.13-21.24 (12.09±5.13)	0.23-0.70 (0.50±0.16)	3.11-11.90 (5.68±2.82)	—	—	4.21-22.46 (11.93±5.27)	—	0.29-1.25 (0.81±0.26)	3.83-17.80 (8.95±4.46)	134-322 (250±72)	7.21-25.68 (14.63±5.28)	—	62
115	11*	—	—	iv 24¹⁴C	8.42-23.81 (14.65±5.13)	0.36-1.04 (0.55±0.21)	5.66-8.68 (7.25±1.50)	—	—	5.97-27.38 (14.74±7.37)	—	0.32-1.66 (0.75±0.42)	4.04-12.92 (9.37±2.63)	—	16.62±4.13	—	56
	2†	—	—	iv 24-¹⁴C	8.79, 8.79	0.41, 0.83	3.66, 7.29	—	—	8.78, 12.64	—	0.48, 1.04	4.94, 13.06	—	8.60, 20.35	—	62
108	10*	—	—	iv 24-¹⁴C	—	—	—	0.55±0.25	—	—	0.40±0.10	0.56±0.16	—	233±84	—	—	—

*Radiolucent stones.
†Pigmented stones.

97

Table 5.1 continued

VI. LIVER DISEASE
(a) Cirrhosis

Reference	Patient description	Age (years)	Weight (kg)	Tracer	Cholic Pool (μmol/kg)	Cholic Pool (g)	Cholic FTR (day⁻¹)	Cholic Synthesis (μmol kg⁻¹ day⁻¹)	Cholic Synthesis (mg/day)
67	12 M	50 (34–67)	—	po 24-¹⁴C	—	0.24–0.72 (0.48±0.15)	0.07–0.38 (0.17±0.09)	—	18–166 (84±48)
68	7 M (mild)	47 (35–58)	—	po 24-¹⁴C	—	0.49±0.06	0.30±0.10	—	91–268 (152±62)
	10 M (adv)	52 (42–67)	—	po 24-¹⁴C	—	0.46±0.17	0.14±0.07	—	18–156 (68±42)
69	2 M	—	—	po 24-¹⁴C	—	0.329, 0.334	0.15, 0.18	—	49, 62
70	5 M	—	—	iv 24-¹⁴C	—	0.225–0.977 (0.513±0.230)	0.09–0.40 (0.21±0.13)	—	42–161 (90±31)
71	3 F	55–66	—	iv 24-¹⁴C	15.1–54.3 (33.9±10.4)	—	0.09–0.30	1.4–16.2	—
72	8 M	49–69	—	iv 24-¹⁴C	—	0.397±0.213	0.10–0.33 (0.19±0.08)	—	38–201 (82±50)

Tracer	Chenodeoxycholic Pool (μmol/kg)	Chenodeoxycholic Pool (g)	Chenodeoxycholic FTR (day⁻¹)	Chenodeoxycholic Synthesis (μmol kg⁻¹ day⁻¹)	Chenodeoxycholic Synthesis (mg/day)	Total Synthesis (μmol kg⁻¹ day⁻¹)	Total Synthesis (mg/day)	Total % Cholic
po 24-¹⁴C	—	0.22–1.26 (0.62±0.27)	0.10–0.50 (0.21±0.11)	—	59–172 (114±36)	—	87–279 (198±68)	42
po 24-¹⁴C	—	0.49±0.20	0.29±0.11	—	85–212 (130±42)	—	176–418 (282±75)	54
po 24-¹⁴C	—	0.67±0.25	0.18±0.06	—	59–172 (117±38)	—	87–272 (185±57)	37
po 2, 4-³H	—	0.492, 1.171	0.30, 0.36	—	178, 348	—	240, 397	17
iv 24-¹⁴C	—	0.239–0.852 (0.477±0.172)	0.13–0.40 (0.28±0.09)	—	95–145 (118±13)	—	184–286 (208±45)	43
—	—	—	—	—	—	—	—	—
iv 24-¹⁴C	—	0.847–0.517	0.08–0.31 (0.18±0.07)	—	76–169 (115±33)	—	127–371 (200±78)	41

Table 5.1 *continued*

(b) Cholestasis

Reference	Patient description	Age (years)	Weight (kg)	Tracer	Pool (μmol/kg)	Synthesis (μmol kg⁻¹day⁻¹)	Cholic Pool (g)	Synthesis (mg/day)	FTR (day⁻¹)	Synthesis (μmol kg⁻¹day⁻¹)	Synthesis (mg/day)	Total Synthesis (μmol kg⁻¹day⁻¹)	Synthesis (mg/day)	% Cholic
71	3F, 1M*	23-59	—	iv 24-^{14}C	21.6-93.2 (56.2±19.8)	—	—	—	0.02-0.29	1.5-15.5	—	—	—	—

Continuation (Chenodeoxycholic / Total) of reference 71:

Tracer	Chenodeoxycholic Pool (μmol/kg)	Pool (g)	FTR (day⁻¹)	Synthesis (μmol kg⁻¹day⁻¹)	Synthesis (mg/day)	Total Synthesis (μmol kg⁻¹day⁻¹)	Synthesis (mg/day)	% Cholic
iv 24-^{14}C	—	—	—	—	—	—	—	—

*Primary biliary cirrhosis, sclerosing cholangitis.

VII. HYPERLIPOPROTEINAEMIA

Reference	Type	Patient description	Age (years)	Weight (kg)	Tracer	Cholic Pool (μmol/kg)	Pool (g)	FTR (day⁻¹)	Synthesis (μmol kg⁻¹day⁻¹)	Synthesis (mg/day)
116		8F, 2M (C)	45-69	49-80	po 24-^{14}C	14.78-83.75	0.320-2.710	0.33	2.86-7.74	65-223
		9 (C+T)	39-70	54-70	po 24-^{14}C	22.41-139.88	0.560-3.080	0.48	7.81-85.82	271-2175
111	IIa	12F, 5M	56	64	po 24-^{14}C	25.85±14.74	0.675±0.385	0.27±0.15	5.74±2.45	150±64
	IIb	6F, 6M	54	70	po 24-^{14}C	30.39±18.03	0.868±0.515	0.28±0.16	6.41±2.66	183±76
	IV	4F, 23M	52	82	po 24-^{14}C	53.38±31.56	1.786±1.056	0.48±0.24	23.25±13.75	778±460
	V	3F, 2M	50	74	po 24-^{14}C	77.70±60.28	2.346±1.820	0.44±0.29	16.76±4.07	506±123
74	IIa	5F	52-61	45-74	po 24-^{14}C	—	320±246	0.30±0.08	—	96±7
	IV.	5M	45-61	73-92	po 24-^{14}C	—	1166±441	0.63±0.11	—	804±306
112	IIa	6F, 4M	41-62	47-96	po 24-^{14}C	—	0.648±0.392	0.44±0.32	—	208±76
	IV	5M	43-53	67-82	po 24-^{14}C	—	1.073±0.356	0.42±0.22	—	385±83

Table 5.1 continued

| | Chenodeoxycholic | | | | | Total | | |
Tracer	Pool (μmol/kg)	Pool (g)	FTR (day⁻¹)	Synthesis (μmol kg⁻¹ day⁻¹)	Synthesis (mg/day)	Synthesis (μmol kg⁻¹ day⁻¹)	Synthesis (mg/day)	% Cholic
po r³H	14.46–159.33	0.3–4.94	—	4.33–9.87	89–306	8.36–15.77	185–497	46
po r³H	12.53–146.45	0.3–3.09	—	4.60–37.45	133–929	15.28–104.39	455–2626	
po r³H	33.60±13.87	0.843±0.348	0.24±0.15	7.13±2.99	179±75	—	329±97	46
po r³H	40.45±13.01	1.110±0.357	0.19±0.06	7.18±3.57	197±98	—	489±154	37
po r³H	26.94±13.19	0.866±0.424	0.33±0.16	7.81±4.11	251±132	—	1029±496	76
po r³H	27.61±2.17	0.801±0.63	0.23±0.09	6.41±2.00	186±87	—	692±37	73
po r³H	—	0.728±0.461	0.24±0.06	—	168±18	—	264±19	36
	—	0.513±0.192	0.43±0.03	—	240±119	—	1044±328	77
po 24-¹⁴C	—	0.725±0.528	0.31±0.32	—	181±85	—	389±152	54
po 24-¹⁴C	—	0.749±0.127	0.36±0.22	—	259±206	—	643±168	60

C = cholesterol; T = triglyceride.

VIII. ENDOCRINE ABNORMALITIES

Reference	Patient description	Age (years)	Weight (kg)	Tracer	Cholic Pool (μmol/kg)	Pool (g)	FTR (day⁻¹)	Synthesis (μmol kg⁻¹ day⁻¹)	Synthesis (mg/day)
117	6F, 1M (hyperthyroid)	52 (33–63)	52 (45–60)	po 24-¹⁴C	24.24–71.77 (43.22±15.23)	0.57–1.37 (0.91±0.27)	0.20–0.63 (0.33±0.11)	9.63–27.63 (13.63±8.08)	196±528 (315±118)
	9F, 1M (hypothyroid)	54 (29–76)	68 (53–93) 167	po 24-¹⁴C	21.29–73.52	0.65–1.90	0.35–1.07	4.80–16.45	103–472

| Chenodeoxycholic | |
Pool (μmol/kg)	Pool (g)
30.3–89.71	0.71–1.71
(54.00±19.04)	(1.14±0.34)
19.35–66.84	0.59–1.73

Table 5.1 *continued*

IX. INTESTINAL DISEASE

Reference	Patient description	Age (years)	Weight (kg)	Tracer	Cholic Pool (μmol/kg)	Cholic Pool (g)	Cholic FTR (day⁻¹)	Cholic Synthesis (μmol kg⁻¹day⁻¹)	Cholic Synthesis (mg/day)
73 1	9F, 8M	30 (17–42)	60 (39–83)	iv 24-^{14}C	28.56 (6.5–52.73)	0.707±0.315	(0.46–4.14) 2.00±1.13	57.12	1414±630
73 2			52 (44–63)	iv 24-^{14}C	21.41 (9.09–45.87)	0.48±0.374	(0.25–1.36) 0.91±47	19.48	437±340

| | Chenodeoxycholic | | | | | Total | | |
Tracer	Pool (μmol/kg)	Pool (g)	FTR (day⁻¹)	Synthesis (μmol kg⁻¹day⁻¹)	Synthesis (mg/day)	Synthesis (μmol kg⁻¹day⁻¹)	Synthesis (mg/day)	% Cholic
iv 11, 12-3H	41.17 (20–87.5)	0.963±0.519	0.81±0.56	32.99	780±420	90.09	2194	64
iv 11, 12-3H	25.23 (8.33–43.33)	0.523±0.351	0.62±0.18	15.64	324±217	35.12	761	57

1 = Ileitis; 2 = ileocolitis.

101

Table 5.2 Total bile acid pool

Reference	Pool (μmol/kg)	Pool (g)
(I) Health		
(a) Normal		
8	—	3.57±0.93
101	—	2.71
102	132.64	3.28
103	—	2.38±0.43
17	—	2.27±0.45
18	69±11.8	1.64±0.36
76	—	2.62±1.21
111	—	1.40±0.63
106	—	1.77±0.18
107	—	1.82±0.51
31	—	2.36
81	70±32	1.85±0.85
66	137.1±36.2	4.2±1.1
108	—	2.25±0.75
109	—	1.8±0.75
47	90±55	—
73	—	3.02±0.63
(b) Formula – Polyunsaturated fat diet		
102	—	3.34
(c) Vegetarian diet		
47	95±48	—
(d) Alterations with drugs		
76 (cholic acid feeding)	—	4.07±2.77
35 (contraceptives)	99.6±22.3	2.19±.49
(II) Disease		
(a) Biliary disease:		
(1) Gallstones		
78	—	1.22±0.32
113	—	1.29±0.25
67	—	0.53–1.76
114	17.87–64.39 (35.89±14.07)	
18	16.3–71.5 (43.6±8.5)	0.40–2.08 (1.24±0.22)
81	51.0–84.6 (68.1±12.8)	
65	51–71.7 (58.5±12.5)	1.79–3.18 (2.45±0.53)
107	—	1.07±0.39
108		2.0±0.9
(2) Post-cholecystectomy		
114 (radiolucent stones)	18.21–50.57 (34.41±10.75)	—
115 (radiolucent stones)	25.33–169.51 36.46±14.64	—
(pigment stones)	19.76,29.52	—
108 (radiolucent stones)		1.65±0.5

Table 5.2   Total bile acid pool

Reference	Pool (μmol/kg)	Pool (g)
(II) Disease continued		
(b) Liver disease:		
(1) Cirrhosis		
67	—	0.72–2.05
		(1.19±0.38)
68 (mild)	—	1.09±0.31
(advanced)		1.17±0.36
(c) Hyperlipoproteinaemia		
116 (cholesterol)	29.24–243.08	0.62–7.65
(cholesterol and triglyceride)	34.94–286.34	0.86–6.17
111 (IIA)	—	1.52±0.60
(IIB)	—	1.99±0.85
(IV)	—	2.65±1.26
(V)	—	3.15±1.76
(d) Endocrine abnormalities		
117 (hyperthyroidism)	69.69–206.33	1.63–3.93
(hypothyroidism)	54.19–187.15	1.65–4.84
(e) Intestinal disease		
73 (ileitis)	90.79±33.41	2.23±1.16
(ileocolitis)	48.73±29.19	1.05±0.73

also been shown, using the technique of isotope dilution, in patients with cirrhosis[67-72].

Increased bile acid synthesis has also been shown using isotope dilution. There is a 5–10-fold increase in synthesis in patients with ileal dysfunction secondary to ileal disease with a normal or decreased pool size[73]. Cholestyramine administration causes increased bile acid synthesis, but little change in exchangeable pool size[74,75].

As noted, in patients with unoperated Crohn's disease the bile acid pool tends to be smaller, and the cholic acid pool is especially decreased[73]. Bile acid turnover is more rapid, but the increased turnover is much greater for cholic than for chenodeoxycholic acid. These findings were interpreted to indicate that jejunal or colonic absorption (or both) of chenodeoxycholic acid contributed to its greater conservation.

Isotope dilution kinetics have also been used to calculate input of exogenously administered chenodeoxycholic acid[18] and cholic acid[76]. For chenodeoxycholic acid, the data were used to infer complete bioavailability of the administered bile acid[18]. However, the validity of the isotope dilution measurements during bile acid feeding has not yet been established.

Secondary bile acids

The input of deoxycholic acid has been measured to define the efficiency of deoxycholic acid absorption in relation to age[77]. It has also been used to define the effect of dietary fibre on the conservation of deoxycholic acid[47].

One study measured the input of lithocholic acid during chenodeoxycholic acid therapy and showed that it was markedly increased[21]. There have been no other studies in man on the effects of drugs on the input of lithocholic acid.

BILE ACID POOL SIZE AND BILE ACID SECRETION

Bile acid secretion refers to the flux of bile acids secreted by the liver. When averaged over the day, it is equal to the bile acids secreted into the intestine, but there are hour-to-hour differences because of the storage and emptying of the gallbladder.

Measurements of bile acid secretion in man preceded measurements of bile acid pool size, but in the early 1970s, when isotope dilution measurements of bile acid kinetics became more frequent, it was assumed that bile acid secretion would be linearly proportional to bile acid pool size[78]. Measurements of bile acid secretion using marker dilution techniques were developed independently by Grundy and Metzger[79] and by the Mayo group[80,81]. The former method featured a continuous infusion of a liquid meal into the intestine; whereas the Mayo approach featured a normal feeding pattern of three liquid meals and an overnight fast.

A number of studies from the Mayo group have presented convincing evidence that secretion is unrelated to the exchangeable pool size; i.e. in subjects with a smaller pool size, there is more frequent cycling of the bile acid pool so that the product of cycling frequency and pool size remains constant[66], but this has not invariably been confirmed by other workers[82].

In contrast, workers using the steady-state infusion technique of Grundy and Metzger have found exactly the opposite, namely that the bile acid secretion rate was directly proportional to bile acid pool size[83]. Specifically, in a group of gallstone subjects with a decreased exchangeable bile acid pool, secretion was lower than that in an age and sex matched control group with a larger exchangeable bile acid pool.

The reason for this discrepancy remains unclarified. It has been reported that the gallbladder does not contract completely in patients studied according to the Grundy–Metzger technique[30], and if so, this would diminish bile acid secretion. On the other hand, this error, if present, should occur in all patients studied. It has also been claimed that perfusion measurements carried out in the non-steady state, as is present in the Mayo technique, are not valid[84].

The matter is not entirely unimportant, as a continuing question regarding the pathogenesis of cholesterol cholelithiasis is whether such patients have decreased bile acid secretion and a normal or sub-normal rate of bile acid synthesis, thus suggesting that such patients have 'inappropriate down-regulation'.

The functions of bile acids in the small intestine are more closely related to bile acid secretion than to pool size. Measurements of secretion would appear to have an important place in the characterization of bile acid metabolism in digestive disease or of the mode of action of agents that alter biliary lipid secretion. Much more experimental work is needed.

Table 5.3 Cholesterol kinetics in health

(A) NORMAL SUBJECTS

| | | | | | | | Daily Cholesterol Input | | Rapid pool | | Slow pool | |
Reference	No. of patients /sex	Age, range (years)	Height, range (cm)	Weight, range (kg)	No. of pools	Length of study (weeks)	Tracer	g	μmol/kg	g	μmol/kg	g	μmol/kg
85	3F, 12M	44	—	74 (49-94)	3	18-24	iv 4^{14}C	(1.10±0.19)	38.4±6.6	24.0±3.2	838±112	84.1±33.1	2937±1156
93	3F, 2M	64 (46-72)	—	65	IOA	10-16	iv 4^{14}C; 1,2^{3}H	0.94 (0.71-1.29)	38.1 (32.8-49.6)	22.8 (16.8-26.5)	940 (692-1312)		
	4F, 4M	56 (41-72)	—	65 (51-81)	IOA	50-66	iv 4^{14}C; 7α^{3}H	1.12 (0.65-1.84)	44.9 (30.9-58.7)	27.2 (15.5-40.2)	1064 (770-1366)	57.3 (42.1-102.2)	2249 (1597-3260)
118	3M	53 (51-54)	180 (175-183)	77 (76-79)	2	12-13	iv 4^{14}C	1.24 (1.17-1.38)	41.8 (38.6-46.9)	26.1 (24.9-28.4)	875 (846-929)	37.9-61.7	1269-2068
94	2F, 1M	38 (22-47)	—	87	2	10-11	iv 1α^{3}H	1.75 (1.10-2.51)	50.2 (39.5-67.6)	18.0 (15.9-21.3)	547 (438-631)		
119	3F, 2M	45-62	—	65-100	2	23-42	iv 7α^{3}H	1.65 (1.03-3.27)		34.4 (26.5-40.1)			

(B) MANIPULATIONS OF DIET OR DRUGS IN NORMALS

Reference		No. of patients /sex	Age, range (years)	Height, range (cm)	Weight, range (kg)	No. of pools	Length of study (weeks)	Tracer	Daily Cholesterol Input g	μmol/kg	Rapid pool g	μmol/kg	Slow pool g	μmol/kg
118	1*	2M	51, 53	175, 183	73, 78	2	12-13	iv 4^{14}C	1.17, 1.43	39.8, 48.6	23.6, 26.8	802, 911	36.2-59.2	1231-2013
	2	2M	53, 54	183, 183	74, 80	2	12-13	iv 4^{14}C	1.09, 1.42	35.65, 48.3	24.4, 27.1	830, 886	36.8-57.8	1225-1926
94	3	1F	47	—	100	2	10-11	iv 1α^{3}H	2.91*(IOA)	75.2	23.3	602		
94	4	1F, 1M	22, 45	—	65, 96	2	10-11	iv 1α^{3}H	1.44, 2.2	57.24, 60.1	19.2, 21.7	518, 864		
119	5	2F, 2M	45, 62	—		IOA	23-42	iv 7α^{3}H	1.47*(IOA) (0.94-2.40)		23.2 (16.1-26.7)			

*IOA = Input-output analysis.
1* = Colestipol hydrochloride, 15 g/day × 5-9 months; 2 = colestipol hydrochloride + clofibrate, 2 g/day × 8 weeks; 3 = cholestyramine, 16 g/day × 1 month; 4 = polyunsaturated diet; 5 = 2 g neomycin × 12-26 weeks.

ISOTOPE DILUTION MEASUREMENT OF CHOLESTEROL KINETICS

When labelled cholesterol is injected intravenously, the specific activity decay curve of plasma declines bi-exponentially for a matter of months[3]. Deconvolution of the curve can be carried out using a complex three-compartment model for simulation[85] or by the input 'stochastic' technique discussed previously[51]. Both give comparable results (Table 5.3). The exact meaning of the transfer coefficients and the fluxes between compartments continues to be debated and will not be discussed here.

To factor out the input of dietary cholesterol from total cholesterol input, one must measure cholesterol absorption by an independent technique. This is usually done by feeding cholesterol tagged with a second isotope and noting the appearance of the administered radioactivity in plasma cholesterol[86,87]. Other methods for measuring cholesterol in the steady state procedure have been discussed by Quintao *et al.*[88] and collated by Sodhi *et al.*[2].

Methods

Cholesterol is administered intravenously to ensure labelling of the pool with a defined dose. The injected cholesterol is known to be taken up by the reticuloendothelial system and to be slowly released. Within a week or so, both the unesterified and esterified cholesterol fractions in serum have achieved identical specific activities. Thus, in practice, serum is saponified and the cholesterol extracted into petroleum hydrocarbon. The cholesterol concentration is determined chemically by a colorimetric, chromatographic, or enzymatic procedure. The radioactivity is determined directly, as radioactivity is present only in the chemical form of cholesterol. Cholesterol may be labelled with either ^3H or ^{14}C, and certain ^3H labels were validated some years ago[89]. Establishment of radiopurity of commercially offered batches of radioactive cholesterol is essential, as radioimpurities may influence the results[90]. The specific activity is converted to % dose per gram (or millimole) cholesterol and plotted on semi-logarithmic paper. Serum samples should be obtained at semi-weekly intervals for the first month and then at bi-weekly intervals for a period of at least 6 months. It is possible for subjects to send their serum surface mail to the analytical laboratory. During this time, the cholesterol intake and diet of the subject should remain as constant as possible.

Validation

The value for the exchangeable cholesterol pool obtained by the isotope dilution technique agrees well with that of total body cholesterol measured chemically in the total carcass of the baboon[91]. Similar validation studies in man have not been carried out for ethical reasons.

The estimates of endogenous synthesis obtained by the isotope dilution method agree acceptably well with those estimated by the sterol balance technique[92].

Alternatives to the isotope dilution technique for estimating cholesterol synthesis in man

An obvious alternative to isotope dilution or sterol balance for measuring cholesterol synthesis rates is to give a radioactive precursor and measure its incorporation into cholesterol. This has been done with acetate, mevalonate, or squalene, but there are vexing and essentially insoluble uncertainties about the extent to which the precursor pool is labelled predictably by the injected tracer[85]. These methods are discussed in some detail by Sodhi *et al.*[2]. In animals, [^{14}C]-octanoate or $^{3}H_2O$ may be used, but only the latter has been reported to give valid estimates of cholesterol synthesis using tissue slices[5]. The Rockefeller University group also reported that cholesterol turnover may be estimated conveniently by a combination of sterol balance and input–output analyses[93].

Application

Use of isotope dilution measurements of cholesterol kinetics have shown that the total exchangeable pool of cholesterol is highly correlated with body weight, as indeed is the rate of cholesterol synthesis. Published data are summarized in Table 5.4.

Cholesterol synthesis has been shown to increase modestly during chole-styramine feeding (Table 5.3; Part B). No difference in cholesterol synthesis was detected during chenodeoxycholic acid or cholic acid feeding in patients with radiolucent gallstones.

Limited measurements of cholesterol synthesis have been carried out in heterozygous and homozygous familial hypercholesterolaemia (Table 5.4; Part C).

Combined measurements of cholesterol and bile acid kinetics have been made by Quarfordt and Greenfield[94]. These have not proved especially helpful, but they do provide information on a key aspect of cholesterol metabolism, i.e., the fraction of synthesized cholesterol which is excreted as neutral sterols and its complement, the fraction which is excreted as bile acids. Similar information can be obtained from the sterol balance technique if one can subtract dietary cholesterol with precision and estimates have been collated by Miettinen[95]. The conclusion of the studies that have been done are in agreement with the sterol balance data, indicating that man is unique among vertebrates in excreting the majority of his cholesterol in the form of neutral sterols, rather than converting it into bile acids. However, this conclusion must be made cautiously, as there has not been any systematic survey of vertebrates, and this fraction may well be influenced by dietary factors such as fibre, which tend to increase bile acid excretion.

Very recently, a series of important papers has been published by Schwartz, Vlahcevic, Swell, and the late Mones Berman[96,97]. These papers detail the kinetics of cholesterol between lipoprotein fractions and report a satisfactory physiological pharmacokinetic model.

Table 5.4 Cholesterol kinetics in disease

(A) BILE ACID FEEDING IN GALLSTONE PATIENTS

Reference	No. of patients /sex	Age range (years)	Height range (cm)	Weight range (kg)	No. of pools	Length of study (weeks)	Tracer	Daily Cholesterol Input		Rapid pool		Slow pool	
								g	μmol/kg	g	μmol/kg	g	μmol/kg
120 1	4F, 4M	57 (44–68)	183 (157–186)	71 (57–85)	IOA	27	iv 26^{14}C	1.15±0.25	41.9±5.9	27.4±6.3	1007±146	41.8±12.3	1499±365
2	4F, 4M	54 (39–68)	168 (144–183)	80 (59–108)	IOA	27	iv 26^{14}C	1.08±0.37	34.4±5.9	32.4±9.8	1060±292	58.9±31.9	1938±1235
3	3F, 4M	54 (43–70)	171 (160–188)	79 (54–117)	IOA	27	iv 26^{14}C	1.09±0.37	35.7±6.2	29.3±10.7	956±136	41.3±19.9	1318±342

IOA = Input–output analysis.

(B) OBESITY

Reference	No. of patients /sex	Age range (years)	Height range (cm)	Weight range (kg)	No. of pools	Length of study (weeks)	Tracer	Daily Cholesterol Input		Rapid pool		Slow pool	
								g	μmol/kg	g	μmol/kg	g	μmol/kg
121	4F, 1M	46 (33–59)	—	139 (102–175)	2		iv 4^{14}C or 1,2α^{3}H	2.37 (1.64–3.37)	44.5 (32.39–59.23)	27.9 (22.51–34.1)	531 (388–662)	100.4 (64.6–126.7)	1885 (1177–2569)
93	6F, 5M	48 (33–59)	—	101 (52–175)	IOA	5–10	iv 4^{14}C 1, 2^{3}H	1.82 (0.87–3.65)	47.0 (32.8–89.7)	24 (15.6–34.1)	693 (315–1104)		

IOA = Input–output analysis.
1 = Placebo; 2 = chenodeoxycholic, 10–25 mg kg⁻¹ day⁻¹ × 6 months; 3 = cholic, 7–30 mg/kg × 6 months.

Table 5.4 continued

(C) HYPERLIPOPROTEINAEMIA

Reference	No. of patients /sex	Age, range (years)	Height, range (cm)	Weight, range (kg)	No. of pools	Length of study (weeks)	Tracer	Daily Cholesterol Input		Rapid pool		Slow pool	
								g	µmol/kg	g	µmol/kg	g	µmol/kg
85	Chol 5F, 5M	54	—	66	3	18–46	iv 4¹⁴C	0.97±0.24	38.0±9.4	30.3±6.9	1186±270	90.6±19.6	3547±767
	Trig 21M	50	—	85	3	18–46	iv 4¹⁴C	1.59±0.49	48.3±14.9	24.2±3.9	736±119	116.3±35.7	3535±1085
	Mixed 2F, 6M	51	—	79	3	18–46	iv 4¹⁴C	1.28±0.32	41.9±10.5	28.7±3.5	939±115	107.4±16.7	3512±546
93	Chol 1F, 1M	30, 36	—	53, 67	2	10–16	iv 4¹⁴C 1, 2³H	0.78, 0.96	37.0, 38.0	26.4, 34.2	1287, 1319		
	Trig 2F	39, 62	—	67, 71	*IOA	10–16	iv 4¹⁴C 1, 2³H	1.06, 1.27	40.9, 46.2	14.7, 25.4	567, 924		
	Mixed 1F, 4M	51 (30–60)	—	68 (58–78)	IOA	10–16	iv 4¹⁴C 1, 2³H	1.18 (0.81–1.80)	44.1 (36.1–59.6)	36 (25.4–51.2)	1395 (991–2294)		
	Chol 1F, 3M	52 (44–58)	—	62 (46–81)	IOA	5–10	iv 4¹⁴C 1, 2³H	0.98 (0.74–1.10)	41.6 (35.1–52.7)	28.9 (15.0–42.5)	1167 (842–1504)		
	Trig 4M	50 (48–52)	—	83 (70–95)	IOA	5–10	iv 4¹⁴C 1, 2³H	1.63 (1.21–2.32)	49.7 (39.9–63.1)	24.3 (18.0–28.9)	753 (596–900)		
	Mixed 1F, 4M	48 (39–58)	—	76 (61–90)	IOA	5–10	iv 4¹⁴C 1, 2³H	1.82 (1.07–2.81)	61.2 (42.5–80.7)	29.6 (25.1–34.3)	1026 (772–1309)		
	Mixed 4F, 5M	49 (18–64)	—	70 (54–92)	IOA	50–66	iv 4¹⁴C 7α3H	1.15 (0.78–1.51)	43.4 (35.6–61.3)	39 (17.1–66.7)	1468 (638–2886)	65.7 (37.1–93.0)	2473 (1712–4450)
118	IIa 1F, 1M	51, 60 (40–61)	168, 180 (145–180)	66, 79 (63–79)	2	12–13	iv 4¹⁴C	1.25, 1.50 (0.91–1.51)	48.6, 49.1 (37.0–49.1)	25.1, 28.5 (22.0–25.7)	934, 976 (804–896)	32.4–54.9	1157–1945
	IV 3M	51	166	73	2	12–13	iv 4¹⁴C	1.21	42.2	23.9	845	33.3–53.2	1169–1861
	IIb 3F	50 (45–55)	161 (160–163)	54 (50–58)	2	12–13	iv 4¹⁴C	0.94 (0.71–1.27)	46.3 (31.9–65.8)	20.4 (17.1–23.4)	994 (767–1212)	27.6–45.6	1334–2210
122	IIa 5M	41 (35–45)	172 (166–176)	72 (62–80)	2	12–21	iv 1, 2³H or iv 1α³H	1.45 (1.32–1.60)	52.4 (47.4–58.2)	30.1 (18.5–36.4)	881 (771–1241)		
	IIb 2F	47, 48	156, 159	60, 64	2	12–21	iv 1α³H or iv 1, 2³H	1.16, 1.37	50.1, 54.9	23.6, 30.4	1020, 1218		
123	Lipids 3F, 19M	39–68	—	72 (53–84)	2	10	iv 4¹⁴C	0.73–1.7	30.5–57.1	14.9–32.7	577–1112	19.8–89.3	817–3028
3	Lipids 2F, 3M	55 (34, 68)	—	—	2	9–10	iv 4¹⁴C	0.98±0.10		25.1±0.9			

*IOA = Input–output analysis.

109

Table 5.4 continued

(D) HYPERLIPOPROTEINAEMIC PATIENTS TREATED WITH LIPID LOWERING DRUGS

Reference	No. of patients /sex	Age, range (years)	Height, range (cm)	Weight, range (kg)	No. of pools	Length of study (weeks)	Tracer	Daily Cholesterol Input g	μmol/kg	Rapid pool g	μmol/kg	Slow pool g	μmol/kg
118 IIa *1	1F, 1M	51, 60	168, 180	66, 79	2	12–13	iv 4^{14}C	2.09, 2.76	81.2, 90.4	21.6, 28.3	839, 926	36.9–86.7	1326–3092
2	1F, 1M	51, 60	168, 180	66, 79	2	12–13	iv 4^{14}C	1.87, 2.76	71.7, 90.1	20.9, 28.0	801, 914	39.8–84.6	1418–2989
IV 1	3M	51 (40–61)	166 (145–180)	73 (63–79)	2	12–13	iv 4^{14}C	2.01 (0.89–2.65)	68.9 (36.2–86.2)	23.8 (22.7–25.4)	844 (784–923)	31.3–64.5	1087–2209
2	1M	40	173	77	2	12–13	iv 4^{14}C	2.35	78.8	23.8	798	38.6–79.7	1294–2671
IIb 1	3F	50 (45–55)	161 (160–163)	54 (50–58)	2	12–13	iv 4^{14}C	1.81 (1.52–2.05)	88.1 (68.2–99.8)	19.6 (16.0–23.7)	958 (718–1227)	25.9–61.9	1244–2987
2	2F	51, 55	160, 163	50, 57	2	12–13	iv 4^{14}C	1.27, 1.59	57.9, 81.7	16.9, 18.3	834, 868	27.4–58.4	1323–2840
122 IIa 3	5M	41 (35–45)	172 (166–176)	72 (62–80)	2	12–21	iv 4^{14}C	2.34 (1.86–3.10)	86.4 (72.8–114.8)	26.1 (20.2–30.5)	932 (842–1019)		
IIb 3 1F		48	156	64	2	12–21	iv 4^{14}C	2.23	96.4	21.9	945		
Lipid 3	2F, 3M	55 (34–68)	—	—	2	9–10	iv 4^{14}C	1.98±0.24		23.5±2.41			

*1 = Colestipol hydrochloride, 15 g/day × 5–9 months; 2 = colestipol hydrochloride + clofibrate, 2 g/day × 8 weeks; 3 = colestipol, 15 g/day × 8 weeks; 4 = cholestyramine, 12 g/day.

Conclusions

Measurement of bile acid kinetics by isotope dilution was originally carried out to define the pool size, hoping that this would give important insights into bile acid metabolism. It seems highly probable that measurement of bile acid secretion is a more physiologically meaningful parameter of bile acid metabolism than measurement of the exchangeable pool size.

The measurement of primary bile acid synthesis by the technique of isotope dilution is a valuable and useful measurement. Similar results can be obtained by chemical measurement of faecal bile acids, but this is considerably more difficult from a methodological standpoint. Whether the measurements of bile acid input obtained by the isotope dilution technique during bile acid feeding are accurate remains unclear.

For secondary bile acids, the isotope dilution technique provides information on the input of newly formed secondary bile acids into the enterohepatic circulation. At the moment, it is not at all clear that the rate of input of deoxycholic acid is important, although limited evidence could be asembled to indicate that if deoxycholic acid input were prevented, the chenodeoxycholic acid pool would expand and bile would become less saturated[98,99].

For lithocholic acid, the importance of measuring input remains unclear. If individuals with defective lithocholic sulphation are identified, then the input of lithocholic acid will be a crucial determinant of whether or not liver disease is induced[100].

As noted, the measurement of cholesterol pool size and synthesis rate by isotope dilution is rather unsatisfactory for several reasons. First, the isotope takes months to equilibrate so that the specific activity decay curve must be defined for at least 6 months. Second, the input of cholesterol derives from not only endogenous synthesis but also absorption of dietary cholesterol. Partitioning of the input between these two fluxes can only be done precisely when the amount of cholesterol absorbed is known; and it can never be known precisely for an interval as long as 6 months. Third, the exchangeable pool has only an approximate physiological meaning, and its constituent pools have mathematical, but not physiological, meaning. Finally, the risk factor for atherosclerosis is considered to be related at least in part to the concentration of cholesterol in various serum lipoprotein fractions; and these are not measured by the isotope dilution technique.

Acknowledgements

The author's work is supported primarily by NIH Grant AM 21506. Additional grants in aid were received from the Falk Foundation and Stokely Van Camp, Inc.

References

1. Hoffman, N. E. and Hofmann, A. F. (1974). Measurement of bile acid kinetics by isotope dilution in man. *Gastroenterology*, **67**, 314
2. Sodhi, H. S., Kudchodkar, B. J. and Mason, D. T. (eds.) (1979). *Clinical Methods in Study of Cholesterol Metabolism*. (Basel: Karger)
3. Goodman, D. S. and Robert, N. (1968). Turnover of plasma cholesterol in man. *J. Clin. Invest.*, **47**, 231
4. Hofmann, A. F. (1976). The enterohepatic circulation of bile acids in man. In Taylor, W. (ed.) *The Hepatobiliary System*. pp. 517-525. (New York: Plenum Press)
5. Turley, S. D. and Dietschy, J. M. (1982). Cholesterol metabolism and excretion. In Arias, I. M., Popper, H., Schachter, D. and Schafritz, D. A. (eds.). *The Liver, Biology and Pathobiology*. pp. 467-492. (New York: Raven Press)
6. Small, D. M. (1977). Bile salts of the blood: High density lipoprotein systems and cholesterol removal. In Bianchi, L., Gerok, W. and Sickinger, K. (eds.). *Liver and Bile*. pp. 89-100. (Lancaster: MTP Press)
7. Bergstrom, S., Rottenberg, M. and Voltz, J. (1953). The preparation of some carboxy-labeled bile acids. Bile Acids and Steroids 2. *Acta Chem. Scand.*, **7**, 481
8. Lindstedt, S. (1957). The turnover of cholic acid in man. *Acta Physiol. Scand.*, **0**, 1
9. Sjovall, J. (1952). Separation of bile acids by paper chromatography. Bile Acids and Steroids 3. *Acta Chem. Scand.*, **6**, 1552
10. Danielsson, H., Eneroth, P., Hellstrom, K., Lindstedt, S. and Sjovall, J. (1963). On the turnover and excretory products of cholic and chenodeoxycholic acid in man. *J. Biol. Chem.*, **238**, 2299
11. Lindstedt, S., Avigan, J., Goodman, D. S., Sjovall, J. and Steinberg, D. (1965). The effect of dietary fat on the turnover of cholic acid and on the composition of the biliary bile acids in man. *J. Clin. Invest.*, **44**, 1754
12. Ali, S. S., Kuksis, A. and Beveridge, J. M. R. (1966). Excretion of bile acids by three men on corn oil and butter fat diets. *Can. J. Biochem.*, **44**, 1377
13. Grundy, S. M., Ahrens, E. H., Jr. and Miettinen, T. A. (1965). Quantitative isolation and gas–liquid chromatographic analysis of total fecal bile acids. *J. Lipid Res.*, **6**, 397
14. Lack, L. and Weiner, I. M. (1961). *In vitro* absorption of bile salts by small intestine of rats and guinea pigs. *Am. J. Physiol.*, **200**, 313
15. Heaton, K. W., Austad, W. I., Lack, L. and Tyor, P. (1968). Enterohepatic circulation of ^{14}C labeled bile salts in disorders of the small bowel. *Gastroenterology*, **55**, 5
16. Wollenweber, J., Kottke, B. A. and Owen, C. A., Jr. (1967). Pool size and turnover of bile acids in six hypercholesterolemic patients with and without administration of nicotinic acid. *J. Lab. Clin. Med.*, **69**, 584
17. Vlahcevic, Z. R., Miller, J. R., Farrar, J. T. and Swell, L. (1971). Kinetics and pool size of primary bile acids in man. *Gastroenterology*, **61**, 85
18. Danzinger, R. G., Hofmann, A. F., Thistle, J. L. and Schoenfield, L. J. (1973). Effect of oral chenodeoxycholic acid on bile acid kinetics and biliary lipid composition in women with cholelithiasis. *J. Clin. Invest.*, **52**, 2809
19. Einarrson, K. and Hellstrom, K. (1974). The formation of deoxycholic acid and chenodeoxycholic acid in man. *Clin. Sci. Mol. Med.*, **46**, 183
20. Cowen, A. E., Korman, M. G., Hofmann, A. F., Cass, O. W. and Coffin, S. B. (1975). Metabolism of lithocholate in healthy man. II. Enterohepatic circulation. *Gastroenterology*, **69**, 67
21. Allan, R. N., Thistle, J. L. and Hofmann, A. F. (1976). Lithocholate metabolism during chenotherapy for gallstone dissolution. II. Absorption and sulfation. *Gut*, **17**, 413
22. Hepner, G. W., Hofmann, A. F. and Thomas, P. J. (1972). Metabolism of steroid and amino acid moieties of conjugated bile acids in man. I. Cholyl glycine (glycocholic acid). *J. Clin. Invest.*, **51**, 1889
23. Hepner, G. W., Hofmann, A. F. and Thomas, P. J. (1972). Metabolism of steroid and amino acid moieties of conjugated bile acids in man. II. Glycine conjugated dihydroxy acids. *J. Clin. Invest.*, **51**, 1898
24. Hepner, G. W., Sturman, J. A., Hofmann, A. F. and Thomas, P. J. (1973). Metabolism of steroid and amino acid moieties of conjugated bile acids in man. III. Cholyl taurine (taurocholic acid). *J. Clin. Invest*, **52**, 433

25. Hellstrom, K. (1981). Bile acid metabolism in hyperlipoproteinemia. In Paumgartner, G., Stiehl, A. and Gerok, W. (eds). *Bile Acids and Lipids*. pp. 5–11. (Lancaster: MTP Press)
26. Hofmann, A. F. (1979). Beaumont Prize Acceptance Speech. *Gastroenterology*, **77**, 955
27. Vantrappen, G., Rutgeerts, P. and Ghoos, Y. (1981). A new method for the measurement of bile acid turnover and pool size by a double label, single intubation technique. *J. Lipid Res.*, **22**, 528
28. Hofmann, A. F., Schoenfield, L. J., Kottke, B. A. and Poley, J. R. (1970). Methods for the description of bile acid kinetics in man. In Olson, R. E. (eds.) *Methods in Medical Research*. pp. 149–180. (Chicago: Yearbook Medical Publishers)
29. Grundy, S. W. (1975). Effects of polyunsaturated fats on lipid metabolism in patients with hypertriglyceridemia. *J. Clin. Invest.* **55**, 269
30. Rutgeerts, P., Ghoos, Y., Vantrappen, G. and Helleman, J. (1981). The fasting bile acid pool size is not equal to the circulating pool size. *Gastroenterology*, **80**, 1266 (abstract)
31. Duane, W. C., Adler, R. D., Bennion, L. J. and Ginsberg, R. L. (1975). Determination of bile acid pool size in man: A simplified method with advantages of increased precision, shortened analysis time, and decreased isotope exposure. *J. Lipid Res.*, **16**, 155
32. Hoffman, N. E., LaRusso, N. F. and Hofmann, A. F. (1976). Sampling intestinal content with a sequestering capsule: A noninvasive technique for determining bile acid kinetics. *Mayo Clin. Proc.*, **51**, 171
33. Hoffman, N. E., LaRusso, N. F. and Hofmann, A. F. (1973). An improved method for faecal collection: the faecal field-kit. *Lancet*, i, 1422
34. DeMark, B. R., Everson, G. T., Klein, P. D., Showalter, R. B. and Kern, F., Jr. (1982). A method for the accurate measurement of isotope ratios of chenodeoxycholic acid and cholic acids in serum. *J. Lipid Res.*, **23**, 204
35. Kern, F., Jr., Everson, G. T., DeMark, B., McKinley, C., Showalter, R., Braverman, D. Z., Szczepanik-Van Leeuwen, P., and Klein, P. D. (1982). Biliary lipids, bile acids, and gallbladder function in the human female: effects of contraceptive steroids. *J. Lab. Clin. Med.*, **99**, 798
36. Fujisawa, K. , Kitahara, T., Ogura, K., Kurihara, N. and Kameda, H. (1980). Studies on the metabolic fate of chenodeoxycholic acid in human. *Gastroenterology*, **79**, 1105 (abstract)
37. Whiting, M. J. and Watts, J. McK. (1980). Prediction of the bile acid composition of bile from serum bile acid analysis during gallstone dissolution therapy. *Gastroenterology*, **78**, 220
38. LaRusso, N. F., Hoffman, N. E. and Hofmann, A. F. (1974). Validity of using 2,4-^{3}H-labeled bile acids to study bile acid kinetics in man. *J. Lab. Clin. Med.*, **85**, 759
39. Ng, P. Y., Allan, R. N. and Hofmann, A. F. (1977). Suitability of 11,12-^{3}H-chenodeoxycholic acid and 11,12-^{3}H-lithocholic acid for isotope dilution studies of bile acid metabolism in man. *J. Lipid Res.*, **18**, 753
40. Einarsson, K., Hellstrom, K. and Kallner, M. (1974). Randomly tritium-labelled chenodeoxycholic acid as tracer in the determination of bile acid turnover in man. *Clin. Chim. Acta*, **56**, 235
41. Panveliwalla, D. K., Persemlidis, D. and Ahrens, E. H., Jr. (1974). Tritiated bile acids: problems and recommendations. *J. Lipid Res.*, **15**, 530
42. Hofmann, A. F., Szczepanik, P. A. and Klein, P. D. (1968). Rapid preparation of tritium labeled bile acids by enolic exchange on basic alumina containing tritiated water. *J. Lipid Res.*, **9**, 707
43. Cowen, A. E., Hofmann, A. F., Hachey, D. L., Thomas, P. J., Belobaba, D. T. E., Klein, P. D. and Tokes, L. (1976). Synthesis of 11,12-^{2}H$_2$- and 11,12-^{3}H$_2$-labeled chenodeoxycholic and lithocholic acids. *J. Lipid Res.*, **17**, 231
44. Dayal, B., Bagan, E., Tint, G. S., Shefer, S. and Salen, G. (1979). Preparation of 3β-^{3}H labeled bile acids and bile alcohols. *Steroids*, **34**, 259
45. Hoffman, N. E. and Hofmann, A. F. (1974). Metabolism of steroid and amino acid moieties of conjugated bile acids in man. IV. Description and validation of a multicompartment model. *Gastroenterology*, **67**, 887
46. Gehan, E. A. and George, S. L. (1970). Estimation of human body surface area from height and weight. *Cancer Chemother. Rep.*, **54**, 225
47. Huijbregts, W. M., van Schaik, A., van Berge Henegouwen, G. P. and van der Werf, D. J.

(1980). Serum lipids, biliary lipid composition, and bile acid metabolism in vegeterians as compared to normal controls. *Eur. J. Clin. Invest.*, **10**, 443

48. Hofmann, A. F., Molino, G., Milanese, M. and Belforte, G. (1983). Description and simulation of a physiological pharmacokinetic model for the metabolism and entero-hepatic circulation of bile acids in man. I. Cholic acid in healthy man. *J. Clin. Invest.* (In press)

49. Cowen, A. E., Korman, M. G., Hofmann, A. F. and Cass, O. W. (1975). Metabolism of lithocholate in man. I. Biotransformation and biliary excretion of intravenously admini-stered lithocholate, lithocholylglycine, and their sulfates. *Gastroenterology*, **69**, 59

50. Low-Beer, T. S., Tyor, M. P. and Lack, L. (1969). Effects on sulfation of taurolithocholic and glycolithocholic acids on their intestinal transport. *Gastroenterology*, **56**, 721

51. Samuel, P. and Lieberman, S. (1973). Improved estimation of body masses and turnover of cholesterol by computerized input–output analysis. *J. Lipid Res.*, **14**, 189

52. Stewart, G. N. (1921). Pulmonary circulation time: Quantity of blood in the lungs and the output of the heart. *Am. J. Physiol.*, **58**, 20

53. Hamilton, W. F., Moore, J. W., Kinsman, J. M. and Spurling, R. G. (1932). Studies on the circulation: IV. Further analysis of the injection method, and of changes in hemo-dynamics under physiological and pathological conditions. *Am. J. Physiol.*, **99**, 534

54. Macdonald, I. A., Hutchinson, D. M. and Forrest, T. P. (1981). Formation of urso- and chenodeoxycholic acids from primary bile acids by *Clostridium Absonum*. *J. Lipid Res.*, **22**, 458

55. Hirano, S., Masuda, N. and Oda, H. (1981). *In vitro* transformation of chenodeoxycholic acid and ursodeoxycholic acid by human intestinal flora, with particular reference to the mutual conversion between the two bile acids. *J. Lipid Res.*, **22**, 735

56. Fromm, H., Farivar, S., Hofmann, A. F., Carlson, G. L. and Amin, P. (1980). Metabolism in man of 7-ketolithocholic acid, a major secondary bile acid. *Am. J. Physiol.*, **239**, G161

57. Danzinger, R. G., Hofmann, A. F., DiPietro, R. A., Ljungwe, E. B. and Barnhart, J. L. (1981). Metabolism and physiological properties of two 7-keto bile acids in the dog. *Hepatology*, **1**, 505 (abstract)

58. Fedorowski, T., Salen, G., Colallilo, A., Tint, G. S., Mosbach, E. H. and Hall, J. C. (1977). Metabolism of ursodeoxycholic acid in man. *Gastroenterology*, **73**, 1131

59. Mok, H. Y. I. and Dowling, R. H. (1975). How well can we measure the bile acid pool size? In Matern, S., Hackenschmidt, J., Back, P. and Gerok, W. (eds.) *Advances in Bile Acid Research*. pp. 315–323. (Stuttgart: Schattauer-Verlag)

60. Dowling, R. H., Hofmann, A. F. and Barbara, L. (eds.) (1979). *Workshop on Ursodeoxy-cholic Acid*. (Baltimore: University Park Press)

61. Pomare, E. W. and Low-Beer, T. S. (1974). Measurement and validation of human bile salt pool size and synthesis. *Clin. Chim. Acta*, **57**, 239

62. McJunkin, B., Fromm, H., Sarva, R. P. and Amin, P. (1981). Factors in the mechanism of diarrhea in bile acid malabsorption: fecal pH – a key determinant. *Gastroenterology*, **80**, 1454

63. Podesta, M. T., Murphy, G. M., Sladen, G. E., Breuer, N. F. and Dowling, R. H. (1979). Fecal bile acid excretion in diarrhea: effect of sulfated and non-sulfated bile acids on colonic structure and function. In Paumgartner, G., Stiehl, A. and Gerok, W. (eds.) *Biological Effects of Bile Acids*. pp. 245–256. (Lancaster: MTP Press)

64. Hutton S. W., Holloway, D. E. and Duane, W. C. (1981). Bile acid synthesis in man determined by isotope dilution versus fecal acidic sterol output. *Hepatology*, **1**, 519 (abstract)

65. LaRusso, N. F., Hoffman, N. E., Hofmann, A. F., Northfield, T. C. and Thistle, J. L. (1975). Effect of primary bile acid ingestion on bile acid metabolism and biliary lipid secretion in gallstone patients. *Gastroenterology*, **69**, 1301

66. LaRusso, N. F., Szczepanik, P. A., Hofmann, A. F. and Coffin, S. B. (1977). The effect of deoxycholic acid ingestion on bile acid metabolism and biliary lipid secretion in normal subjects. *Gastroenterology*, **72**, 132

67. Vlahcevic, Z. R., Juttijudata, P., Bell, C. C., Jr. and Swell, L. (1972). Bile acid metabolism in patients with cirrhosis. II. Cholic and chenodeoxycholic acid metabolism. *Gastro-enterology*, **62**, 1174

68. McCormick, W. C., Bell, C. C., Jr., Swell, L. and Vlahcevic, Z. R. (1973). Cholic acid synthesis as an index of the severity of liver disease in man. *Gut*, **14**, 895
69. Stiehl, A., Earnest, D. L. and Admirand, W. H. (1975). Sulfation and renal excretion of bile salts in patients with cirrhosis of the liver. *Gastroenterology*, **68**, 534
70. Stiehl, A., Ast, E., Czygan, P., Frohling, W., Raedsch, R. and Kommerell, B. (1978). Pool size, synthesis, and turnover of sulfated and non-sulfated cholic acid and chenodeoxycholic acid in patients with cirrhosis of the liver. *Gastroenterology*, **74**, 572
71. Engelking, L. R., Barnes, S., Hirschowitz, B. I., Dasher, C. A., Spenney, J. G. and Naftel, D. (1980). Determination of the pool size and synthesis rate of bile acids by measurements in blood of patients with liver disease. *Clin. Sci.*, **58**, 485
72. Patteson, T. E., Vlahcevic, Z. R., Schwartz, C. C., Gustaffsson, J., Danielsson, H. and Swell, L. (1980). Bile acid metabolism in cirrhosis. VI. Sites of blockage in the bile acid pathways to primary bile acids. *Gastroenterology*, **79**, 620
73. Rutgeerts, P., Ghoos, Y. and Vantrappen, G. (1982). Kinetics of primary bile acids in patients with non-operated Crohn's disease. *Eur. J. Clin. Invest.*, **12**, 135
74. Einarsson, K., Hellstrom, K. and Kallner, M. (1974). The effect of cholestyramine on the elimination of cholesterol as bile acids in patients with hyperlipoproteinemia type II and IV. *Eur. J. Clin. Invest.*, **4**, 405
75. Andersen, E. (1979). The effect of cholestyramine on bile acid kinetics in healthy controls. *Acta Med. Scand.*, **643**, 657
76. Einarsson, K., Hellstrom, K. and Kallner, M. (1973). Feedback regulation of bile acid formation in man. *Metabolism*, **22**, 1477
77. van der Werf, S. D. J., van Berge Henegouwen, G. P. and van Tongeren, J. H. M. (1982). Absorption of endogenous deoxycholate in relation to biliary bile acid composition and cholesterol saturation in man. *Gastroenterology*, **82**, 1202 (abstract)
78. Swell, L., Bell, C. C., Jr. and Vlahcevic, Z. R. (1971). Relationship of bile acid pool size to biliary lipid excretion and the formation of lithogenic bile in man. *Gastroenterology*, **61**, 716
79. Grundy, S. M. and Metzger, A. L. (1972). A physiologic method for estimation of hepatic secretion of biliary lipids in man. *Gastroenterology*, **62**, 1200
80. Brunner, H., Northfield, T. C., Hofmann, A. F., Go, V. L. W. and Summerskill, W. H. J. (1974). Gastric emptying and secretion of bile acids, cholesterol, and pancreatic enzymes during digestion: duodenal perfusion studies in healthy subjects. *Mayo Clin. Proc.*, **49**, 851
81. Northfield, T. C. and Hofmann, A. F. (1975). Biliary lipid output during three meals and an overnight fast. I. Relationship to bile acid pool size and cholesterol saturation of bile in gallstone and control subjects. *Gut*, **16**, 1
82. Mok, H. Y. I., von Bergmann, K. and Grundy, S. M. (1977). Regulation of pool size of bile acids in man. *Gastroenterology*, **73**, 684
83. Shaffer, E. A. and Small, D. M. (1977). Biliary lipid secretion in cholesterol gallstone disease. The effect of cholecystectomy and obesity. *J. Clin. Invest.*, **59**, 828
84. Levitt, M. D. and Bond, J. (1977). Use of the constant perfusion technique in the non-steady state. *Gastroenterology*, **73**, 1450 (editorial)
85. Goodman, D. S., Smith, F. R., Seplowitz, A. H., Ramakrishnan, R. and Dell, R. B. (1980). Prediction of the parameters of whole body cholesterol metabolism in humans. *J. Lipid Res.*, **21**, 699
86. Zilversmit, D. B. (1972). A single blood sample dual isotope method for the measurement of cholesterol absorption in rats. *Proc. Soc. Exp. Biol. Med.*, **140**, 862
87. Samuel, P., McNamara, D. J., Ahrens, E. H. Jr., Crouse, J. R. and Parker, T. (1982). Further validation of the plasma isotope ratio method for measurement of cholesterol absorption in man. *J. Lipid Res.*, **23**, 480
88. Quintao, E., Grundy, S. M. and Ahrens, E. H. Jr. (1971). An evaluation of four methods for measuring cholesterol absorption by the intestine in man. *J. Lipid Res.*, **12**, 221
89. Wood, P. D. S., Myers, D., Lee, Y. L., Shioda, R. and Kinsell, L. (1967). 1,2-^{3}H-Cholesterol as a tracer in studies of human cholesterol metabolism. *J. Lipid Res.*, **8**, 406
90. Davidson, N. O, Ahrens, E. H. Jr., Bradlow, H. L., McNamara, D. J., Parker, T. S. and Samuel, P. (1980). Unreliability of tritiated cholesterol: studies with [1,2-^{3}H] cholesterol and [24,25-^{3}H] cholesterol in humans. *Proc. Natl. Acad. Sci. USA*, **4**, 2255

91. Wilson, J. D. (1970). The measurement of the exchangeable pools of cholesterol in the baboon. *J. Clin. Invest.*, **49**, 655

92. Grundy, S. M. and Ahrens, E. H. Jr. (1969). Measurements of cholesterol turnover, synthesis and absorption in man, carried out by isotope kinetic and sterol balance methods. *J. Lipid Res.*, **10**, 91

93. Samuel, P., Lieberman, S. and Ahrens, E. H. Jr., (1978). Comparison of cholesterol turnover by sterol balance and input–output analysis, and a shortened way to estimate total exchangeable mass of cholesterol by the combination of the two methods. *J. Lipid Res.*, **19**, 94

94. Quarfordt, S. H. and Greenfield, M. F. (1973). Estimation of cholesterol and bile acid turnover in man by kinetic analysis. *J. Clin. Invest.*, **52**, 1937

95. Miettinen, T. A. (1973). Clinical implications of bile acid metabolism in man. In Nair, P. P. and Kritchevsky, D. (eds.) *The Bile Acids.* pp. 191–239. (New York: Plenum Press)

96. Schwartz, C. C., Vlahcevic, Z. R., Berman, M., Meadows, J. G., Nisman, R. M. and Swell, L. (1982). Central role of high density lipoprotein in plasma free cholesterol metabolism. *J. Clin. Invest.*, **70**, 105

97. Schwartz, C. C., Berman, M., Vlahcevic, Z. R. and Swell, L. (1982). Multicompartmental analysis of cholesterol metabolism in man. A quantitative kinetic evaluation of precursor sources and turnover of high density lipoprotein cholesterol ester. *J. Clin. Invest.* (in press)

98. Hofmann, A. F., Grundy, S. M., Lachn, J. M., Lan, S. P., Baum, R. A., Hanson, R. F., Hersh, T. and Hightower, N. *et al.* (1983). Pretreatment biliary lipid composition in white patients with radiolucent gallstones in the National Cooperative Gallstone Study. *Gastroenterology* (in press)

99. Low-Beer, T. S. and Pomare, E. W. (1975). Can colonic bacterial metabolites predispose to cholesterol gallstones? *Br. Med. J.*, **i**, 438

100. Marks, J. W., Sue, S. O., Pearlman, B. J., Bonorris, G. G., Varady, P., Lachin, J. M. and Schoenfield, L. J. (1981). Sulfation of lithocholate as a possible modifier of chenodeoxycholic acid-induced elevations of serum transaminase in patients with gallstones. *J. Clin. Invest.*, **68**, 1190

101. Hellstrom, K. (1965). On the bile acid and neutral fecal steroid excretion in man and rabbits following cholesterol feeding. *Acta Physiol. Scand.*, **63**, 21

102. Hellstrom, K. and Lindstedt, S. (1966). Studies on the formation of cholic acid in subjects given standardized diet with butter or corn oil as dietary fat. *Am. J. Clin. Nutr.*, **18**, 46

103. Vlahcevic, Z. R., Buhac, I., Farrar, J. T., Bell, C. C. Jr. and Swell, L. (1971). Bile acid metabolism in patients with cirrhosis. I. Kinetic aspects of cholic acid metabolism. *Gastroenterology*, **60**, 491

104. Danzinger, R. G., Hofmann, A. F. and Schoenfield, L. J. (1971). Measurement of bile acid kinetics in man using stable isotopes: Application to cholelithiasis. *Gastroenterology*, **60**, 192 (abstract)

105. Vlahcevic, Z. R., Bell, C. C. Jr., Gregory, D. H., Buker, G., Juttijudata, P. and Swell, L. (1972). Relationship of bile acid pool size to the formation of lithogenic bile in female Indians of the Southwest. *Gastroenterology*, **62**, 73

106. Hepner, G. W. (1975). Effect of decreased gallbladder stimulation on enterohepatic cycling and kinetics of bile acids. *Gastroenterology*, **68**, 1574

107. Pedersen, L. and Arnfred, T. (1975). Kinetics and pool size of chenodeoxycholic acid in cholesterol gallstone patients. *Scand. J. Gastroenterol.*, **10**, 557

108. Roda, E., Aldini, R., Mazzella, G., Roda, A., Sama, C., Festi, D., and Barbara, L. (1978). Enterohepatic circulation of bile acids after cholecystectomy. *Gut*, **19**, 640

109. Duane, W. (1978). Simulation of the defect of bile acid metabolism associated with cholesterol cholelithiasis by sorbitol ingestion in man. *J. Lab. Clin. Med.*, **91**, 969

110. Duane, W., Holloway, D. E., Hutton, S. W., Corcoran, P. J. and Haas, N. A. (1982). Comparison of bile acid synthesis determined by isotope dilution versus fecal acidic sterol output in human subjects. *Lipids*, **17**, 345

111. Einarsson, K., Hellstrom, K. and Kallner, M. (1974). Bile acid kinetics in relation to sex, serum lipids, body weights, and gallbladder disease in patients with various types of hyperlipoproteinemia. *J. Clin. Invest.*, **54**, 1301

112. Einarsson, K., Hellstrom, K. and Leijd, B. (1977). Bile acid kinetics and steroid balance

during nicotinic acid therapy in patients with hyperlipoproteinemia types II and IV. *J. Lab. Clin. Med.*, **90**, 613

113. Vlahcevic, Z. R., Bell, C. C. Jr., Buhac, I. Farrar, J. T. and Swell, L. (1970). Diminished bile acid pool size in gallstones. *Gastroenterology*, **59**, 165

114. Almond, H. R., Vlahcevic, Z. R. Bell, C. C. Jr., Gregory, D. H. and Swell, L. (1973). Bile acid pools, kinetic and biliary lipid composition before and after cholecystectomy. *N. Engl. J. Med.*, **289**, 1213

115. Kimball, A., Pertsemidis, D. and Panveliwalla, D. (1976). Composition of biliary lipids and kinetics of bile acids after cholecystectomy in man. *Dig. Dis. Sci.*, **21**, 776

116. Kottke, B. A. (1969). Differences in bile acid excretion. Primary hypercholesterolemia compared to combined hypercholesteremia and hypertriglyceridemia. *Circulation*, **XL**, 13

117. Hellstrom, K. and Lindstedt, S. (1964). Cholic-acid turnover and biliary bile-acid composition in humans with abnormal thyroid function. *J. Lab. Clin. Med.*, **63**, 666

118. Goodman, D. S., Noble, R. P. and Dell, R. B. (1973). The effects of colestipol resin and of colestipol plus clofibrate on the turnover of plasma cholesterol in man. *J. Clin. Invest.*, **52**, 2646

119. Samuel, P., Holtzman, C. M., Meilman, E. and Perl, W. (1968). Effect of neomycin on exchangeable pools of cholesterol in the steady state. *J. Clin. Invest.*, **47**, 1806

120. Hoffman, N. E., Hofmann, A. F. and Thistle, J. L. (1974). Effect of bile acid feeding on cholesterol metabolism in gallstone patients. *Mayo Clin. Proc.*, **49**, 236

121. Nestel, P. J., Schreibman, P. H. and Ahrens, E. H. Jr. (1973). Cholesterol metabolism in human obesity. *J. Clin. Invest.*, **52**, 2389

122. Miller, N. E., Clifton-Bligh, P. and Nestel, P. J. (1973). Effects of colestipol, a new bile-acid-sequestering resin, on cholesterol metabolism in man. *J. Lab. Clin. Med.*, **82**, 876

123. Nestel, P. J., Whyte, H. M. and Goodman, D. S. (1969). Distribution and turnover of cholesterol in humans. *J. Clin. Invest.*, **48**, 982

6
Biliary lipid secretion – sterol balance

K. von BERGMANN

Studies of the enterohepatic circulation (EHC) of bile acids and cholesterol are physiologically important and clinically relevant to gallstone formation and gallstone dissolution. Therefore, several methods have been developed for quantitative measurements of partial function of the EHC of biliary lipids. The analysis of cholesterol, bile acids and phospholipids in fasting gallbladder bile has given useful information on biliary lipid composition. With this method it has been demonstrated that cholesterol gallstones in man are frequently associated with supersaturated bile, i.e. bile that contains more cholesterol than can be solubilized by the bile acids and/or phospholipid content[1]. Administration of chenodeoxycholic (CDCA) or ursodeoxycholic acid (UDCA) reduces the molar percentage of cholesterol in bile and might thereby induce cholesterol gallstone dissolution[2-4]. Stone dissolution appears to be associated with a reduction in lithogenicity of bile, i.e. a reduction in concentration of cholesterol relative to the solubilizing lipids – bile acids and phospholipids. Measurement of the lithogenicity of bile before and during treatment with CDCA or UDCA as well as looking for cholesterol crystals[5] will help to select patients with cholesterol gallstones for therapy and is important for dose adjustment[6]. Although the analysis of the biliary composition of fasting gallbladder bile is important and has given relevant information in this field, it does not define the underlying mechanism of cholesterol gallstones development by which administration of CDCA or UDCA reduces the lithogenicity of bile.

This review will summarize the method of measuring biliary lipid secretion rates, which give more information of the pathophysiology of cholesterol gallstone formation and the effect of bile acid feeding on these parameters. In addition it will deal with studies which were performed in Dr Grundy's laboratory where faecal excretion of bile acids and neutral steroids were measured along with biliary lipid outputs. From these measurements of partial functions of the EHC, daily synthesis and secretion of bile acid and cholesterol as well as intestinal absorption of bile acids and cholesterol may be estimated. Pool size of bile acids can be measured simultaneously with estimation of biliary outputs by using an isotope dilution principle[7].

In 1972 Grundy and Metzger[8] described a physiological method for estimation of hepatic secretion of biliary lipids in man. This method employs duodenal intubation with a triple lumen tube the evening before the study. The next morning the tube is positioned under X-ray guidance so that the two proximal outlets are located opposite the ampulla of Vater and the third 10 cm distally at the ligamentum of Treitz (Figure 6.1). A liquid formula is infused continuously through the one proximal lumen; beta-sitosterol is also infused as a non-absorbable dilution marker. After allowing 4 h for gallbladder contraction and for stabilization of hepatic bile secretion, hourly samples are obtained by slow and continuous aspiration from the proximal and distal outlet. Less than 5% of duodenal content passing these outlets are withdrawn and hourly outputs of biliary lipids remains constant up to 24 hours[8]. Since the infusion rate of beta-sitosterol was known with precision, measurement of cholesterol and beta-sitosterol recovery at the distal port

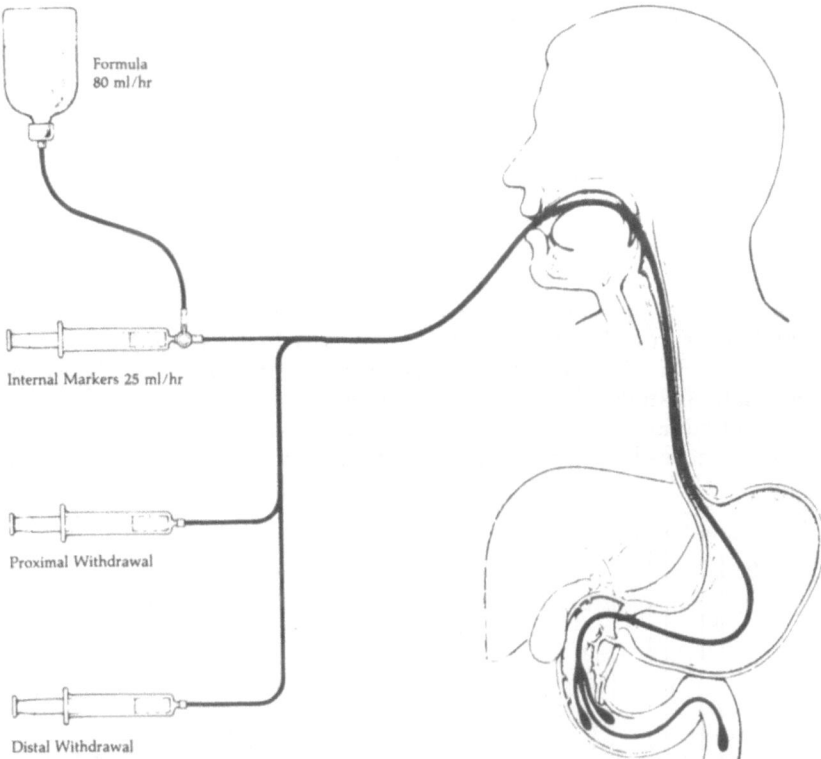

Formula
80 ml/hr

Internal Markers 25 ml/hr

Proximal Withdrawal

Distal Withdrawal

Figure 6.1 Measurement of biliary lipid secretion by means of a tube having three lumens with perforated olives. The tube is swallowed by the patient the evening before the study. In the morning the position of the tube is controlled by X-ray guidance. A liquid formula (34 kcal/h) plus beta-sitosterol as a recovery marker is infused through the most proximal lumen. After allowing 4 hours for stabilization of hepatic bile secretion and gallbladder contraction hourly samples were obtained from the second proximal and the distal outlets by slow and continuous aspiration. Less than 5% of passing intestinal content is aspirated through this procedure. Thus, the EHC of biliary lipid is not interrupted

gave the rate of cholesterol secretion. Measurements of concentrations of bile acids and phospholipids relative to cholesterol at the proximal outlet permit calculation of the hourly secretion rates of bile acids and phospholipids:

$$\text{Biliary cholesterol (mg/h)} = \frac{\text{Cholesterol}}{\text{Sitosterol}} \times \text{sitosterol (mg/h)} \qquad (1)$$

$$\text{Biliary bile acids (mg/h)} = \frac{\text{Bile acids}}{\text{Cholesterol}} \times \text{cholesterol (mg/h)} \qquad (2)$$

$$\text{Biliary phospholipids (mg/h)} = \frac{\text{Phospholipids}}{\text{Cholesterol}} \times \text{cholesterol (mg/h)} \qquad (3)$$

The results of cholesterol secretion in equations (2) and (3) are derived from equation (1). Equations with corrections for cholesterol and phospholipid contents of formula diets are given in the original paper of Grundy and Metzger[8].

A similar method for measurement of biliary lipid secretion has been used by Shaffer and Small[9]. However, they used sulphobromophthalein as non-absorbable dilution marker and infused an essential amino acid solution to contract the gallbladder and provide a source of calories during the study instead of a full-formula diet which contains fat, carbohydrates and protein. On the other hand, Hofmann and co-workers[10] recommended that measurements be made over 24 hours during which subjects ingest three liquid meals in order to simulate more closely man's feeding pattern. For comparison and interpretation of data from the various laboratories, it is important to know whether biliary secretion rates during constant infusion of a full-liquid formula or an essential amino acid solution and during intermittent feeding using three liquid meals and an overnight fast are the same.

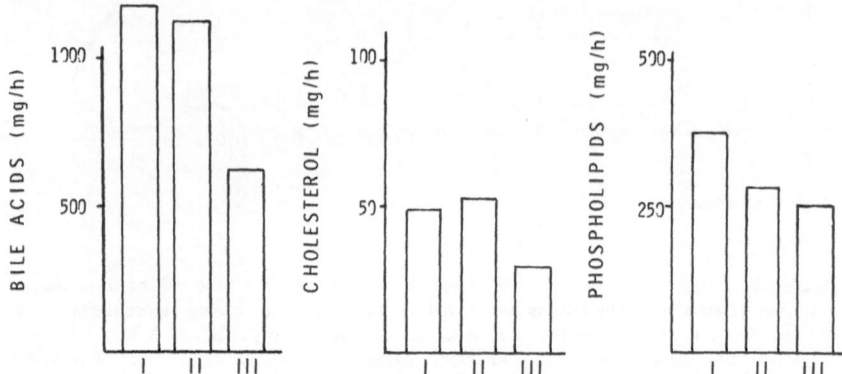

Figure 6.2 Comparison of mean hourly outputs of bile acids, cholesterol and phospholipids in three comparable groups of patients by three different groups of investigators (I = reference 11; II = reference 10; III = reference 9.)

Figure 6.2 summarizes the results from comparable control groups published from the three different laboratories (the data were derived from references[9-11]). The results of the different studies indicate that similar results are obtained for average hourly secretion rates of biliary lipids whether the diet is given continuously into the duodenum or is fed orally as three meals per day. Indeed, an intraindividual comparison in nine patients using both the methods of Grundy and Metzger and Hofmann and co-workers shows a good agreement when the results are expressed in terms of mg/h outputs (Table 6.1). In contrast to the similarity in results by the two methods, the biliary secretion rates measured by Shaffer and Small[9] are different from those from Grundy and co-workers[11] and Hofmann and co-workers[10]. However, recent studies from Kern and co-workers (personal communication) have demonstrated that an essential amino acid solution infusion into the duodenum does not tonically contract the gallbladder in contrast to a full-liquid formula. Therefore, the biliary secretion rates are lower and the bile acid pool circulates less often in the EHC. Whereas the bile acids pool circulates 9.4 and 6.4 per day in control subjects from Grundy's and Hofmann's groups, respectively, the cycling frequency was only 4.6 per day in the control subjects from Shaffer and Small[9].

Table 6.1 Mean hourly biliary lipid secretion in nine subjects during constant infusion of a liquid formula into the duodenum and intermittent feeding of three equicaloric meals and an overnight fast*

| | Biliary lipid secretion | | |
	Cholesterol (mg/h)	Bile acids (mg/h)	Phospholipids (mg/h)
Intermittent	48	794	304
Continuous	46	769	308

*Data derived from reference 12.

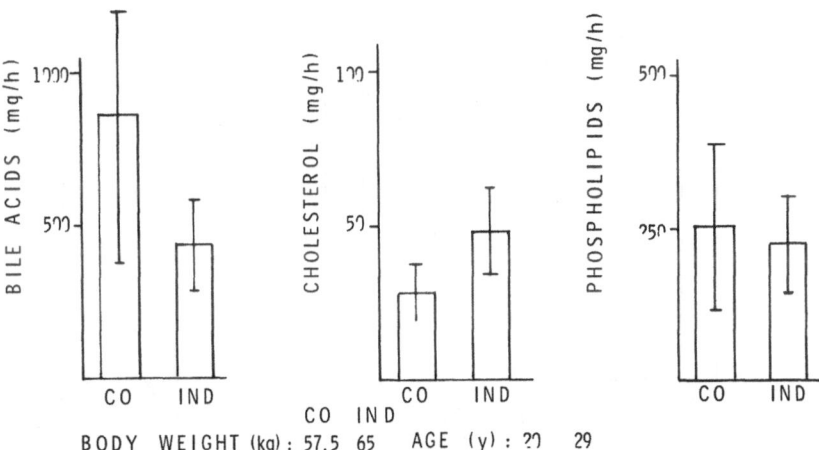

BODY WEIGHT (kg) : 57.5 65   AGE (y) : 27 29

Figure 6.3 Comparison of mean hourly outputs of bile acids, cholesterol and phospholipids in Caucasian women without gallstones (CO) and Indian women with gallstones (IND). Bile acid secretion was significantly higher in Caucasian women without gallstones, and cholesterol secretion was significantly higher in Indian women with gallstones. (From reference 16.)

121

It is currently believed that the primary defect in cholesterol gallstone formation is an abnormal hepatic secretion of biliary lipids[13-16]. Grundy and co-workers[16] have measured the biliary lipid secretion rates in American Indian women who are particularly prone to development of cholesterol gallstone[17]. These authors compared their results obtained in Indian women with gallstones with Caucasian women without gallstones. The results are summarized in Figure 6.3. Their results demonstrated that Indian women with stones have two abnormalities leading to the production of bile which is supersaturated with cholesterol; not only was bile acid secreted at a reduced rate by the liver, but also, outputs of cholesterol were increased. Therefore, production of supersaturated bile in these Indian women with gallstones was due to a combined defect in hepatic secretion of biliary lipids. Another group of patients with a high risk of cholesterol gallstone formation are obese subjects[18]. Bennion and Grundy[19] measured the biliary output in very obese patients and compared the results with normal weight subjects (Figure 6.4). These authors concluded that obesity is characterized by excessive hepatic secretion of cholesterol which results in lithogenic bile. However, not all patients with cholesterol gallstone are obese or American Indians. It was therefore of interest to compare the biliary lipid output in normal weight subjects matched for age, sex and weight with patients with radiolucent gallstones.

The results obtained from different groups are controversial. Whereas Northfield and Hofmann[20] could not find any difference in total biliary lipid output between gallstone and contol subjects (Figure 6.5), a significant lower bile acid and phospholipid secretion in cholesterol gallstone subjects could be demonstrated by Shaffer and Small[9] (Figure 6.6). Comparable results could

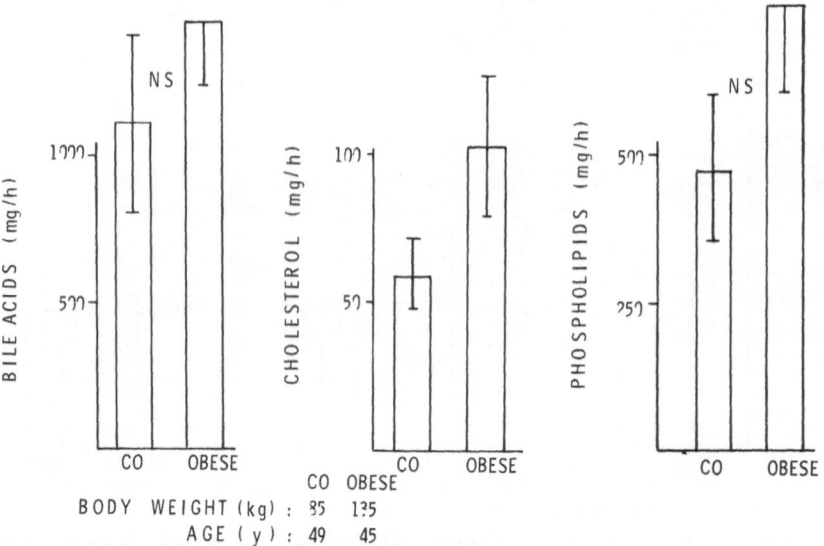

Figure 6.4 Comparison of mean hourly outputs of bile acids, cholesterol and phospholipids in control subjects (CO) and very obese patients (OBESE). Cholesterol secretion was significantly higher in obese patients. (NS=not significant; from reference 19.)

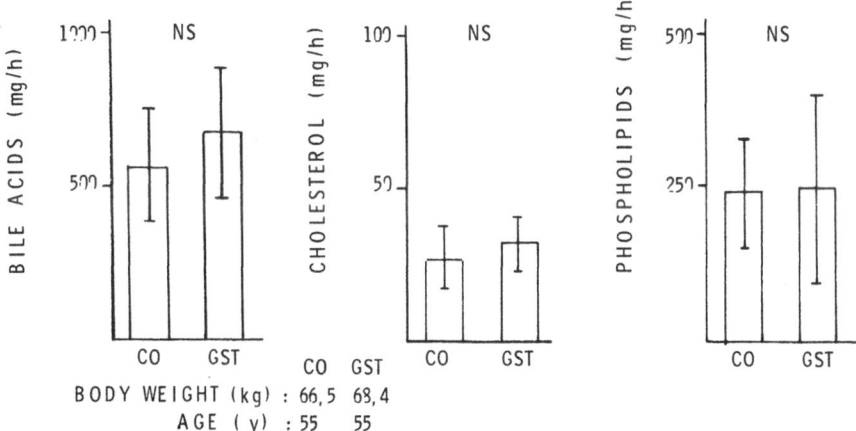

Figure 6.5 Comparison of mean hourly outputs of bile acids, cholesterol and phospholipids in control subjects (CO) and patients with gallstones (GST). (NS = Not significant; from reference 20.)

be obtained by Dowling and co-workers (personal communication). However, it must be mentioned that these results obtained by these two groups of investigators were performed with the infusion of an essential amino acid solution into the duodenum, which does not tonically contract the gallbladder. On the other hand, this method might be more sensitive to small differences in hepatic lipid output. More studies have to be performed to define the underlying mechanism in the difference of biliary lipid secretion in normal weight subjects with and without gallstones.

As mentioned before, oral administration of CDCA and UDCA has been shown to promote cholesterol gallstone dissolution in man [2-4], and stone dissolution appears to be associated with a reduction in lithogenicity of bile.

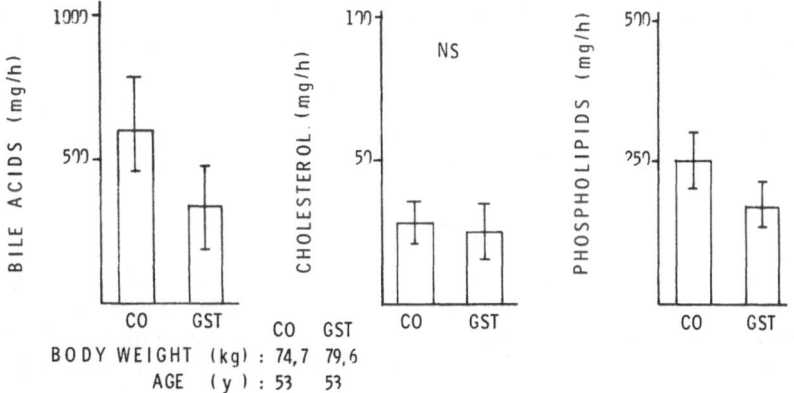

Figure 6.6 Comparison of mean hourly outputs of bile acids, cholesterol and phospholipids in control subjects (CO) and patients with gallstones (GST). (NS = not significant; bile acid and phospholipids secretion was significantly lower in patients with cholesterol gallstones; from reference 9.)

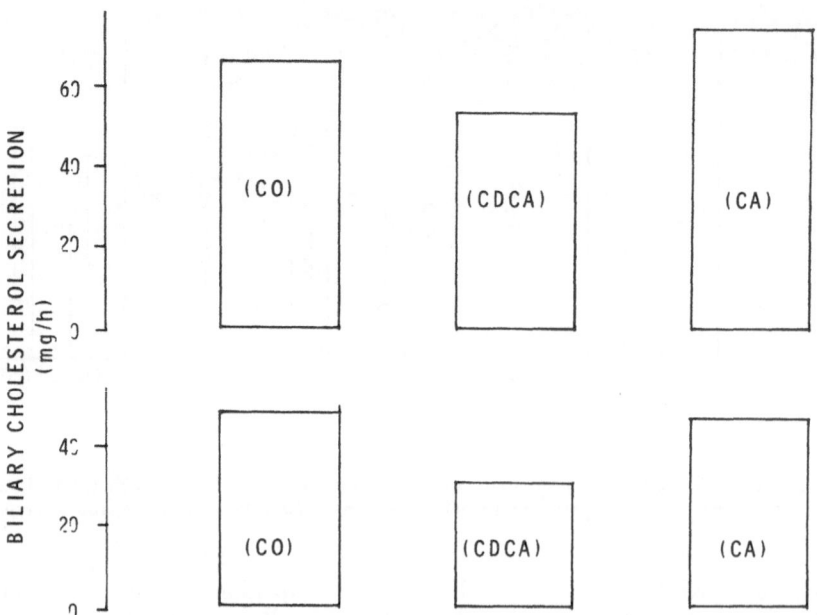

Figure 6.7 Comparison of hourly secretion rate of biliary cholesterol during a control period (CO), chenodeoxycholic (CDCA) and cholic acid administration (CA). The results of the upper part of the figure are derived from the data of LaRusso et al.[22] and in the lower part from Adler et al.[21]

Theoretically, a decrease in supersaturated bile could be achieved by several mechanisms: an increase in hepatic secretion of bile acids and/or phospholipids, a decrease in secretion of cholesterol, or by all three mechanisms. Adler et al.[21] and LaRusso et al.[22] measured the biliary lipid secretion before and during CDCA and cholic acid (CA) administration. Both investigators demonstrated that CDCA but not CA reduces biliary cholesterol secretion significantly (Figure 6.7). Whereas Adler et al.[21] using a low dose of CDCA could not find a difference in bile acid or phospholipid secretion, LaRusso et al.[22] using a higher dose of CDCA depicted a slight but not significant increase in bile acid and phospholipid secretion. Later, Mok et al.[23] could demonstrate an increased bile acid secretion during feeding of CDCA in obese subjects undergoing weight reduction and Tangedahl et al.[24] depicted an increased bile acid secretion in hypercholesterolaemic subjects during CDCA administration. Studies performed in our laboratory[25,26] in 10 non-obese patients with radiolucent gallstones using CDCA and UDCA in a fixed dose of 1 g/day in a crossover design, revealed that bile acid decreases biliary secretion of cholesterol and increases bile acid and phospholipid secretion. The results of this study are summarized in Figure 6.8. The effect of UDCA on depression of hepatic secretion of cholesterol is more pronounced than the effect of CDCA. This confirms previous results from Stiehl and co-workers[27], that UDCA reduces the lithogenicity of fasting gallbladder bile more than an equimolar dose of CDCA.

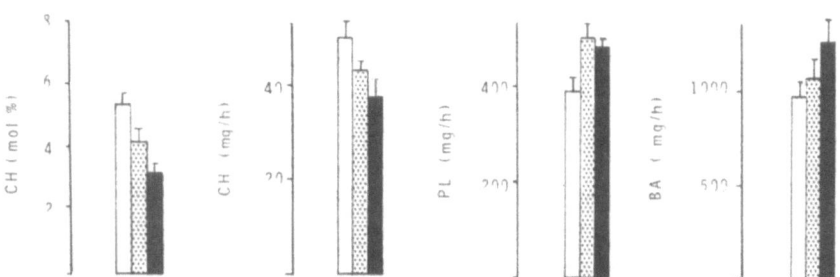

Figure 6.8 Comparison of mol % of cholesterol (CH), biliary secretion of cholesterol, phospholipids (PL) and bile acids (BA) in normal weight patients with radiolucent gallstones before (open bars) and during chenodeoxycholic acid (shaded areas) and ursodeoxycholic acid (black areas) administration. (1 g/day; from references 25 and 26.)

Since it has been demonstrated that similar results are obtained for average hourly secretion rates of biliary lipids whether the formula is given continuously into the duodenum or is fed orally in three meals per day, measurements of daily biliary lipid output may be accomplished in a shorter time. Thus, the combination of measurement of biliary lipid secretion and quantitative measurement of neutral and acidic steroids in faeces[28,29] can give further useful results in respect of intestinal cholesterol and bile acid absorption. In addition this method can differentiate between the mass and percentage of cholesterol and bile acid absorption. Several previous attempts have been made to measure cholesterol absorption in man; however, most of the techniques developed thus far estimate absorption of exogenous cholesterol only[30-36]. Since the bulk of cholesterol which enters the intestinal tract is of biliary origin[7,8,19] change in biliary cholesterol secretion as well as change in dietary cholesterol must influence the mass or percentage of cholesterol absorption. Using the combination of biliary lipid secretion and faecal excretion of bile acids and neutral steroids von Bergmann et al.[12] and Mok et al.[37] could demonstrate that absorption of bile acids was highly efficient (mean 97.5%), similar to values quoted in the literature. In addition their results indicate that absorption of cholesterol was surprisingly high (mean 60%). Earlier studies have generally given lower values of cholesterol absorption[32,33,35,36]. The method of measurement of cholesterol absorption was further evaluated when cholesterol absorption was measured in eight subjects by an intestinal perfusion method[38] and the combined biliary outputs and sterol balance. No difference in percentage of cholesterol absorption could be detected using the direct (intestinal perfusion) and the indirect method (combined biliary outputs and sterol balance).

The usefulness of measuring cholesterol absorption by this method is demonstrated by an example from the literature. Adler and co-workers[21] measured in their subjects before and during CDCA administration not only biliary lipid secretion rates along with the faecal excretion of neutral steroids but also cholesterol absorption by the method of Quintao[33]. At this time these authors were not aware that biliary cholesterol secretion using continuous formula infusion for 8 hours gave valid estimation of overall

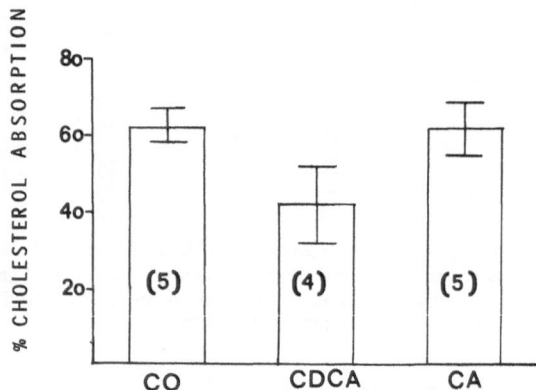

Figure 6.9 Comparison of cholesterol absorption during a control period (CO) and cheno-deoxycholic (CDCA) and cholic acid (CA) administration. Cholesterol absorption was significantly lower during CDCA administration. Data are derived from Adler et al.[21]. The results were calculated according to the equation of von Bergmann et al.[12]. Number in parentheses represents number of patients studied

daily secretion rates of biliary cholesterol. Their results on cholesterol absorption using the double isotope method of Quintao et al.[33] could not demonstrate any difference between the control period and CDCA as well as CA period (mean cholesterol absorption during the control, CDCA and CA period was 36%, 33% and 46%, respectively). However, recalculation of cholesterol absorption using the combined biliary outputs and sterol balance method revealed a significant reduction of cholesterol absorption during CDCA administration (Figure 6.9). Although the effect of CDCA on cholesterol absorption is still controversial in the literature[39-41], this discrepancy in the results using two different methods demonstrates the importance of comparison methods from different laboratories. On the other hand, change in either dietary or biliary cholesterol must be followed by a change either in percentage or in mass of cholesterol absorption.

References

1. Admirand, W.H. and Small, D.M. (1968). The physicochemical basis of cholesterol gallstone formation in man. *J. Clin. Invest.*, **47**, 1043
2. Danzinger, R.G., Hofmann, A.F., Schoenfield, L.J. and Thistle, J.L. (1972). Dissolution of cholesterol gallstones by chenodeoxycholic acid. *N. Engl. J. Med.*, **286**, 1
3. Bell, G.D., Whitney, B. and Dowling, R.H. (1972). Gallstone dissolution in man using chenodeoxycholic acid. *Lancet*, **ii**, 1213
4. Makino, I., Shinozaki, K., Nakagawa, K. and Yoshino, S. (1975). Dissolution of cholesterol gallstones by long-term administration of ursodeoxycholic acid. *Jpn. J. Gastroenterology*, **72**, 690
5. Sedaghat, A. and Grundy, S.M. (1980). Cholesterol crystals and the formation of cholesterol gallstones. *N. Engl. J. Med.*, **302**, 1274

6. Mok, H. Y. I., Bell, G. D. and Dowling, R. H. (1974). Effect of different doses of cheno-deoxycholic acid on bile-lipid composition and on frequency of side-effects in patients with gallstones. *Lancet*, ii, 253
7. Grundy, S. M. (1975). Effects of polyunsaturated fats on lipid metabolism in patients with hypertriglyceridemia. *J. Clin. Invest.*, 55, 269
8. Grundy, S. M. and Metzger, A. L. (1972). A physiological method for estimation of hepatic secretion of biliary lipids in man. *Gastroenterology*, 62, 1200
9. Shaffer, E. A. and Small, D. M. (1977). Biliary lipid secretion in cholesterol gallstone disease. *J. Clin. Invest.*, 59, 828
10. Northfield, T. C. and Hofmann, A. F. (1973). Biliary lipid secretion in gallstone patients. *Lancet*, i, 747
11. Von Bergmann, K., Mok, H. Y. I., Hardison, W. G. M. and Grundy, S. M. (1979). Cholesterol and bile acid metabolism in moderately advanced, stable cirrhosis of the liver. *Gastroenterology*, 77, 1183
12. Von Bergmann, K., Mok, H. Y. I. and Grundy, S. M. (1976). Effects of intermittent and continuous feeding on biliary lipid secretion in man. In Paumgartner, G. and Stiehl, A. (eds.) *Bile Acid Metabolism in Health and Disease*, pp. 191–196. (Lancaster: MTP Press)
13. Swell, L., Bell, C. C. and Vlahcevic, Z. R. (1971). Relationship of bile acid pool size to biliary lipid excretion and the formation of lithogenic bile in man. *Gastroenterology* 61, 716
14. Schoenfield, L. J. (1972). Animal models of gallstone formation. *Gastroenterology*, 63, 189
15. Small, D. M. (1972). Gallstones: diagnosis and treatment. *Postgrad. Med.*, 51, 187
16. Ahlberg, J., Angelin, B., Einarsson, K., Hellstroem, K. and Leijd, B. (1977). Influence of deoxycholic acid on biliary lipids in man. *Clin. Sci. Mol. Med.*, 53, 249
17. Sampliner, R. E., Bennett, P. H., Comess, L. J., Rose, F. A. and Burch, T. A. (1970). Gallbladder disease in Pima Indians. Demonstration of high prevalence and early onset by cholecystography. *N. Engl. J. Med.*, 283, 1358
18. Friedman, G. D., Kannel, W. B. and Dawber, T. R. (1966). The epidemiology of gallbladder disease: observation in the Frammingham Study. *J. Chron. Dis.*, 19, 273
19. Bennion, L. J. and Grundy, S. M. (1975). Effects of obesity and caloric intake on biliary lipid metabolism in man. *J. Clin. Invest.*, 55, 996
20. Northfield, T. C. and Hofmann, A. F. (1975). Biliary lipid output during three meals and an overnight fast. I. Relationship to bile acid pool size and cholesterol saturation of bile in gallstone and control subjects. *Gut*, 16, 1
21. Adler, R. D., Bennion, L. J., Duane, W. C. and Grundy, S. M. (1975). Effects of low dose chenodeoxycholic acid feeding on biliary lipid metabolism. *Gastroenterology*, 68, 326
22. LaRusso, N. F., Hoffman, N. E., Hofmann, A. F., Northfield, T. C. and Thistle, J. L. (1975). Effect of primary bile acid ingestion on bile acid metabolism and biliary lipid secretion in gallstone patients. *Gastroenterology*, 69, 1301
23. Mok, H. Y. I., von Bergmann, K., Course, J. R. and Grundy, S. M. (1979). Biliary lipid metabolism in obesity. Effects of bile acid feeding before and during weight reduction. *Gastroenterology*, 76, 556
24. Tangedahl, T. N., Hofmann, A. F. and Kottke, B. A. (1979). Biliary lipid secretion in hypercholesterolemia. *J. Lipid Res.*, 20, 125
25. Von Bergmann, K., Gutsfeld, M. Schulze-Hagen, K. and von Unruh, G. (1978). Effects of ursodeoxycholic acid on biliary lipid secretion in patients with radiolucent gallstones. In Paumgartner, G., Stiehl, A., and Gerok, W. (eds.) *Biological Effects of Bile Acids. Falk Symposium 26*, pp. 61–66. (Lancaster: MTP Press)
26. Leiss, O., Bosch, T. and von Bergmann, K. (1981). Effects of bile acid feeding on lipo-protein concentration, change in cholesterol synthesis and biliary lipid secretion in patients with radiolucent gallstones. In Paumgartner, G., Stiehl, A. and Gerok, W. (eds.) *Bile Acids and Lipids*. pp. 247–253. (Lancaster: MTP Press)
27. Stiehl, A., Czygan, P., Kommerell, B., Weis, H. J. and Holtermueller, K. H. (1978). Urso-deoxycholic acid versus chenodeoxycholic acid. Comparison of their effects on bile acid and bile lipid composition in patients with cholesterol gallstones. *Gastroenterology*, 75, 1016
28. Miettinen, T. A., Ahrens, E. H. and Grundy, S. M. (1965). Quantitative isolation and

gas–liquid chromatographic analysis of total dietary and fecal neutral steroids. *J. Lipid Res.*, **6**, 411

29. Grundy, S. M., Ahrens, E. H. and Miettinen, T. A. (1965). Quantitative isolation and gas–liquid chromatographic analysis of total fecal bile acids. *J. Lipid Res.*, **6**, 397
30. Wilson, J. D. and Lindsay, C. A. (1965). Studies on the influence of cholesterol on cholesterol metabolism in the isotopic steady state in man. *J. Clin. Invest.*, **44**, 1805
31. Grundy, S. M. and Ahrens, E. H. Jr. (1969). Measurement of cholesterol turnover, synthesis and absorption in man, carried out by isotope kinetic and sterol balance methods. *J. Lipid Res.*, **10**, 92
32. Borgstroem, B. (1969). Quantification of cholesterol absorption in man by fecal analysis after the feeding of a single isotope-labeled meal. *J. Lipid Res.*, **10**, 91
33. Quintao, E., Grundy, S. M. and Ahrens, E. H. (1971). An evaluation of four methods for measuring cholesterol absorption by the intestine in man. *J. Lipid Res.*, **12**, 221
34. Zilversmit, D. B. (1972). A single blood sample dual isotope method for the measurement of cholesterol absorption in rat. *Proc. Soc. Exp. Biol. Med.*, **140**, 862
35. Kudchodkar, B. J., Sodhi, H. S. and Harlick, L. (1973). Absorption of dietary cholesterol in man. *Metabolism*, **22**, 155
36. Connor, W. E. and Lin, D. S. (1974). The intestinal absorption of dietary cholesterol by hypercholesterolemic (Type II) and normocholesterolemic humans. *J. Clin. Invest.*, **53**, 1062
37. Mok, H. Y. I., von Bergmann, K. and Grundy, S. M. (1979). Effects of continuous and intermittent feeding on biliary lipid outputs in man: application for measurements of intestinal absorption of cholesterol and bile acids. *J. Lipid Res.*, **20**, 389
38. Grundy, S. M. and Mok, H. Y. I. (1977). Determination of cholesterol absorption in man by intestinal perfusion. *J. Lipid Res.*, **18**, 263
39. Mok, H. Y. I. and Grundy, S. M. (1980). Cholesterol and bile acid absorption during bile acid therapy in obese subjects undergoing weight reduction. *Gastroenterology*, **78**, 62
40. Einarsson, K. and Grundy, S. M. (1980). Effects of feeding cholic acid and chenodeoxycholic acid on cholesterol absorption and hepatic secretion of biliary lipids in man. *J. Lipid Res.*, **21**, 23
41. Ponz de Leon, M. M., Carulli, N. and Loria, P. (1979). The effect of chenodeoxycholic acid (CDCA) on cholesterol absorption. *Gastroenterology*, **77**, 223

7
Bile in the stomach

C. J. FIMMEL AND A. L. BLUM

HISTORICAL PROLOGUE: WILLIAM BEAUMONT AND DUODENOGASTRIC REFLUX

In his celebrated book entitled *Experiments and Observations on the Gastric Juice and the Physiology of Digestion*[1] William Beaumont precisely describes duodenogastric reflux of bile. While observing the stomach of his patient and experimental subject, Alexis St. Martin, across a gastric fistula, Beaumont noted: 'on lying him horizontally on his back, pressing the hands upon the hepatic region, agitating a little and at the same time turning him to the left side, bright yellow bile appears to flow freely through the pylorus, and passes out through the tube. Sometimes it is found mixed with the gastric juice, without this operation. This is, however, seldom the case unless it has been excited by some other cause.' Anger, while reducing the secretion of gastric acid, 'causes an influx of bile into the stomach which impairs its solvent properties.' 'Irritation of the pyloric extremity of the stomach with the end of the elastic tube or the bulb of the thermometer, generally occasions a flow of bile into this organ.' 'I have observed that when the use of fat or oily food has been persevered in for some time, there is generally the presence of bile in the gastric fluids. Whether this be a pathological phenomenon, induced by the peculiarly indigestible nature of oily food; or whether it be a provision of nature, to assist a chymification of this particular kind of diet, I have not yet satisfied myself.' 'With the exception that I have mentioned, it (bile) is never found in the gastric cavity, in a state of health; and it is only in certain morbid conditions that it is found there.' Six years later Beaumont had the opportunity to re-examine his subject after he had 'been drinking ardent spirits, pretty freely, for 8 or 10 days past.' Beaumont noted 'considerable erythema and some aphthous patches' and 'extracted about an ounce of gastric fluid, consisting of ropy mucus, some bile.' These signs disappeared within a few days of abstinence of alcoholic drinks.

150 years later, Beaumont's description remains unsurpassed, and only minor modifications are necessary.

DOES BILE REFLUX CAUSE ULCERS?

Arguments in favour

The authors quoted in Table 7.1 feel, with one exception[7], that bile reflux causes gastric ulcers because in their series ulcer patients had, on average, higher bile salt concentrations in their stomachs than healthy subjects. The highest intragastric bile salt concentrations were found in patients after distal gastric resection. Black *et al.* argued that reflux causes ulcers and not vice versa, because patients with active ulcers, healing ulcers, and healed ulcers had similar bile salt concentrations in their gastric juice[4,5].

Table 7.1 Bile acids in the stomach

	Reference	Bile acids in gastric juice (mmol/l)		
		Fasting	Postprandial	
Normal stomach	2	Range = 0.02–2.0 Mean (±SD) = 0.8±0.5		
	3	Range = 0.01–0.33	Mean Maximum	= 0.06 = 0.69
	4, 5	Range = 0–0.12	Range	= 0–0.48
	6	Mean (±SD) before IMC* = 0.6±0.4 Mean (±SD) after IMC* = 0.2±0.1		
	7	Median = 0.06 Range = 0.05–0.10	Median Range	= 0.30 = 0.07–0.38
Gastric ulcer	2	Range = 0.4–10.6 Mean (±SD) = 4.6±3.4		
	3	Range = 0.03–3.17	Mean	= 1.1±0.3
	4, 5	Range = 0–3.2	Range	= 0.1–7.4
After distal gastric resection	8	Asymptomatic range = 0–1	Asymptomatic range	= 0.6–11.5
		Symptomatic range = 2–4	Symptomatic range	= 2–16
	7	Range = 2.5–32 Median = 4	Range Median	= 0.6–11.5 = 2

*Describes bile salt concentrations before and after phase III of the interdigestive myoelectrical complex.

Arguments against

Intragastric bile salts may, at least in part, be biologically inactive. For example, Duane and Wegand found in patients after gastric surgery that almost half of the intragastric bile salts were insoluble[7].

Even the high bile salt concentrations found in gastric ulcer patients may be too low to cause mucosal damage. It should be noted that it is impossible to give a threshold dose for damaging concentrations of bile salts by merely measuring bile salt concentrations. Micellar bile salts are more potent than non-micellar bile salts[7], dehydroxylated secondary bile salts cause more damage than primary bile salts; bile salts in acid solution are more potent than in neutral solution[9]. The damaging effect is enhanced by the addition of lysolecithin[7a] or pancreatic juice; a secreting mucosa may be less vulnerable than a resting mucosa; ischaemia renders the stomach vulnerable; and a second bile salt exposure may be less effective than the first challenge. All these factors should be taken into consideration before concluding that a certain bile salt concentration measured in the human stomach is high enough to damage the mucosa.

With a few exceptions, bile reflux does not produce ulcers in animal models; in fact, during prolonged exposure of the stomach to bile, an increased resistance has been noted[10]. We measured the damaging effect of human gastric juice in a simple model using its haemolytic effect on human erythrocytes. Haemolytic activity was expressed with a lysolecithin standard. The lytic effect was similar in patients with peptic lesions and in subjects with a normal gastrointestinal tract. We were unable to observe an increased duodenogastric reflux in patients with gastric ulcer.

Authors who observed increased concentrations of bile salts in the stomachs of gastric ulcer patients also observed an increased concentration in duodenal ulcers, where a pathogenetic role of intragastric bile is unlikely. Finally, even the authors in favour of the bile salt theory (Table 7.1) were able to measure elevated bile salt concentrations only in a minority of their gastric ulcer patients (Figure 7.1).

QUANTITATIVE MEASUREMENTS OF DUODENOGASTRIC REFLUX

Most of the many methods so far proposed to measure duodenogastric reflux depend on the use of a duodenogastric tube. This tube might, however, affect duodenogastric reflux. Recently some methods have been proposed to measure reflux in the absence of a transpyloric tube. These methods depend on the appearance within the stomach of a labelled hepatic excretion marker. Reflux is assessed by scintigraphic measurements.

We have developed a method which allows simultaneous measurements of gastric secretion, gastric emptying, and duodenogastric reflux and avoids transpyloric intubation. Duodenogastric reflux is measured by abdominal scanning of an intravenously infused hepatic excretion marker (^{99m}Tc). ^{51}CrCl is used as a gastric volume marker. Duodenogastric reflux rate, gastric emptying rate, and the rate of gastric volume secretion are calculated using a set of differential equations.

Figure 7.2 shows gastric emptying rate and duodenogastric reflux rate in healthy volunteers, studied in the upright and supine position during an infusion of atropine. Atropine slowed gastric emptying and increased duodenogastric reflux. Postprandial reflux was not higher than fasting reflux. Figure 7.3 shows gastric emptying rates and duodenogastric reflux rates in healthy controls and subjects with endoscopically proved active gastric ulcer. No difference was observed between controls and ulcer patients.

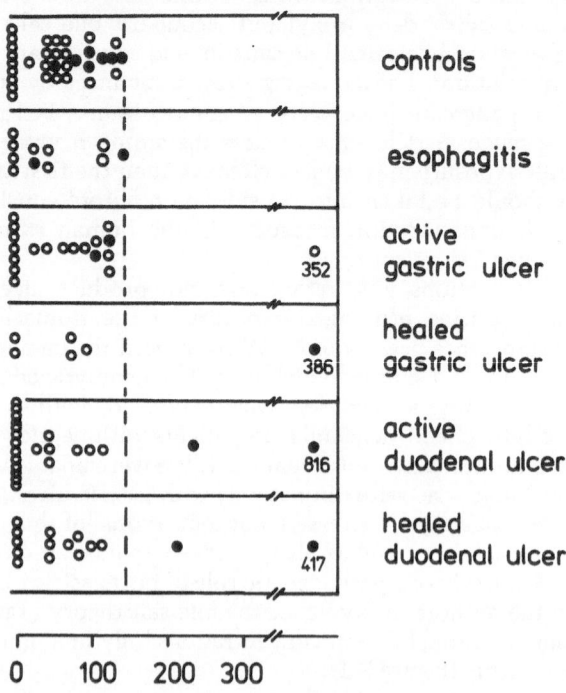

Figure 7.1 Bile salt concentrations in groups of patients

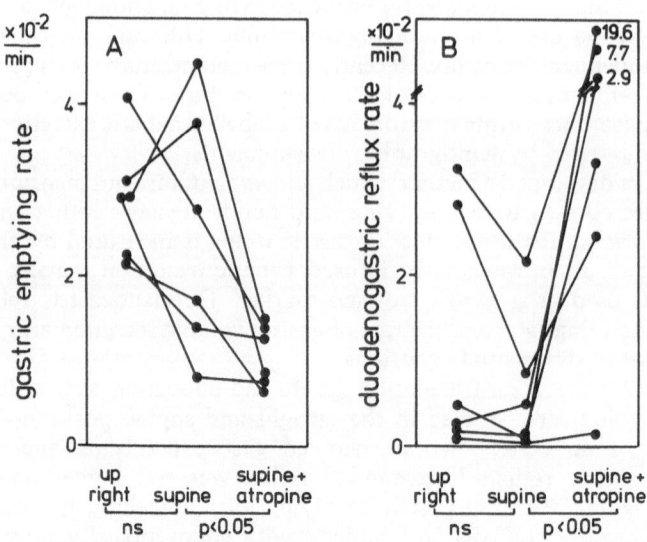

Figure 7.2 Gastric emptying rates and duodenogastric reflux rates in healthy volunteers during atropine infusion. (NS=not significant)

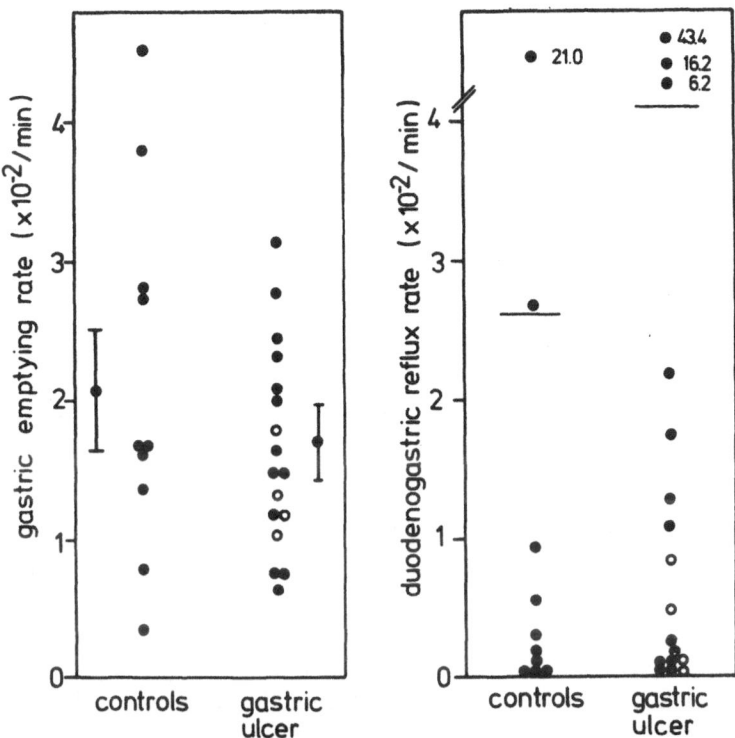

Figure 7.3 Gastric emptying rates and duodenogastric reflux rates in healthy controls and in subjects with endoscopically proved gastric ulcer

In a second series of experiments, the effect of the pylorus on duodeno-gastric reflux was examined. Trained, unrestrained dogs were used. They had either an intact pylorus, or had undergone pyloroplasty, or pylorec-tomy. A duodenal fistula was constructed with an isoperistaltic jejunal loop. In addition, a Komarov type oesophagostomy was constructed that did not interfere with food and fluid intake. Fasting reflux rate was similar in dogs with an intact pylorus and in those with pyloroplasty or pylorectomy. In all three types of dogs, a transpyloric tube caused a five-fold increase of the reflux rate. A low dose of apomorphine that did not produce vomiting increased the reflux rate ten-fold, irrespective of whether the pylorus was intact. Administration of a meal increased reflux. This rise was more pronounced in dogs with pylorectomy or pyloroplasty than in dogs with a normal pylorus, and it was higher after a lipid meal than after a protein meal (Figure 7.4). A fatty meal increased reflux. This rise was more marked in dogs with pylorectomy or pyloroplasty than in dogs with a normal pylorus.

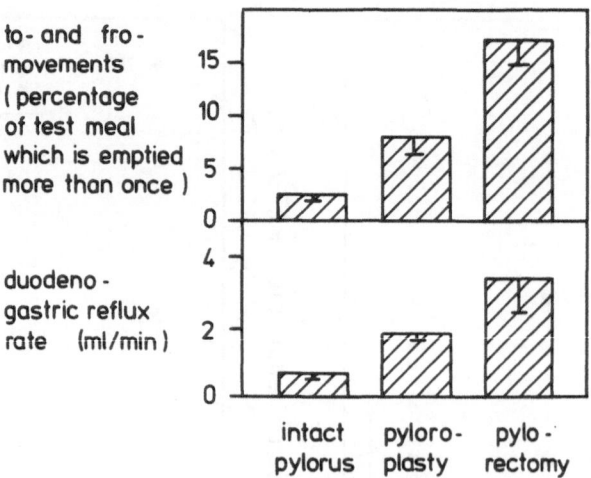

Figure 7.4   Results showing effect of pylorus on duodenogastric reflux

Our studies demonstrate that in animals the pylorus is an anti-reflux barrier: a compromised pylorus allows reflux to increase, and complete pyloric destruction leads to a marked increase of reflux. Since we did not observe increased duodenogastric reflux in gastric ulcer patients, it appears unlikely that in these patients pyloric dysfunction was responsible for the development of ulcers. In view of the known heterogeneity of gastric ulcer disease, however, our negative results do not necessarily apply to other ulcer patients. Furthermore, our results do not rule out pyloric dysfunction, duodenogastric reflux and an impairment of gastric emptying of solid meals.

MECHANISMS OF GASTRIC MUCOSAL DAMAGE INDUCED BY BILE SALTS

Figures 7.5–7.7 show a schematic representation of the gastric mucosa before, during, and after bile salt attack. The following sections discuss the mechanisms of attack.

Dissolution of mucosal lipids

This is probably the major mechanism by which bile salts disrupt the mucosal barrier. Duane et al.[7] showed that micellar bile salts release phospholipid and cholesterol from the plasma membrane. In addition, experiments with isolated gastric cells have shown that during incubation with 5 mmol/l sodium taurocholate, the prostaglandin 6-keto-PGF was also released from the plasma membrane[11-13]. Non-micellar bile salts did not break the barrier and did not release membrane lipids. These findings are corroborated by histological examinations: after a 30-minute exposure to

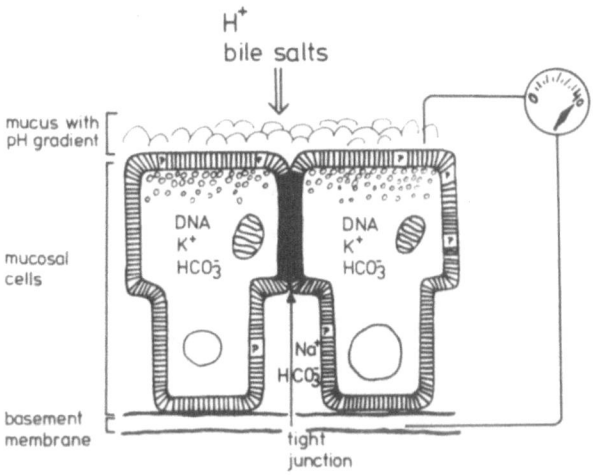

Figure 7.5 Gastric mucosa before bile salt attack. Two surface cells of the gastric mucosa are schematically represented. The cell membranes are shown to contain lipids and prostaglandins (P). The cells contain mucus granules (top), mitochondria (middle) and a nucleus (bottom). Cellular constituents (DNA, K^+, HCO_3^-) and interstitial constituents (NA^+, HCO_3^-), which play a role during damage, are shown. Electrical potential difference is $-40\,mV$.

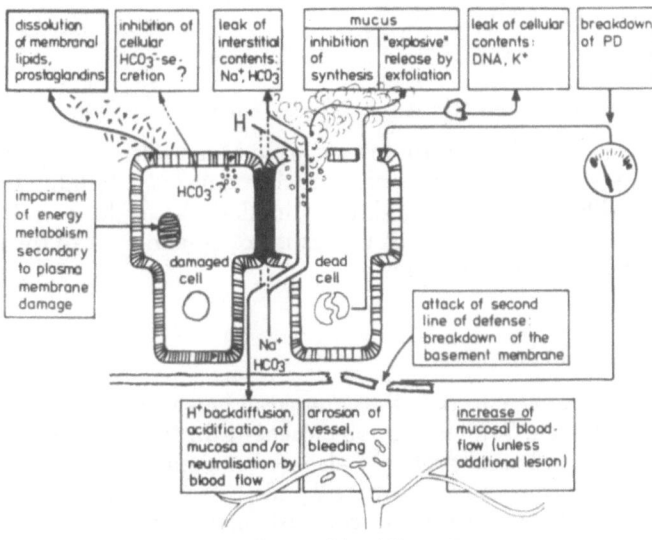

Figure 7.6 Gastric mucosa during bile salt attack

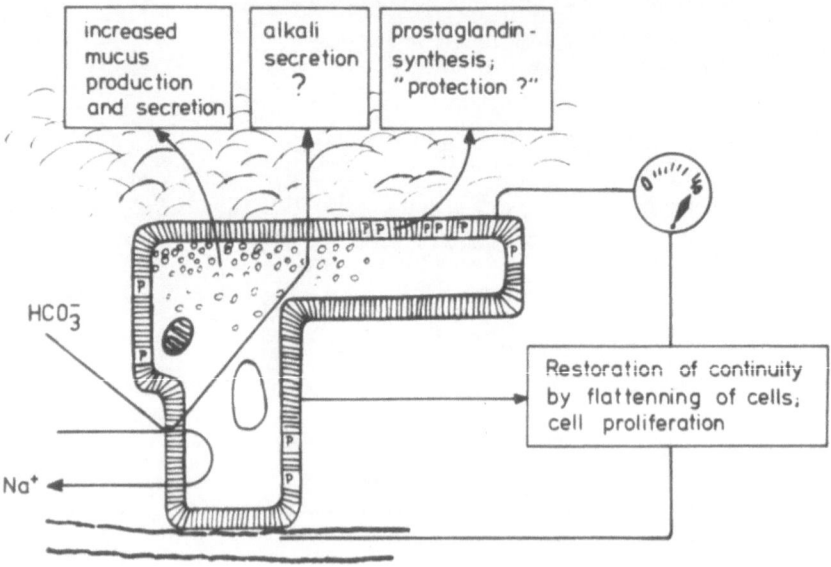

Figure 7.7 Gastric mucosa after bile salt attack

deoxycholate, the histological signs of mucosal damage are limited to the apical cell surface. On the other hand, Duane could recently show that bile acids probably disrupt the mucosal barrier by an uptake of bile acids. Under these circumstances, micelle formation is not required for the disruption of the barrier (Duane, 1980).[7]

Inhibition of mucus biosynthesis

Sticky mucus is thought to form an unstirred layer with a pH gradient[14]. Barrier breakers such as aspirin and probably taurocholate inhibit mucus biosynthesis. Bile salts may in addition stimulate the explosive release of mucus by total cell extrusion. This mucus is not able to stick to the gastric mucosa and floats off into the lumen.

Sodium and bicarbonate loss

An early sign of damage to the gastric mucosal barrier is the entry of Na^+ into the gastric lumen. Sodium is a constituent of the interstitial fluid which leaks across dead cells and probably also across damaged tight junctions. Amphibian gastric mucosa *in vitro* responds to sodium taurocholate by turning off its alkali production. In contrast, mammalian mucosa *in vivo* releases large amounts of alkali when exposed to sodium taurocholate. The source of this alkaline tide is the interstitial fluid[15]. It is not known whether the mammalian gastric mucosa actively secretes alkali.

Breakdown of the transmucosal electrical potential difference

The gastric mucosa maintains a transmucosal electrical potential difference of about 40–50 mV. This potential difference breaks down soon after exposure to bile salts. A typical example is shown in Figure 7.8. Here, a human stomach has been exposed for 15 minutes to 5 mmol/l sodium taurocholate. The breakdown of the potential difference is followed by an outpouring of the cellular contents. Figure 7.9 shows the effect of increasing concentrations of sodium taurocholate on potential difference at pH 3. The threshold dose is 5 mmol/l.

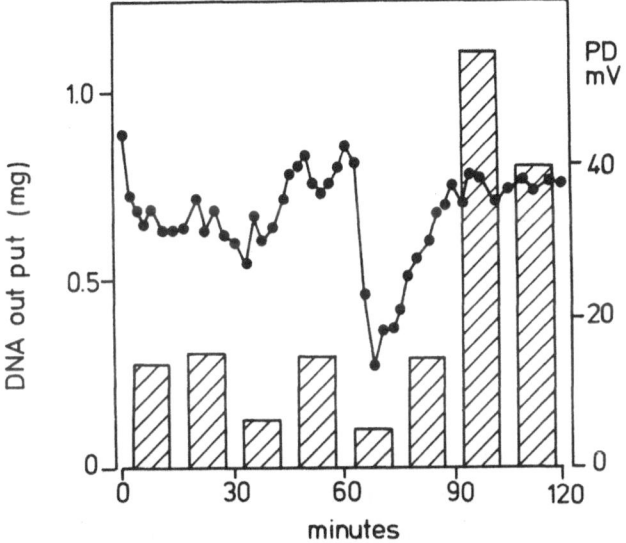

Figure 7.8 Changes in transmucosal potential difference (PD, black dots) and DNA output striated bars after exposure to taurochloric acid solution (5 mmol/l) in a normal human volunteer.

Changes in electrical potential difference should be interpreted with care because they depend on the secretory status of the mucosa and on physical factors such as intragastric pH and fluid volume. It should also be noted that certain damaging agents such as intravenous aspirin produce severe gastric lesions without affecting the electrical potential difference[16].

Impairment of energy metabolism

Some authors have suggested that bile salt damage starts by an impairment of energy metabolism after absorption of the bile salts. It is more likely, however, that these events are the consequence of apical membrane damage. Other damaging agents such as bile acids, lysolecithin[17], aspirin[18] and in particular ethanol[9] may directly attack intracellular metabolism.

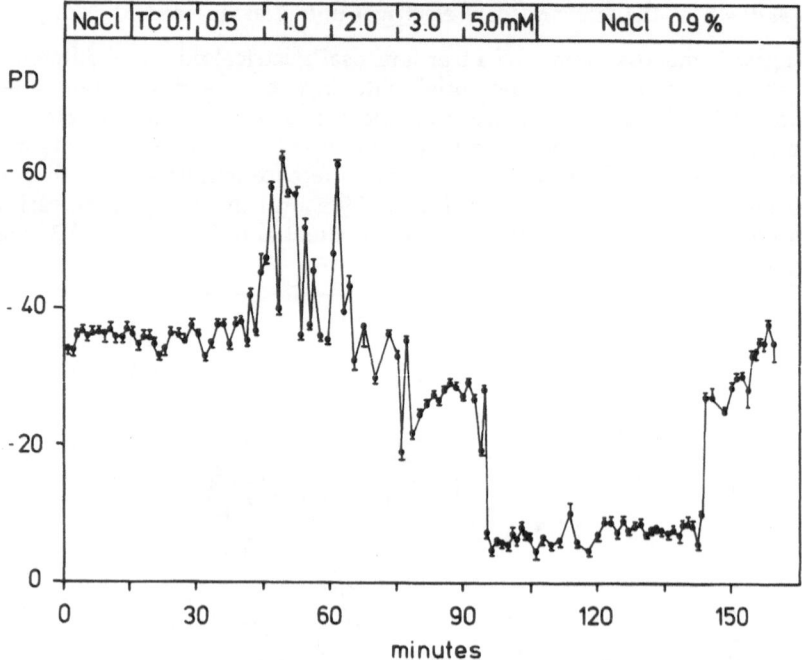

Figure 7.9 Effect of sodium taurocholate concentration on transmucosal potential difference at pH 3

Cell death; extrusion of cellular content

When isolated, dispersed gastric cells were preloaded with ^{86}Rb and then exposed to 5 mmol/l of sodium taurocholate, there was an immediate leakage of [86]Rb. In this experiment, Rb was used as a marker of potassium fluxes (Figure 7.8). In man, bile salt exposure leads to a similar potassium loss which is paralleled by a loss of deoxyribonucleic acid (Figure 7.8).

Acid back diffusion

The physiological intramucosal pH is about 7.4. Marked acid back diffusion is noted as soon as the disruption of cells becomes manifest on histological examination[19]. This may lead to mucosal acidification, which in turn produces massive destruction of cells and even gross mucosal lesions. It is, however, not possible to estimate the degree of mucosal acidification by simply measuring the rate of back diffusion, because intramucosal pH depends on gastric mucosal blood flow and blood pH: there is little change of intramucosal pH even in the presence of a high back diffusion rate, provided that gastric mucosal blood flow is high or the blood is alkalotic. Thus, intramucosal pH is the result of acid back diffusion, acid neutralization by plasma bicarbonate and acid removal by circulation.

Mucosal blood flow

Together with the basement membrane, mucosal blood vessels are the second line of defence. Bile salts are potent barrier breakers, but they produce only minor macroscopic damage, probably because they stimulate mucosal blood flow. When bile salts are given in a state of reduced mucosal blood flow, they produce severe lesions[20,21]. Other barrier breakers such as aspirin and indomethacin reduce basal gastric mucosal blood flow[22]. This reduction may be the cause for the severe damaging effects of these agents.

Other effects

It is questionable whether bile salts affect gastric acid secretion[23]. They might, by destroying the chief cells, increase pepsin output, but this is not likely to be of major importance.

An inhibition of cell proliferation is known to lead to mucosal damage. An inhibition of cell proliferation by bile salts has not been described.

PROTECTION FROM THE BILE SALT ATTACK

Mucus secretion

The protective properties of mucus are discussed above. It has been suggested but has not been proved that the stimulation of mucus secretion is a protective' mechanism. Some prostaglandins increase the production of mucus[24] and the mucus layer covering the mucosa (A. Garner, personal communication). They also stimulate cyclic AMP-synthesis in mucus-cell fractions[25]. When given for several weeks, prostaglandins also increase the number of mucin-producing cells (F. Halter, personal communications).

Stimulation of bicarbonate secretion

Theoretically, bicarbonate may improve mucosal protection by creating a pH-gradient within the mucus layer. PGE_2 and its analogues stimulate bicarbonate secretion in the amphibian stomach and duodenums[26-28]. A chloride carrier may be involved in this mechanism[29]. High serosal bicarbonate concentration protects both amphibian and mammal gastric mucosa[30,31].

In the mammal, gastric bicarbonate secretion is controversial. Some authors claim that the human fundic mucosa actively secretes bicarbonate and that this secretion may be stimulated by prostaglandins of the E series, but the reported technique of measuring secretion is open to question (C. Johansson, personal communication). Swiercyek *et al.* have shown that in the dog conventional doses of prostaglandins do not stimulate bicarbonate secretion, whereas high doses lead to a marked outpouring of bicarbonate as a consequence of membrane damage[15].

Inhibition of acid secretion

Many cytoprotective prostaglandins and prostacyclins inhibit gastric acid secretion, probably by inhibiting the cyclic AMP formation in parietal cells[32]. However, the threshold dose for protection is claimed to be below the threshold dose for secretory inhibition.

Under certain experimental conditions secretory inhibitors such as histamine antagonists and anticholinergics are 'protective'. On the other hand, recent work has shown that histamine H_1- and H_2-blockade has no protective effect against a 20 mmol/l sodium taurocholate challenge in the dog Heidenhain pouch[28]. The secreting mucosa may even be more resistant than a non-secreting stomach[34].

Blood flow

Increased blood flow protects against barrier breakers, and some cytoprotective agents such as prostacyclin increase mucosal blood flow. Other types of protective agents, however, such as PGE_2, have no effect on blood flow at low concentrations and, when given at higher doses, even reduce blood flow in parallel with their inhibition of acid secretion[35]. Thus, blood flow does not explain the protective effect of many of the prostaglandins.

Bicarbonate content of plasma

An important mechanism of protection is a high bicarbonate content of plasma. Metabolic acidosis was, in our own study (unpublished observation), shown to promote stress lesions during haemorrhagic shock. When metabolic acidosis was corrected by bicarbonate, stress lesions were prevented. Bicarbonate probably acts directly on the mucosa by neutralizing acid after back-diffusion from the lumen into the mucosa.

Other mechanisms which might protect the mucosa

It is not known whether prostaglandins have a direct effect on membrane resistance. Bowen et al. found a stimulation of cellular sodium extrusion by PGE_2 that might prevent the sodium accumulation and osmotic swelling induced by barrier breakers[36]. In our experiments with isolated rat gastric cells, PGE_2 did not prevent sodium influx after taurocholate administration[11-13].

Prostaglandins in high doses accelerate gastric emptying[37] and may thus shorten the contact of the mucosa with barrier breakers. This mechanism cannot explain the protective effect of low-dose prostaglandins, which do not affect gastric motility[38].

140

Are endogenous prostaglandins protective?

Many barrier breakers inhibit prostaglandin synthesis[37,40]. Mucosal prostaglandin concentrations are found to be subnormal in gastric ulcer[39], but not in duodenal ulcer[40]. There is circumstantial evidence that mechanisms which increase the prostaglandin formation of the mucosa are protective. There is, however, no proof that prostaglandin deficiency is a cause of decreased resistance or that simulation of prostaglandin synthesis is directly responsible for protection.

Does protection by prostaglandins really work?

When we perfused human stomachs with a 5 mmol/l sodium taurocholate solution, the drop of electrical potential difference could not be prevented by instillation of PGE_2. The elusiveness of a mode of action is not only a characteristic of prostaglandins but also of other 'protective' agents, for example carbenoxolone. Some prostaglandin experiments look like witchcraft[38] and may raise some doubt about 'cytoprotection'. In a careful histological study, the only clear-cut effect of prostaglandin protection was the prevention of ethanol-induced haemorrhage[41].

CONCLUSIONS

150 years after Beaumont's observations, his description of bile salts in the stomach remains unsurpassed. Two minor corrections of his pathophysiological concept have had to be made:

(1) The healthy gastroduodenal junction is not completely 'tight' – some reflux occurs even in healthy individuals in the fasting state and after a meal.

(2) A physiological role of intragastric bile salts has never been defined. On the contrary, we know that they in fact damage the gastric mucosa. Some mechanisms of bile salt damage have been experimentally elucidated, for instance membrane disruption, bicarbonate loss, breakdown of transmucosal electrical potential difference, and impairment of cellular energy metabolism. There is even a considerable body of knowledge about the possible ways by which the stomach defends itself against damaging agents.

Nevertheless, Beaumont's most important question has not been answered: Do bile salts produce gastric diseases by their own action or do they merely accompany or aggravate the effect of other pathophysiological mechanisms?

Acknowledgements

Supported by Swiss National Foundation Grant No. 3.940.0.80.

References

1. Beaumont, W. (1833). *Experiments and Observations on the Gastric Juice and the Physiology of Digestion.* (Plattsburgh: F. P. Allen)
2. Du Plessis, D. J. (1965). Pathogenesis of gastric ulceration. *Lancet*, i, 974
3. Rhodes, J., Barnardo, D. E., Phillips, S. F., Roverstad, R. A. and Hofmann, A. F. (1969). Increased reflux of bile into the stomach in patients with gastric ulcer. *Gastroenterology*, 57, 241
4. Black, R. B., Hole, D. and Rhodes, J. (1971). Bile damage to the gastric mucosal barrier: the influence of pH and bile acid concentration. *Gastroenterology*, 61, 178
5. Black, R. B., Roberts, G. and Rhodes, J. (1971). The effect of healing on bile reflux in gastric ulcer. *Gut*, 12, 552
6. Keane, F. B., Dimagno, E. P., Malagelada, J. R. (1981). Duodenogastric reflux in humans: its relationship to fasting antroduodenal motility and gastric, pancreatic, and biliary secretion. *Gastroenterology*, 81, 726
7. Duane, W. C. and Wiegand, D. M. (1980). Mechanism by which bile disrupts the gastric mucosa barrier in the dog. *Clin. Invest.*, 66, 1044
8. Hoare, A. M., Keighley, R. B., Starkey, B. and Alexander-Williams, J. Measurement of bile acids in gastric aspirates: an objective test for bile reflux after gastric surgery. *Gut*, 19, 166
9. Eastwood, G. L. and Kirchner, J. D. V. (1974). Changes in the fine structure of mouse gastric epithelium, produced by ethnol and urea. *Gastroenterology*, 67, 71
10. Scheurer, V., Schlegel, J. and Kelly, D. (1977). *Gastroenterology*, 72, 1127
11. Müller-Lissner, S. A., Fimmel, C. J., Sonnenberg, A., Peskar, B., Fischer, J. A. and Blum, A. L. (1980). The effect of prostaglandins on isolated rat gastric cells. *Scand. J. Gastroenterol.*, 16, 229
12. Müller-Lissner, S. A., Schattenmann, G., Schenker, G., Sonnenberg, A., Hollinger, A., Siewert, J. R. and Blum, A. L. (1981). Duodenogastric reflux in the fasting dog: role of pylorus and duodenal motility. *Am. J. Physiol.*, 214, G159
13. Müller-Lissner, S. A. Sonnenberg, A. Müller-Duysing, W., Will, N., Heinzel, F. and Blum, A. L. (1981). Quantitative measurement of duodenogastric reflux in man. *Scand. J. Gastroenterol.*, 16, 43
14. Allen, A. and Garner, A. (1980). Mucus and bicarbonate secretion in the stomach and their possible role in mucosal protection. *Gut*, 21, 249
15. Swierczek, J. S. and Konturek, S. J. (1981) *Am. J. Physiol.* 241, G509
16. Bugat, R., Thompson, M. R., Aures, D. and Grossman, M. I. (1976). Gastric mucosal lesions produced by intravenous infusion of aspirin in cats. *Gastroenterology*, 71, 754
17. Kivilaakso, E., Fromm, D. and Silen, W. (1978). Effects of lysolecithin on isolated gastric mucosa. *Surgery*, 84, 616
18. Hingson, D. J. and Ito, S. (1971). Effect of aspirin and related compounds on the fine structure of mouse gastric mucosa. *Gastroenterology*, 61, 156
19. Kelly, D. G., Code, C. F., Lechage, J., Bugajski, J. and Schlegel, J. E. (1969). Physiological and morphological characteristics of progressive disruption of the canine gastric mucosal barrier. *Dig. Dis. Sci.*, 24, 424
20. Chueng, L. Y. (1980). Topical effects of 16, 16-dimethyl prostaglandin E_2 on gastric blood flow in dogs. *Am. J. Physiol.*, 238, G154
21. Ritchie, W. P. (1975). Acute gastric mucosal damage induced by bile salts, acid and ischemia. *Gastroenterology*, 68, 699
22. Kauffman, G. L., Aures, D. and Grossman, M. I. (1980). Intravenous indomethacin and aspirin reduce basal gastric mucosal blood flow in dogs. *Am. J. Physiol.*, G151
23. Thomas, E. W. G. (1980). Functional changes in acid secretion produced by duodeno-gastric reflux. *Gut*, 21, 413
24. Domschke, W., Domschke, S., Homig, D. and Damling, C. (1978). Prostaglandin-stimulated gastric mucus secretion in man. *Acta Hepatogastroenterol.*, 25, 292
25. Garner, A. and Heylings, J. R. (1979). Stimulation of alkaline secretion in amphibian-isolated gastric mucosa by 16, 16-dimethyl PGE_2 and PGF_2. *Gastroenterology*, 76, 497
26. Kivilaakso, E. (1981). High plasma HCO_3- protects gastric mucosa against acute ulceration. *Gastroenterology*, 80, 1193

27. Garner, A., Flemström, G. and Heylings, J. R. (1979). Effects of antiinflammatory agents and prostaglandins on acid and bicarbonate secretions in the amphibian-isolated gastric mucosa. *Gastroenterology*, 77, 451
28. Gurl, N. J. *et al.* (1982). Histamine H_1 and H_2 blockade does not maintain electrochemical gradients across canine gastric mucosa exposed to bile salt. *Dig. Dis. Sci.*, 27, 538
29. Takeuchi, K. and Silen, W. (1980). Effect of changes in (C1) and (HCO_3) of bathing solutions on luminal alkalinization in frog fundic mucosa. *Gastroenterology*, 80, 1299
30. Chueng, L. Y. and Porterfield, G. (1979). Protection of gastric mucosa against acute ulceration by intravenous infusion of sodium bicarbonate. *Am. J. Surg.*, 137, 106
31. Kivilaakso, E. (1981). Effect of ambient HCO_3- on intracellular pH of isolated amphibian gastric mucosa. *Gastroenterology*, 80, A41
32. Nompleggi, D., Myers, L., Castell, D. and Dubois, A. (1980). Effect of a prostaglandin E_2 analog on gastric emptying and secretion in rhesus monkeys. *J. Pharmacol. Exp. Ther.*, 212, 491
33. Soll, A. H. and Whittler, B. J. R. (1979). Activity of prostacyclin, a stable analogue, 6 $-PGI_1$ and 6-oxo-PGF_{1a} on canine isolated parietal cells. *Br. J. Pharmacol.* 66, 97P
34. Smith, P., O'Brien. P., Fromm, D. and Silen, W. (1977). Secretory state of gastric mucosa and resistance to injury by exogenous acid. *Am. J. Surg.*, 133, 81
35. Francis, H. P. and Smy, J. R. (1978). Comparison of intravenous and close arterial infusions of prostaglandins E_1 and E_2 on gastric acid secretion and mucosal blood flow in anaesthetized cats. *Am. J. Physiol.*, 285, 38
36. Bowen, J. C., Kuo, Y. J., Pawlik, W., William, D., Shanbour, L. L., and Jabobson, E. D. (1975). Electrophysiological effects of burimamide and 16, 16-dimethyl prostaglandin E_2 on the canine gastric mucosa. *Gastroenterology*, 68, 1480
37. Konturek, S. J., Kwiecien, N., Obtulowicz, W., Sito, E., Olesky, J. and Dembinska-Kiec, A. (1981). Generation of prostaglandins (PGs) in gastrointestinal mucosa of healthy subjects and duodenal ulcer (DU) patients. *Gastroenterology*, 80, 1196
38. Robert, A., Nezamis, J. E., Lancaster, C. and Hanchar, A. J. (1979). Cytoprotection by prostaglandins in rats. *Gastroenterology*, 77, 433
39. Wright, J. P., Young, G. O., Klaff, L. J., Weers, L. A., Price, S. K. and Marks, I. N. (1982). Gastric mucosal prostaglandin E levels in patients with gastric ulcer disease and carcinoma, *Gastroenterology*, 82, 263
40. Konturek, S. J., Piastucki, I., Brzozowski, T., Radecki, T., Dembinska, A., Zmuda, A. and Gryglewski, R. (1981). Role of prostaglandins in the formation of aspirin-induced gastric ulcers. *Gastroenterology*, 80, 4
41. Lacy, E. R., and Ito, S. (1980). Cytology of prostaglandin treated rat gastric mucosa damaged by absolute ethanol. *Gastroenterology*, 80, 1201

8
Motility of the human biliary tree

A. TORSOLI, E. CORAZZIARI AND E. De MASI

The mechanical activity of the human biliary tree has been rather neglected by motilists for a long time, and this is mainly because of the difficulties encountered in introducing their recording devices into the gallbladder and the bile ducts. Specific motor events, however, take place along the entire biliary tract, and the related disorders have a great relevance in both clinical medicine and surgery.

Emptying of the gallbladder, the movements of the common bile duct and the choledocho-duodenal junction will be discussed.

EMPTYING OF THE GALLBLADDER

In physical terms, the gallbladder can be defined as a pressure condenser in parallel with the common duct. There is evidence of this after gallbladder removal, when stimuli producing transient obstruction of the common bile duct critically increase its intraluminal pressure and easily produce pain.

In physiological terms, the motor function of the gallbladder consists in collecting, retaining and releasing bile. Limited amounts of bile may be delivered on fasting, following different stimuli after a glass of water (Figure 8.1) or even with no apparent stimulation at all; the main emptying is, however, related to the ingestion of food.

There has been a long debate, in the past, on the nature of this emptying, whether active or passive. Some animal species have in fact a non-contractile gallbladder[1]. In man, as well as in the dog and the cat, the great emptying was finally proved to be active by showing that CCK-stimulated reduction in volume of the gallbladder was associated with a definite increase in its intraluminal pressure[2].

Pressure curves indicate a tonic type of contraction, with no phasic or peristaltic events, which is longer and stronger than the spontaneous contractions of the interdigestive period. The pressure peak does not usually exceed the pressure of liver secretion[3], but higher values can be observed when obstruction occurs at the cystic duct.

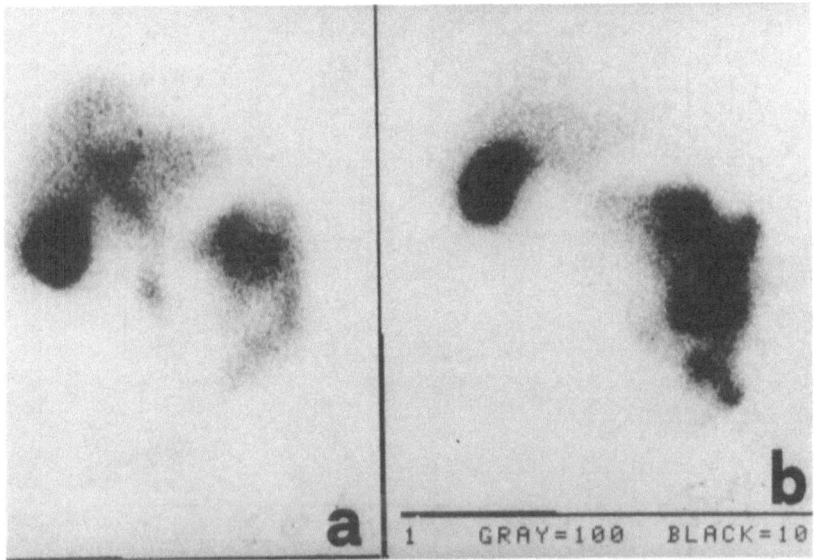

Figure 8.1 Cholescintigraphy. (a) basal conditions; (b) visible contraction of the gallbladder after ingestion of a glass of water

The outflow, generally ranging from 40 to 70%, begins shortly after the onset of gallbladder contraction, when the pressure reaches and overcomes the resistance offered by the cholecysto-cystic junction. This resistance is greater from the gallbladder to cystic duct than in the opposite direction[4], and has been seen to increase after abrupt distension of the gallbladder or administration of morpine and then to decrease with amyl nitrite. Amyl nitrite re-opens the junction and re-establishes bile flow[5].

This suggests not only a valve- but also a sphincter-like mechanism. It may explain why in some cases the junction is occluded even in the absence of stones or obvious organic alterations. However, anatomical data in this area are conflicting and require further investigation.

Gallbladder emptying appears to be primarily controlled by hormones, but the hormones concerned and their role in the process have not yet been defined. Cholecystokinin (CCK) has a direct myogenic effect, which can be blocked by a specific receptor antagonist, dibutyryl – cGMP[6] and a second target on cholinergic neurones has recently been reported[7].

Besides CCK, many other GI peptides and neuropeptides may interfere with gallbladder motility. A plasma motilin increase has been shown to be associated with water-stimulated gallbladder contraction[8] and the contractile effect of bombesin in man has been shown[9] (Figure 8.2). Vasoactive Intestinal Peptide (VIP) *in vivo* and *in vitro*, relaxes the gallbladder when contracted by CCK[10,11]. Pancreatic polypeptide and somatostatin also produce relaxation[12,13], but the significance of these various effects remains unclear.

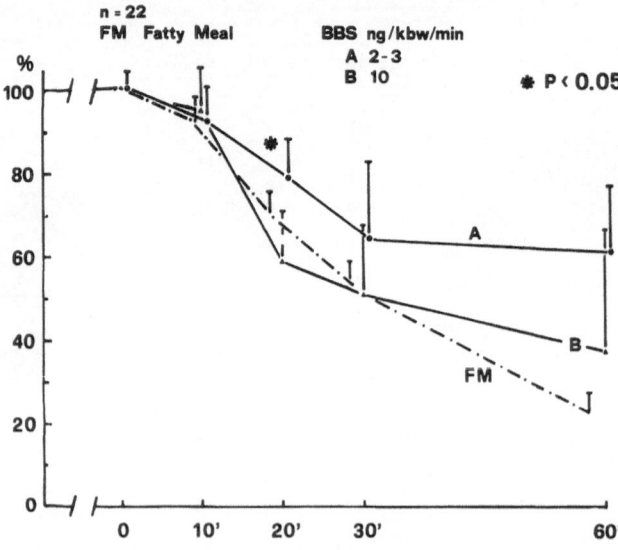

Figure 8.2 Planimetric variations of the gallbladder area during bombesin infusion. 2–3, 10 indicate the infusion rate of the polypeptide in $ng\,kg^{-1}\,min^{-1}$. FM refers to the conventional two-egg meal

CCK and caerulein, when administered in adequate doses, reduce the volume of the gallbladder to the same degree and at the same rate as a conventional fatty meal[2,14].

There is also evidence that postprandial gallbladder emptying may be regulated by nerves. Adrenergic alpha- and beta-receptors, cholinergic and peptidergic receptors have been demonstrated in the gallbladder muscle tissue.

Adrenergic innervation seems to be mainly inhibitory; postgangliar vagal innervation includes cholinergic as well as peptidergic neurones, and at this level enkephalin is likely to play a contractile role, whereas VIP has an inhibitory effect.

Acetylcholine and other parasympathetic agents increase gallbladder tone and motility, while truncal vagotomy, but not selective vagotomy, produces significant increase in volume of the gallbladder at rest which may be interpreted as evidence of atony of the viscus. Vagotomy does not alter gallbladder response to a fatty meal, except by increasing the sensitivity threshold of the muscle. This has been interpreted as a denervation-induced super-sensitivity, but could perhaps reflect the presence of VIPergic neurones in vagal innervation.

THE MOVEMENTS OF THE COMMON BILE DUCT

The movements of the common bile duct have also been the subject of a long-lasting discussion concerning the role of the duct in bile transport. X-ray evidence of peristaltic contractions has been reported in man, despite the fact that in the human bile duct there is no continuous longitudinal and circular muscle: and this is a *sine qua non* condition for the occurrence of peristalsis. Indeed, no phasic pressure variations in a coherent time–space sequence have ever been recorded in man.

The radiological changes considered as peristaltic, probably represent the elastic wall reaction to pressure variations related to sphincter movements[15,16].

The common bile duct pressure usually increases after cholecystokinin when the gallbladder is functioning, and decreases after its removal.

THE MOVEMENTS OF THE CHOLEDOCHODUODENAL JUNCTION

Although Oddi's work on the choledocho-duodenal junction has been questioned for almost a century most of the acquisitions about the anatomy of this area are derived from his studies[17,18]. Boyden studying the sphincter in different species was able to demonstrate its embryological and anatomical independence[19,20]. He also showed that the superior segment of the sphincter

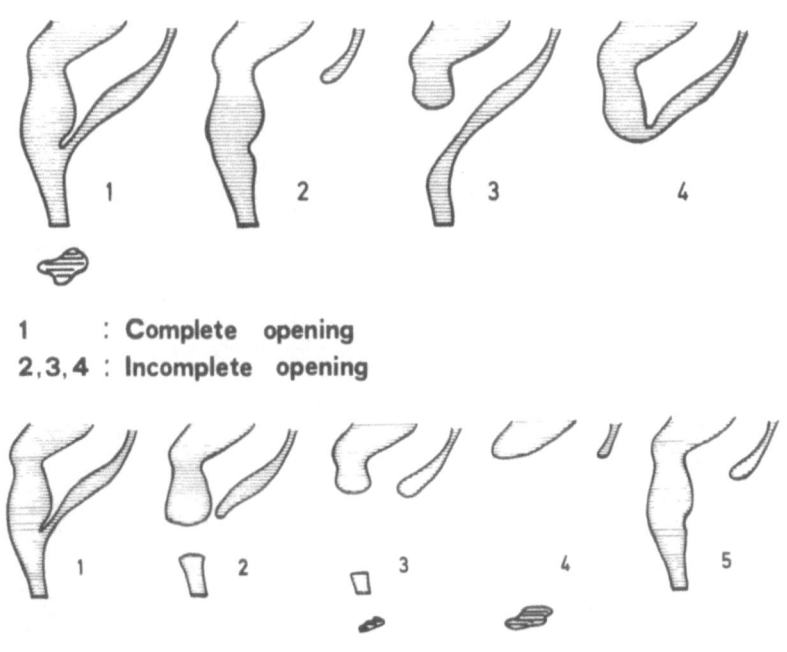

1 : Complete opening
2, 3, 4 : Incomplete opening

1, 2, 3, 4 : Complete closure
5 : Incomplete closure

Figure 8.3 Schematic drawings from cinefluorographic images concerning opening and closing movements of the human choledocho-duodenal junction

147

muscle is partially extramural and that the longitudinal muscle is only represented by two lateral fascicles. Comparative studies also indicate that the sphincter is usually lacking in species without a gallbladder, and this suggests that its primary function lies in promoting gallbladder filling and perhaps in regulating its emptying.

Cinefluorography has for a long time recorded rapid opening and closing movements of the choledoco-duodenal junction in man. Opening consists in a progressive dilatation from the proximal to the distal part of the sphincter segment, 0.5–2 seconds in duration, followed by flow of bile into the duodenum. The closing movement, 1–3 seconds in duration, begins as a ring-like contraction at about half-way of the sphincter. Then, the upper part contracts from below upwards, obstructing the duct, while the lower part contracts from above downwards and empties the ampulla (Figure 8.3). So, bile actually flows into the duodenum during both contraction and decontraction of the sphincter.

More recently, by using pull-through manometry with a triple-lumen catheter[21] introduced via a duodenoscope, it has been possible to identify a high-pressure segment $(22 \pm 2.8\,\text{mmHg})$ about 6–12 mm in length, corresponding to the sphincter. Phasic pressure variations, sometimes, rhythmic, other times irregular, measuring 90–100 mmHg in amplitude, 3.5 per minute in frequency and of 5–6 seconds in duration, are usually superimposed on the basal pressure (Figure 8.4).

A proximally (Figure 8.5) and/or distally (Figure 8.6) propagating pattern of the phasic contractions may be occasionally observed.

Which kind of relationship, if any, between this activity and the movements detected by cinefluorography, remains to be established. Considering that the external diameter of the catheter almost equals the

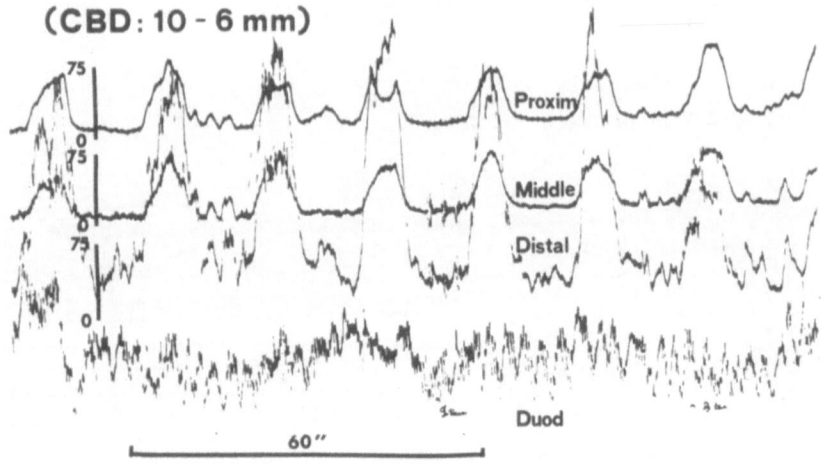

Figure 8.4 Manometric recordings with a triple-lumen catheter (proximal, middle, distal) from the sphincter of Oddi and with a single-lumen catheter from the duodenum (Duod). Simultaneous phasic contractions at three levels of the sphincter of Oddi. Calibration in mmHg

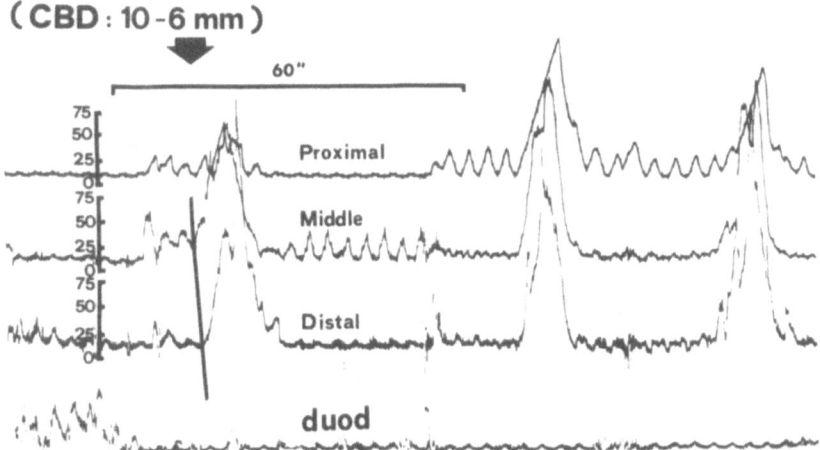

Figure 8.5 Manometric recording with a triple-lumen catheter (proximal, middle, distal) from the sphincter of Oddi and with single-lumen catheter from the duodenum (duod). On the left phasic contractions propagating distally

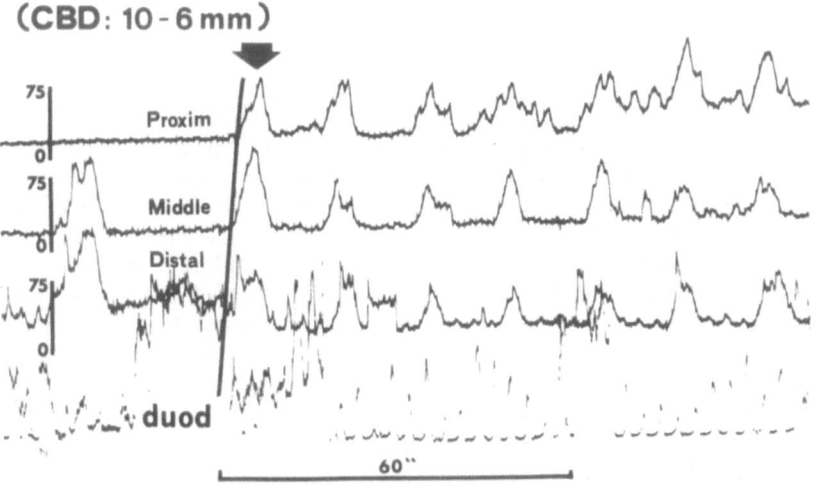

Figure 8.6 Manometric recording with a triple-lumen catheter (proximal, middle, distal) from the sphincter of Oddi and with a single-lumen catheter from the duodenum (duod). On the left, phasic contractions propagating proximally

internal diameter of the sphincter, further studies are necessary to determine to which extent the above-mentioned phasic pressure variations are related to the presence of the catheter within the sphincter.

CCK, caerulein (Figure 8.7) and glucagon depress this activity and dilate the sphincter. There is evidence of the physiological role of the CCK in

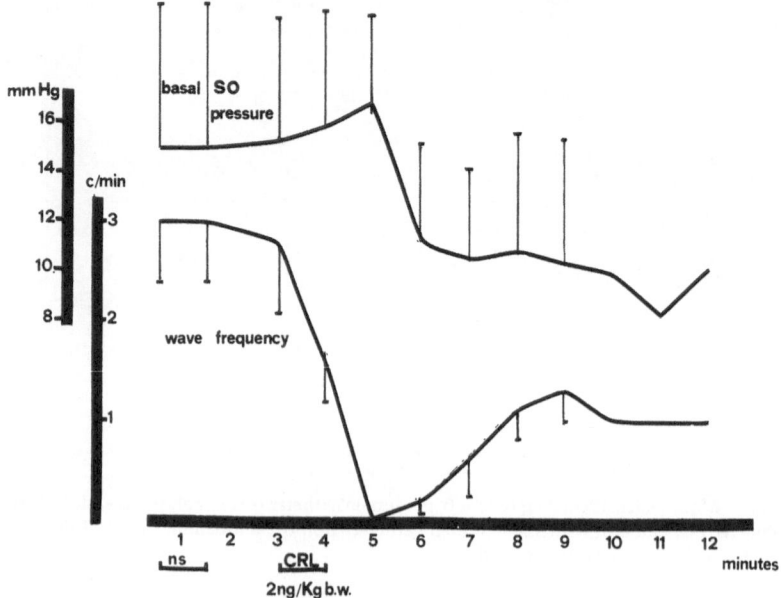

Figure 8.7 Basal sphincter of Oddi pressure tone (upper line) and phasic wave frequency (lower line) before, during and after administration of normal saline (ns) and caerulein (CRL). Significant reduction of wave frequency 2 min after the end of CRL infusion

inhibiting the sphincter. CCK inhibition seems to be the net result of two effects: a direct myogenic effect producing contraction, and a neurogenic effect, consisting of the activation of a VIP, intrinsic neurone resulting in relaxation. The neurogenic effect seems to predominate in man, whereas the myogenic effect would be prevalent in other species, like the rabbit[22].

The sphincter muscle also possesses receptors for different peptides, such as alpha-endorphine and enkephalins, in addition to cholinergic and alpha- and beta-adrenergic receptors. Parasympathomimetic drugs and vagal stimulation increase flux resistance, while the effects of adrenergic stimulation remain controversial.

Many questions still await an answer. But the sphincter can no longer be considered a 'somewhat mythical entity'. On the contrary, it appears to be a well-established reality, unique in its structure and function.

References

1. Magee, D. F. (1965). Physiology of gallbladder emptying. In Taylor, W. (ed.) *The Biliary System.* pp. 233–247. (Oxford: Blackwell Scientific Publications)
2. Torsoli, A., Ramorino, M. L. and Carratù, R. (1973). On the use of cholecystokinin in the roentgenological examination of the extrahepatic biliary tract and intestines. In Jorpes and Mutt (eds.) Secretin, cholecystokinin–pancreozymin and gastrin. *Handb. Exp. Pharm.* 34, 247
3. Jordan, P. H. (1964). Physiology of bile secretion. *Am. J. Surg.*, 107, 367

4. Caroli, J., Varay, A. and Gilles, E. (1945). Le functionment du sphincter vesiculaire chez l'homme: observation d'une double intubation. *Arch. Mal. Appl. Dig.*, **34**, 350
5. Torsoli, A. Ramorino, M.L. and Alessandrini, A. (1970). Motility of the biliary tract. *Rend. Gastroenterol.*, **2**, 67
6. Poitras, P., Iacino, D. and Walsh, J.H. (1980). Dybutyril-cGMP: inhibitor of the effect of cholecystokinin and gastrin on the guinea pig gallbladder *in vitro*. *Biochem. Biophys. Res. Commun.*, **96**, 476
7. Behar, J. and Biancani, P. (1980). Effect of cholecystokinin and the octapeptide on the feline sphincter of Oddi and gallbladder. Mechanism of action. *J. Clin. Invest.*, **66**, 1231
8. Svenberg, G.T., Christofides, N.D., Fitzpatrick, M.L., Bloom, S.R. and Wellbourn, R.B. (1981). Biliary output in man is associated with a rise in plasma motilin. *Gut*, **22**, A870
9. Corazziari, E., Torsoli, A., Melchiorri, P. and Delle Fave, G. (1974). Effect of bombesin on human gallbladder emptying. *Rend. Gastroenterol.*, **6**, 52
10. Ryan, J. and Cohen, S. (1977). Effect of vasoactive intestinal polypeptide basal and cholecystokinin induced gallbladder pressure. *Gastroenterology*, **73**, 870
11. Said, S.I. and Makhlouf, G.M. (1977). VIP spectrum of biological actions. In Chey, Y. and Brooks, F.P. (eds.) *Endocrinology of the Gut*, pp. 83–87. (New Jersey: CB Slack)
12. Greenberg, G.R., McCloy, R.F., Chadwick, V.S., Adrian, T.E., Baron, J.H. and Bloom, S.R. (1979). Effect of bovine pancreatic polypeptide on basal pancreatic and biliary outputs in man. *Dig. Dis. Sci.*, **24**, 11
13. Patel, Y.C., Zingg, H.H., Fitzpatrick, D. and Srikant, C.B. (1981). Somatostatin: some aspects of its physiology and pathophysiology. In Bloom, S.R. and Polak, J.M. (eds.) *Gut Hormones*. 2nd edn., pp. 339–349. (Edinburgh: Churchill-Livingstone)
14. Carratu, R., Arcangeli, G. and Pallone, F. (1971). Effects of caerulein on the human biliary tract. *Rend. Gastroenterol.*, **3**, 28
15. Nebesar, R.A., Pollard, J.J. and Potsaid, M.S. (1966). Cinecholangiography: some physiological observations. *Radiology*, **86**, 475
16. Stassa, G. and Graffe, W.B. (1968). The cineradiographic evaluation of the biliary tract after drug therapy following cholecystectomy, sphincterotomy, and vagotomy. *Radiology*, **91**, 297
17. Oddi, R. (1887). *Di una speciale disposizione a Sfintere dello Sbocco del Coledoco.* Santucci ed. (Perugia: Ann Università Libera Perugia)
18. Oddi, R. (1888). Sulla tonicità dell sfintere del coledoco. *Arch. Sci. Med.*, **12**, 333
19. Boyden, E.A. (1937). The sphincter of Oddi in man and certain representative mammals. *Surgery*, **1**, 25
20. Boyden, E.A. (1951). The anatomy of the choledochoduodenal junction in man. *Surg. Gynecol. Obstet.*, **104**, 641
21. Toouli, J., Geenen, J.E., Hogan, W.J., Dodds, W.J. and Arndorfer, R.C. (1982). Sphincter of Oddi motor activity: a comparison between patients with common bile duct stones and controls. *Gastroenterology*, **82**, 111
22. Sarles, J.C., Bidart, J.M., Devaux, M.A., Echinard, C. and Castagnini, A. (1976). Action of cholecystokinin and caerulein on the rabbit sphincter of Oddi. *Digestion*, **14**, 415

9
Gallbladder contraction: hormonal regulation

V. S. CHADWICK, P. N. MATON AND A. C. SELDEN

Several circulating (endocrine) gut peptide hormones and non-circulating (paracrine and neurocrine) gut peptides have effects on gallbladder motility or function, when tested in *in vitro* or *in vivo*. Many of these reported effects are 'pharmacological' and the criteria for attributing a 'physiological' role to many of these peptides have not been fulfilled.

In order to demonstrate a 'physiological' role in regulation of gallbladder contraction or relaxation, a reliable radioimmunoassay for the hormone in plasma is essential. If a physiological stimulus (e.g. a meal) produces both gallbladder contraction and an increase in circulating levels of the peptide hormone, and if the same response is obtained by infusion of the pure hormone to achieve comparable plasma levels, then a physiological role for that hormone is probable. In some cases, however, the activity of a hormone may be potentiated or inhibited by another (e.g. secretin potentiation of chole-cystokinin (CCK)) or the hormone may exist in several molecular forms with differing bioactivities so that by infusing a single molecular form of a hormone one is not simulating the true physiological situation.

MEASUREMENT OF GALLBLADDER CONTRACTION

Several techniques are suitable for studying gallbladder contraction and relaxation (or storage) in man, including various imaging techniques – for example, ultrasound[1], and hepatobiliary scanning with [^{99}Tc]HIDA[2] and the duodenal perfusion techniques where changes in gallbladder storage or emptying are inferred from changes in the duodenal recovery of either endogenous bilirubin[3] or exogenously administered indocyanine green[4,5] (ICG). In the perfusion techniques, plasma levels of the marker should be monitored to detect changes in hepatic uptake, while pancreatic secretion must be monitored to detect altered activity of the sphincter of Oddi. Furthermore, studies may have to be performed in cholecystectomized subjects before attributing observed effects in normals to an effect on the gallbladder rather than the extrahepatic biliary tree. Using these techniques gallbladder storage and emptying patterns during fasting and in response to luminal (e.g. fatty acids, amino acids and bile acids) stimuli or exogenous (e.g. CCK–secretin infusions) stimuli can be determined and the effects of other peptide hormones monitored.

CHOLECYSTOKININ

CCK-secreting cells are located in the upper small intestine[6,7]. Although intravenous infusions of CCK or the synthetic decapeptide analogue caerulein are known to cause gallbladder contraction and pancreatic enzyme secretion, knowledge about the role of CCK in normal physiology and disease states is limited because of difficulties in measuring levels of this hormone in blood. Radioimmunoassays have proved to be uniquely difficult in the case of CCKs since most anti-CCK antibodies cross-react with gastrins, and use of a single antibody to measure 'total CCK levels' does not distinguish between the various molecular forms (those with 4, 8, 12, 33 and 39 amino acid residues), each of which differ in bioactivity.

In our laboratories we have developed a high-pressure liquid chromatographic (HPLC) method[8,9] of processing plasma samples which concentrates and separates the various CCK peptides. Each of the forms may then be measured in appropriate column fractions using a simple assay recognizing the common carboxyl terminal of all CCKs. This approach overcomes most of the problems of measuring CCK levels and has been applied to the study of the different molecular forms of circulating CCKs during fasting in response to the ingestion of fat[10].

Ten healthy volunteers underwent an overnight fast and then took a breakfast of 100 ml of an emulsion of peanut oil. This stimulus produces prompt gallbladder contraction (within 20 minutes). Blood samples for CCK measurements were taken at 5-minute intervals after the fat meal. In five subjects the study was repeated after pretreatment with atropine 0.6–0.9 mg.

Fasting levels of CCK 8 and CCK 33/39 were less than 3 and less than 6 pmol/l, respectively. After oral fat both CCK 8 and CCK 33/39 levels rose promptly with peak levels of 15 ± 4.4 pmol/l at 30 minutes for CCK 8 and two peaks of 14.3 ± 4.2 pmol/l at 15 minutes and 20.2 ± 9.4 pmol/l at 90 minutes for CCK 33/39. The biphasic profile for combined CCK levels was evident with the small forms predominating between 5 and 30 minutes and the larger forms between 60 and 120 minutes. Pretreatment with atropine reduced CCK 8 levels by 50% and CCK 33 levels by 66%. These results show that both large and small forms of CCKs are released into the circulation following ingestion of a liquid fat meal. The gallbladder exhibits prompt and progressive contraction for the first 40 minutes following such a stimulus and since 5–10 pmol/l of CCK 8 or CCK 33 are probably sufficient for a biological response these data are consistent with a physiological role for CCK in promoting gallbladder contraction in response to oral fat. Cholinergic mechanisms are probably involved in CCK release as indicated by the effects of atropine.

PANCREATIC POLYPEPTIDE (PP)

Pancreatic polypeptide secreting cells are localized in the pancreas[11] and this hormone is released into the circulation following ingestion of protein or fat, by vagal stimulation and by endocrine stimulation[12] (CCK infusions). Intravenous infusions of bovine pancreatic polypeptide (BPP) in man to achieve plasma levels comparable with those observed after meals result in gallbladder relaxation and storage[13,14]. PP levels remain elevated for several hours following meals and these observations are consistent with a possible role for this hormone in promoting gallbladder storage between meals.

MOTILIN

Motilin is localized in the enterochromaffin cells of the duodenum and jejunum[15] and is released following mixed meals or oral fat[16]. During fasting partial gallbladder emptying occurs and is associated in time with an increase in circulating plasma motilin levels. Similarly ingestion of water stimulates partial gallbladder emptying and motilin release[17]. Intravenous infusion of motilin, however, although known to increase gallbladder pressure in animals had no significant effect on gallbladder emptying in man[18]. These data suggest that changes in endogenous motilin levels associated with gallbladder emptying are consequential rather than causal.

EFFECTS OF OTHER GUT PEPTIDES

Substance 'P' stimulates gallbladder contraction in the dog[19] and bombesin causes gallbladder contraction in both dog and man[20] though this may be mediated indirectly via stimulation of CCK release. Vasoactive intestinal polypeptide (VIP)[21] and somatostatin cause gallbladder relaxation[22], the latter possibly by inhibiting CCK release[23]. The role of these peptides in the physiological regulation of gallbladder function is not yet clear. At 'physiological' plasma levels gastrin, secretin, gastric inhibitory peptide (GIP) and neurotensin have no apparent effect on the gallbladder though secretin may potentiate the effects of CCK[24].

CONCLUSION

Cholecystokinins (CCK 8 and CCK 33/39) are probably the most important hormones mediating gallbladder contraction in response to meals. Pancreatic polypeptide may have a role in promoting gallbladder storage and opposing the effects of CCK. The release of both of these hormones is influenced by the cholinergic nervous system.

Several other peptide hormones may modulate the effects of these hormones either by stimulating or inhibiting their release or by modifying the target organ response. Although theoretically under- or over-secretion of gut peptides would be associated with abnormalities of gallbladder contraction there is little experimental evidence for this at present.

References

1. Wiener, I., Kazutoma, I., Fagan, C.J., Lilja, P., Watson, L.C. and Thompson, J.C. (1981). Release of cholecystokinin in man: Correlation of blood levels with gallbladder contraction. *Archiv. Surg.*, **194**, 321
2. Spellman, S.J., Shaffer, E.A. and Rosenthall, L. (1979). Gallbladder emptying in response to cholecystokinin. A cholescintigraphic study. *Gastroenterology*, **77**, 115
3. Greenberg, G.R., McCloy, R.F., Chadwick, V.S., Adrian, T.E., Baron, J.H. and Bloom, S.R. (1979). Effect of bovine pancreatic polypeptide on basal pancreatic and biliary outputs in man. *Dig. Dis. Sci.*, **24**, 11
4. Van Berge-Henegouwen, G.P. and Hofmann, A.F. (1978). Nocturnal gallbladder storage and emptying in gallstone patients and healthy subjects. *Gastroenterology*, **78**, 879
5. Bjornsson, O.G., Maton, P.N. and Chadwick, V.S. (1982). Effects of duodenal perfusion with sodium taurocholate on biliary and pancreatic secretion in man. *Eur. J. Clin. Invest.*, **12**, 97
6. Polak, J.M., Pearse, A.G.E., Bloom, S.R., Buchan, A.M., Rayford, P.L. and Thompson, J.C. (1975). Identification of cholecystokinin-secreting cells. *Lancet*, ii, 1016
7. Buffa, R., Solcia, E. and Go, V.L.W. (1976). Immunohistochemical identification of the cholecystokinin cell in the intestinal mucosa. *Gastroenterology*, **70**, 528
8. Maton, P., Selden, C., Murphy, R. and Chadwick, V.S. (1980). High pressure liquid chromatography (HPLC) analysis and bioassay of cholecystokinins. Proceedings of the 3rd International Symposium on GI hormones. *Reg. Peptides Suppl.*, **1**, 573
9. Selden, A.C., Maton, P.N., Murphy, R. and Chadwick, V.S. (1981). HPLC and bioassay of cholecystokinins. *Hormone Metab. Res.*, **13**, 363
10. Maton, P.N., Selden, A.C. and Chadwick, V.S. (1982). Measurement of multiple forms of cholecystokinin in plasma using high pressure liquid chromotography and radio-immunoassay: Effects of oral fat and atropine. *Reg. Peptides*, **3**, 76
11. Adrian, T.E., Bloom, S.R., Bryant, M.G., Polak, J.M., Hertz, Ph. and Barnes, A.J. (1976). Distribution and release of human pancreatic polypeptides. *Gut*, **17**, 940
12. Adrian, T.E., Bloom, S.R., Besterman, H.S., Barnes, A.J., Cooke, T.J.C., Russell, R.C.G. and Faber, R.G. (1977). Mechanism of pancreatic polypeptides release in man. *Lancet*, i, 161
13. Greenberg, G.R., Adrian, T.E., Baron, J.H., McCloy, R.F., Chadwick, V.S. and Bloom, S.R. (1978). Inhibition of pancreas and gallbladder by pancreatic polypeptide. *Lancet*, ii, 1280
14. Bjornsson, O.G., Adrian, T.E., Dawson, J., McCloy, R.F., Greenberg, G.R., Bloom, S.R. and Chadwick, V.S. (1979). Effects of gastrointestinal hormones on fasting gallbladder storage patterns in man. *Eur. J. Clin. Invest.*, **9**, 293
15. Pearse, A.G.E., Polak, J.M., Bloom, S.R., Adams, C., Dryburgh, J.R. and Brown, J.C. (1974). Enterochromaffin cells of the mammalian intestine as the source of motilin. *Virchows Arch. B. Cell Pathol.*, **16**, 111
16. Mitzregg, P., Bloom, S.R., Christofides, N.D., Besterman, H., Domschke, W., Domeschke, S., Wunsch, E., Jolger, E. and Demling, L. (1976). Release of motilin in man. *Scand. J. Gastroenterol.*, **11**, Suppl. **39**, 53
17. Svenberg, T., Christofides, N.D., Fitzpatrick, M.L., Bloom, S.R. and Welbourn, R.B. (1981). Biliary output in man is associated with a rise in plasma motilin. *Gut*, **22**, A870
18. Svenberg, T., Christofides, N.D. Fitzpatrick, M.L., Bloom, S.R. and Welbourn, R.B. (1982). Plasma motilin and biliary output in man. *Clin. Sci.*, **62**, 20
19. Thulin, L. and Holm, I. (1976). Effect of substance P on the flow of hepatic bile and pancreatic juice. In *Substance P. Proceedings of Nobel Symposium.* (New York: Raven Press)
20. Colazziari, E., Torsoli, A., Melchiorri, P. and Delle Fave, G.F. (1974). Effect of bombesin on human gallbladder emptying. *Rendic Gastroenterologica*, 6 52
21. Said, S.I. (1975). Vasoactive intestinal polypeptide (VIP). Current status. In Thompson, J.C., (ed.) *Gastrointestinal Hormones*. pp. 591-598. (Austin: University of Texas Press)
22. Creutzfeldt, W., Lankisch, P.G. and Folsch, U.R. (1975). Hemmung der sekretin-und cholezystokinin-pankreozymin-induzierten Saft-und Enzym-sekretion des Pankreas und der Gallenblasen-kontraktion beirn Menschen durch Somatostatin. *Dtsch. Med.*

Wochenschr., **100**, 1135
23. Schlegel, W., Raptis, S., Dollinger, H. C. and Pfeiffer, E. F. (1977). Inhibition of secretin pancreozymin and gastrin release and their biological activities by somatostatin. pp. 361-377. In *Hormonal Receptors in Digestive Tract Physiology.* (Amsterdam: Elsevier/North Holland. Biomedical Press)
24. Hubel, K. A. (1972). Secretin: A long progress note. *Gastroenterology*, **62**, 318

10
Bile acids in constipation and diarrhoea

R. HERMON DOWLING

INTRODUCTION

The idea that bile might be an important regulator of intestinal function is not new: in the sixteenth century, Andreas Vesalius suggested that 'the biting quality of bile irritates the intestines and propels the refuse'[1]. Over the past 20 years the concept that when the active transport system for bile acids is affected by ileal disease or resection, bile acids spill into the colon and diarrhoea results, has become well established[2]. The story was consolidated some 15 years ago when George Rowe, a cardiologist, noted for the first time that bile-acid-mediated diarrhoea might be relieved by treatment with the bile acid binding agent cholestyramine[3].

The evidence that bile acids influence normal colonic function, however, is largely indirect and comes from observations that bile-acid excess causes diarrhoea[4,5] while bile-acid deficiency may lead to constipation[6,7] (Table 10.1). The cathartic effect of the di-hydroxy bile acids, such as chenodeoxycholic (CDCA) and deoxycholic (DCA) acids, is greater than that of the tri-hydroxy bile acid, cholic acid; and from the studies of Chadwick et al., on

Table 10.1 Evidence that bile acids influence normal colonic function

Bile acid excess in colon causes diarrhoea	Bile acid deficiency from colon causes constipation
Ileal resection or by-pass	Treatment with bile acid binding agents: Cholestyramine
Ileal disease: e.g. Crohn's disease Ileocaecal TB Radiation ileitis	Aluminium hydroxide Congenital bile acid deficienty[6,7]
Defects in active ileal bile acid transport[4,5]	
CDCA treatment in some gallstone patients	

structure/activity relationships[8], we now know that the two hydroxyl groups must be in the alpha configuration. When bile acids such as these spill into the colon, water and electrolyte transport are inhibited and colonic motility is increased. This happens, for example, after ileal resection and during the treatment of some gallstone patients with CDCA. Conversely, constipation is seen in patients treated with bile acid binding agents, such as the anion-exchange resin cholestyramine and the antacid aluminium hydroxide.

BILE ACID-MEDIATED DIARRHOEA

The diarrhoea of CDCA treatment

If, arbitrarily, we define diarrhoea as more than two loose bowel actions per day in patients who had previously had normal bowel function, the overall incidence of diarrhoea in CDCA-treated patients is about 40%. However it is dose related, increasing from 33% in patients given less than 13 mg $CDCA \, kg^{-1} day^{-1}$, to 50% when the dose exceeds $16 \, mg \, kg^{-1} day^{-1}$. Fortunately, in most cases it is easily controlled. It frequently remits spontaneously and if not, it usually responds to a reduction in the CDCA dose and only rarely requires anti-diarrhoeal medication[9].

But why should some cheno-treated patients develop diarrhoea whilst others do not? To study this problem, Podesta and colleagues[10] looked at the relationship between the stool weight (g/day) and total faecal bile acid output (mg/day). They found a reasonably close linear relationship between these two variables ($y = 0.10x + 78$; $n = 52$; $r = 0.62$; $p < 0.001$) so that the

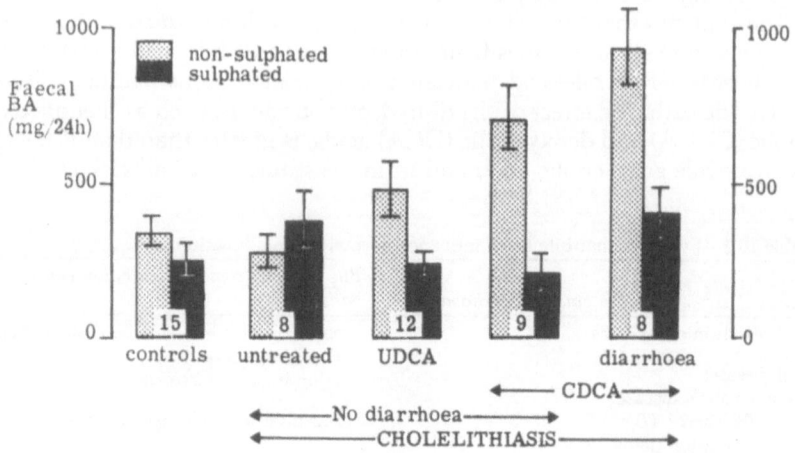

Figure 10.1 Sulphated and non-sulphated faecal bile acid excretion plotted in mg/day for control subjects, untreated gallstone patients, gallstone patients given UDCA and those given CDCA, where the results are sub-divided into those for patients with and without diarrhoea[10]

higher the faecal bile acid excretion, the greater was the stool weight. They went on to measure faecal bile acid excretion in different patient groups – controls, untreated gallstone patients, those given urso and those given cheno, with and without diarrhoea. And in each group, faecal bile acid output was subdivided into the sulphated and non-sulphated fractions (Figure 10.1). These results were based on differences in faecal bile acid excretion between the solvolysed and non-solvolysed material and for technical reasons, there was considerable controversy about Podesta's findings when they were first presented[10]. Other investigators found lower quantities of sulphated bile acids in the stools[11–14]. But whatever the *magnitude* of the sulphated fraction, it is obvious from Podesta's results that in patients with diarrhoea both the sulphated and non-sulphated faecal bile acid fractions increase. It was far from clear, however, whether the sulphated or the non-sulphated fraction was the most important in the pathogenesis of the bile-acid-mediated diarrhoea.

The effect of sulphated and non-sulphated bile acids on the colon

To study this further, Breuer *et al.*[15] used an *in vivo*, single-pass, colonic perfusion model in conscious restrained rats to measure changes in net water and electrolyte transport and in the output of protein and DNA into the effluent fluid after perfusing 5–15 mmol/l solutions of sulphated or non-sulphated bile acids through the colon. Their perfusion medium was an isotonic electrolyte solution containing the non-absorbable marker, polyethylene glycol (molecular weight 4000) made up to simulate the ileal effluent. They used a 30 min equilibration period followed by 5×10 min collection periods (a total perfusion time of 80 min) starting with the electrolyte solution alone and followed by a test solution containing either the sulphated or the non-sulphated bile acid or a mixture of the two (perfused for a further 80 min period).

5 mmol/l sulphated or non-sulphated deoxycholate

Table 10.2 shows the effect of DCA on net mucosal transport of water and sodium, and compares the results found when the electrolyte solution alone was perfused during both 80 min perfusion periods, when the electrolyte solution was followed by 5 mmol/l non-sulphated DCA and when the electrolyte solution was followed by 5 mmol/l sulphated DCA[15].

With the control solution alone, there was net water absorption $(+14.3 \pm 1.13 \,\mu l\, cm^{-1} (10\ min)^{-1})$ during the first 80 min perfusion period and net transport improved slightly during the second 80 min period (to $+16.6 \pm 1.34 \,\mu l\, cm^{-1} (10\ min)^{-1}$). In keeping with the results of many previous studies, net water absorption changed to net secretion $(-12.8 \pm 1.96 \,\mu l\, cm^{-1} (10\ min)^{-1}; p < 0.001)$ after perfusing the non-sulphated DCA. In contrast, there was no such 'cathartic' effect with the sulphated bile acid where the pattern of results was similar to that seen when the electrolyte solution alone was perfused during both perfusion periods.

Table 10.2 Effect of perfusing 5 mmol/l non-sulphated and 5 mmol/l sulphated DCA through the colon on net mucosal water and sodium transport and on the outputs of protein and DNA into the effluent fluid. Results are mean values ± SEM[15]

	Control period electrolyte solution	Test period electrolyte solution	Control period electrolyte solution	Test period 5 mmol/l non-sulphated DCA	Control period electrolyte solution	Test period 5 mmol/l sulphated DCA
Net water transport (μl cm^{-1} (10 min)$^{-1}$)	+14.3±1.13	+16.6±1.34 ($p < 0.05$)	+12.6±1.32	−12.8±1.96 ($p < 0.001$)	+10.1±0.91	+12.3±1.04 ($p < 0.05$)
Net sodium transport (μEq cm^{-1} (10 min)$^{-1}$)	+3.7±0.59	+3.8±0.48 (NS)	+3.6±0.43	−5.3±0.80 ($p < 0.002$)	+2.6±0.75	+3.4±0.47 (NS)
Protein output (μg cm^{-1} (10 min)$^{-1}$)	13.2±1.62	5.7±0.97 ($p < 0.02$)	8.2±1.5	139.2±18.1 ($p < 0.001$)	8.2±1.36	10.8±1.21 ($p < 0.001$)
DNA output (μg cm^{-1} (10 min)$^{-1}$)	0.89±0.16	0.22±0.06 ($p < 0.02$)	0.68±0.06	39.4±4.1 ($p < 0.001$)	0.54±0.09	1.76±0.28 (NS)

NS = Not significant.

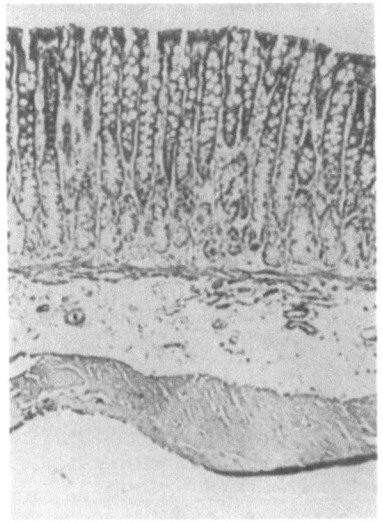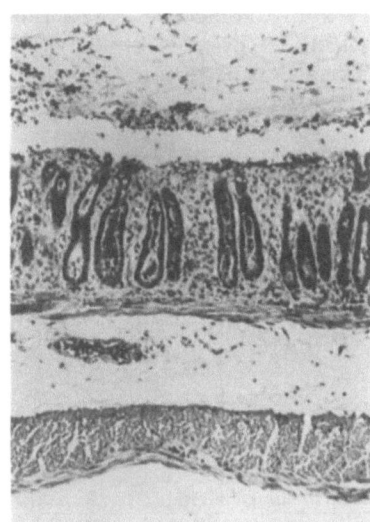

Figure 10.2 Colonic mucosal histology after 2×80 min perfusion periods, with the control (electrolyte) solution alone (left panel) or the control solution followed by a test solution containing 5 mmol/l non-sulphated DCA[15]. The mucosa on the left shows oedema in the submucosa and lamina propria, but is otherwise normal. The mucosa on the right shows, in addition to oedema, goblet cell depletion and an inflammatory infiltrate in the lamina propria, epithelial cell damage, surface ulceration and epithelial and inflammatory cells trapped in the excess surface mucus

A similar pattern of results was seen for sodium transport (Table 10.2). In other words, there was a slight increase in net sodium absorption from perfusion period 1 to perfusion period 2, with both the electrolyte solution alone and the 5 mmol/l sulphated DCA. But as with water transport, perfusion with the non-sulphated bile acid again changed net sodium absorption $(+3.6\pm0.43\,\mu\mathrm{Eq\,cm^{-1}(10\,min)^{-1}})$ to net secretion $(-5.3\pm0.80;\ p\langle0.002\rangle)$.

At the same time, there were striking changes in colonic mucosal histology. Figure 10.2 shows the appearance of the colon after perfusion with the electrolyte solution alone which resulted in a normal, albeit slightly oedematous, mucosa free from inflammation and showing normal crypts packed with goblet cells. In contrast, after perfusion with 5 mmol/l non-sulphated DCA, the mucosa became highly abnormal with an inflammatory cell infiltrate in the lamina propria, goblet cell depletion and desquamation of the epithelial cells which were trapped in the surface mucus.

These morphological changes were associated with striking changes in protein and DNA output into the perfusion effluent (Table 10.2). With the electrolyte solution alone, protein output decreased slightly between the first and second perfusion periods, but with the non-sulphated DCA there was a 16-fold increase in mean protein output and only a modest, although statistically significant, change with the sulphated bile acid. Similarly, there was a 57-fold increase in DNA output into the effluent after perfusion with the 5 mmol/l non-sulphated DCA solution but again only a very modest change after perfusion with the 3-mono-sulphate ester.

POSSIBLE MECHANISMS FOR THE CHANGES IN COLONIC MUCOSAL STRUCTURE AND FUNCTION DURING BILE-ACID PERFUSION

The possible mechanisms for the changes described during the experimental animal studies and, indeed, the mechanism for the diarrhoea seen in patients given CDCA treatment and in other types of bile acid-mediated diarrhoea, are poorly understood but have been summarized in Table 10.3.

Table 10.3 Possible mechanisms whereby excess bile acids in the colonic lumen cause diarrhoea.

Increased colonic motility	Decreased net water and electrolyte transport
Kirwan et al.[16]	Changes in:
Falconer et al.[17]	(i) The adenylate cyclase/cyclic AMP system[19-22]
Flynn et al.[18]	(ii) The guanylate cyclase/cyclic GMP system[22]
	(iii) The sodium/potassium dependent ATPase system[23]
	(iv) Mucosal permeability – reversible[24]
	(v) Prostaglandin metabolism[26]
	(vi) Mucosal damage or epitheliolysis[8,25]

First, there are changes in colonic motility and the results of several studies[16-18] have suggested that when excess amounts of di-hydroxy bile acids spill into the colon, colonic transport becomes more rapid than normal. Secondly, as illustrated above, there are changes in net water and electrolyte transport and, in turn, there are at least six possible explanations for this phenomenon:

(1) Changes in the adenylate cyclase/cyclic AMP system[19-22].
(2) Changes in the guanylate cyclase/cyclic GMP system[22].
(3) Changes in the sodium/potassium dependent ATP-ase system[23].
(4) Changes in mucosal permeability, which are believed to be reversible[24].
(5) Mucosal damage or epitheliolysis[8,25] as illustrated in Figure 10.2.
(6) Changes in prostaglandin metabolism[26].

The first five of these hypothetical mechanisms have been discussed many times before and are not reviewed further here, but for several reasons the sixth mechanism is discussed in more detail.

The role of prostaglandins in bile-acid-mediated diarrhoea

Prostaglandins are known to be 'cathartic' to the small intestine[27-30] and possibly also to the colon. Secondly, both bile acids and prostaglandins stimulate the adenylate cyclase/cyclic AMP system[31,32] which, as shown classically with the cholera toxin model, provokes marked increases in net intestinal secretion. Thirdly, bile acids and prostaglandins may also produce intestinal mucosal damage[33]; and fourthly, recent studies by Rampton and colleagues from our unit[26] have shed new light on this subject. Rampton *et al.*[26] compared the effect of DCA alone, of PGE_2 alone (chosen because it is the most stable and predominant prostaglandin in the colon) and DCA alone in animals pre-treated with prostaglandin synthesis inhibitor, indomethalin, on colonic mucosal water and electrolyte transport and on the output of immunoreactive PGE_2, into the perfusion effluent.

Figure 10.3 shows the effect of DCA alone in 1, 2 and 5 mmol/l concentrations, on delta water transport plotted above and below the zero line where the delta value refers to the difference between the first and second 80 min perfusion periods. The results illustrated in the Figure confirm the well-known fact that there is a clear-cut, dose–response effect so that the higher the concentration of deoxycholate in the perfusion medium, the greater is the net secretion of water.

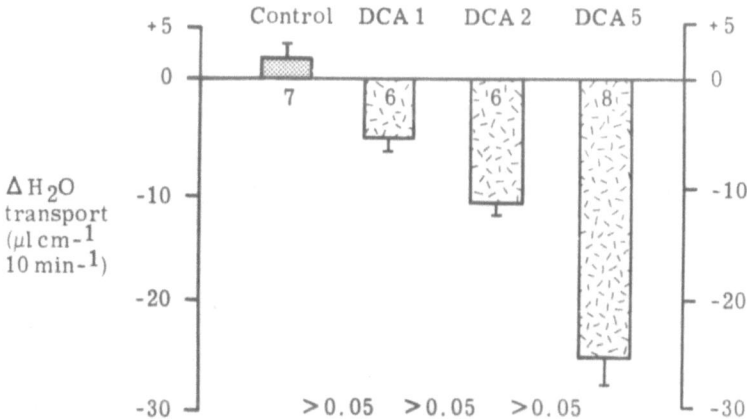

Figure 10.3 Effect of perfusing an electrolyte solution alone (control) or electrolyte solutions containing 1, 2, or 5 mmol/l non-sulphated DCA through the colon, on delta (Δ) water transport

Figure 10.4 shows the effect of perfusing 1, 2 and 5 mmol/l DCA through the colon, on PGE_2 output into the perfusion effluent. During the control perfusion (electrolyte solution alone), the mean output of PEG_2-like material was $23\,fmol\,cm^{-1}\,(10\,min)^{-1}$ but after perfusion with 5 mmol/l DCA, there was a 270-fold increase in prostaglandin output to a mean of $6260\,fmol\,cm^{-1}$ $(10\,min)^{-1}$ ($p < 0.005$). Again, this was a dose-related phenomenon with an 8-fold increase in PEG_2 output after perfusion with a 1 mmol/l non-sulphated DCA solution and a 10-fold increase after 2 mmol/l DCA (Figure 10.4).

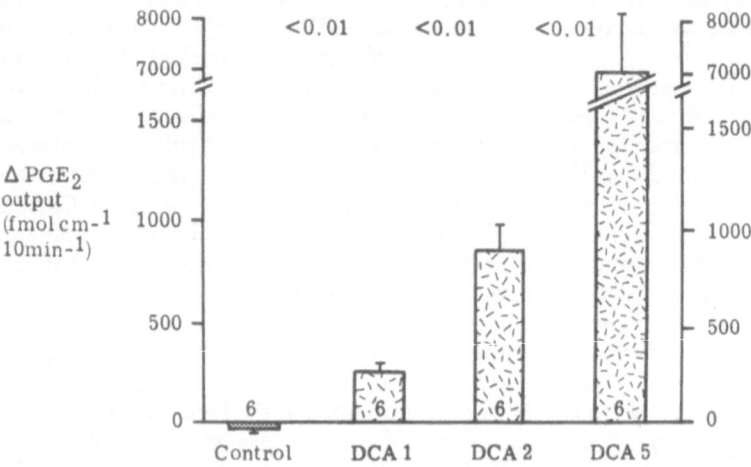

Figure 10.4 Effect of perfusing an electrolyte solution alone (control) or electrolyte solutions containing 1, 2, or 5 mmol/l non-sulphated DCA through the colon on delta (Δ) PGE_2 output into the perfusion effluent

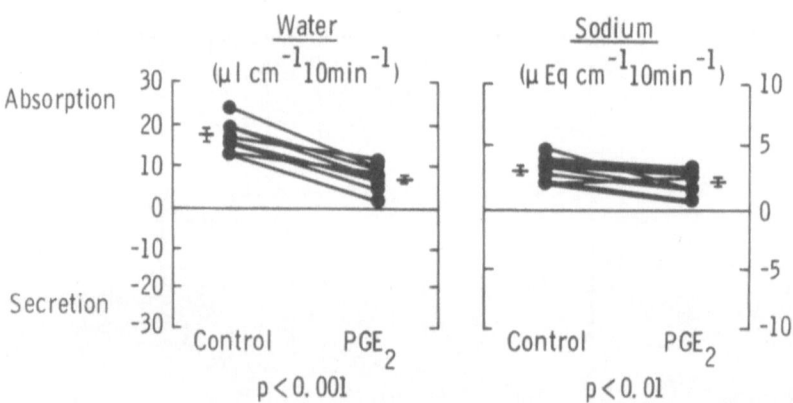

Figure 10.5 Effect of perfusing an electrolyte solution containing PGE_2 (100 μg/ml or 0.28 mmol/l) through the colon on net mucosal water and sodium transport

Does this mean that prostaglandins mediate the bile-acid induced effects on water and electrolyte transport? Figure 10.5 shows the effects of perfusing PEG_2, in a concentration of 100 μg/ml, through the colon on net mucosal transport of water and sodium. When compared with the control (electrolyte solution alone) perfusion, the PGE_2 perfusion did indeed lead to small, but significant, reductions in both Δwater (-11.2μl cm^{-1}(10 min)$^{-1}$) and Δsodium (-9μEq cm^{-1}(10 min)$^{-1}$) absorption but it never induced secretion. It is worth emphasizing that this PGE_2 concentration is considerably

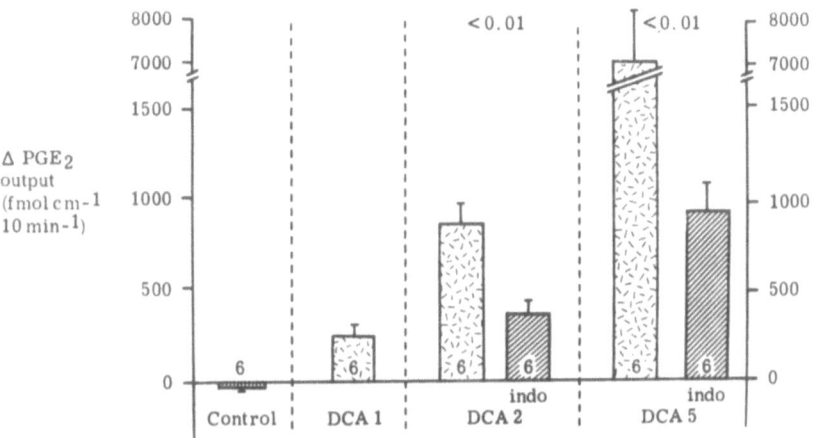

Figure 10.6 Effect of perfusing electrolyte solutions containing 1, 2 or 5 mmol/l non-sulphated DCA on delta (Δ) PGE$_2$ output into the perfusion effluent in untreated animals (stippled bars) and in rats pre-treated with indomethacin (cross-hatched bars)

higher than that found in the effluent fluid after perfusing the highest concentration of deoxycholate. This suggests, therefore, that although high concentrations of luminal prostaglandins *can* reduce colonic water and electrolyte transport, this effect does not occur after perfusion with concentrations of prostaglandins found in the perfusion effluent after 5 mmol/l DCA. And since we never induced net secretion, it seems unlikely, on this evidence at least, that prostaglandins are major mediators of bile acid-induced colonic secretion. Further support for this conclusion comes from studies with the prostaglandin synthesis inhibitor, indomethacin.

Figure 10.6 shows the effect of perfusing 1, 2, and 5 mmol/l concentrations of deoxycholate, on Δ prostaglandin output before, and after pre-treatment, with 10 mg indomethacin/kg body weight given subcutaneously 16 h and again 1 h before the study. As Figure 10.6 shows, indomethacin treatment does indeed have a marked effect on PGE$_2$ output. In other words, by using the prostaglandin synthetase inhibitor, we achieved our original aim of inhibiting prostaglandin synthesis and output. But what of the corresponding changes in Δwater transport?

Figure 10.7 (upper panel) shows, on the left, Δ PGE$_2$ output (as already illustrated, in part, in Figure 10.6) and on the right, the corresponding changes in Δwater transport after perfusing 2 mmol/l non-sulphated DCA through the colon, in rats with and without indomethacin pre-treatment. Despite the significant reduction in PGE$_2$ output after indomethacin, there was no corresponding change in Δwater transport. In fact, if anything, the 2 mmol/l DCA produced a greater change in water transport after indomethacin than before. Conversely, if we compare the results of ΔPGE$_2$ output after perfusing 5 mmol/l deoxycholate in animals pre-treated *with* indomethacin, with those found after perfusing 2 mmol/l DCA *without* indomethacin

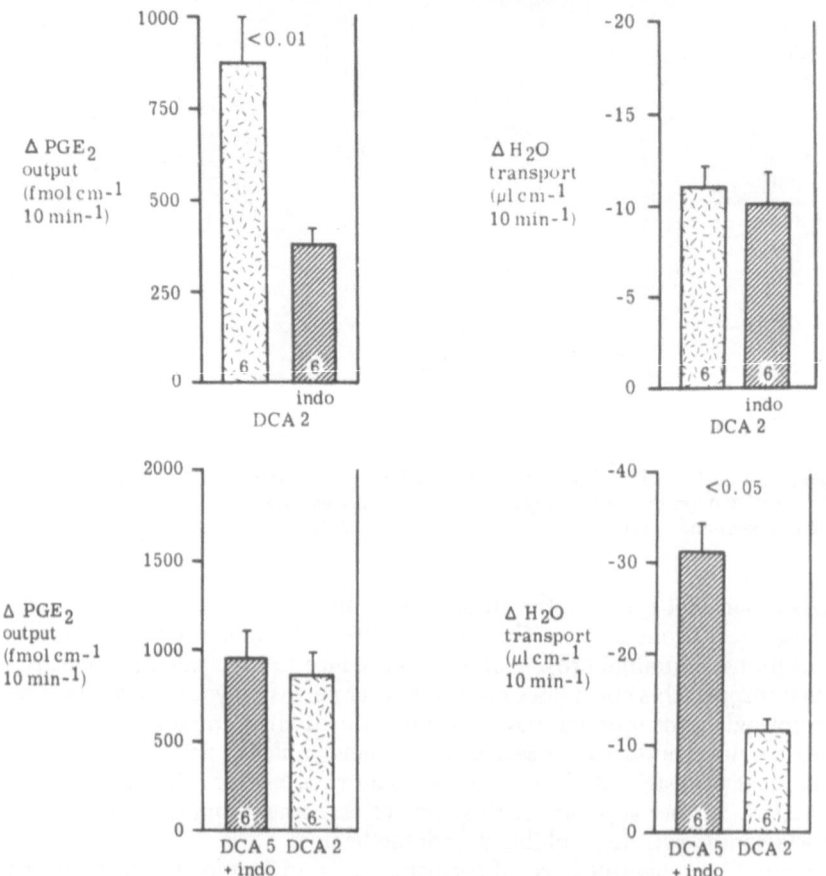

Figure 10.7 Selected results illustrating the dissociation between delta (Δ) PGE_2 output and Δwater transport in rats perfused with 2 mmol/l non-sulphated DCA with (cross-hatched bars) and without (stippled bars) indomethacin pre-treatment – upper panel – or with 5 mmol/l DCA in treated rats and 2 mmol/l DCA in untreated rats – lower panel

(Figure 10.7, lower panel), it can be seen that ΔPGE_2 output was virtually identical, but Δwater transport was strikingly different.

Comment

This dissociation between prostaglandin synthesis and release on the one hand, and electrolyte transport on the other, confirmed and consolidated our belief that prostaglandins are unlikely to be important mediators of deoxycholate-induced changes in colonic water and electrolyte absorption. If we can extrapolate from these findings in animals to man and particularly to patients with bile-acid-mediated diarrhoea, our results suggest that these patients should not respond to treatment with drugs such as indomethacin (or to beta-blockers such as propranolol). Indeed, despite the results of elegant animal studies by Conley, Schoenfield and colleagues[34] and by Binder et al.[35], most clinical investigators find that neither indomethacin nor propranolol are helpful in the treatment of patients with bile acid-related diarrhoea.

BILE ACID DEFICIENCY ASSOCIATED WITH CONSTIPATION

The evidence that bile acid deficiency may lead to constipation is summarized in Table 10.1.

Normal man excretes up to 500–600 mg of bile acids each day in the stools[10], and it has been suggested that this normal colonic throughput of bile acids may act as a physiological laxative. The fact that bile-acid binding agents, such as aluminium hydroxide and cholestyramine, may lead to constipation has already been discussed but several years ago, studies by Iser et al.[6] in a unique patient with congenital bile acid deficiency, provided a further link in the chain of evidence that lack of bile acids might cause constipation.

Case report

At the time of study, the patient was a healthy looking woman aged 29 – even if she was somewhat small in stature at 1.5 m (4'11").

Previous history

From the age of 3, the patient had had documented steatorrhoea, but despite this she had been constipated and on clinical grounds was thought to have been suffering from coeliac disease. Then in 1953, when she was aged 10, she was investigated by Ross and colleagues from Birmingham[7], who suggested that she probably had bile acid deficiency. They based this conclusion on the fact that she had low concentrations of cholic acid in duodenal samples, and that her steatorrhoea could be partly corrected by oral replacement therapy with the desiccated ox-bile preparation 'Desibyl'.

Present history

Without treatment, the patient was markedly constipated, opening her bowels only once every 3–6 weeks. The Desibyl treatment had been of some help, and whilst taking it she opened her bowels about once every 2 weeks; but the only way she could maintain anything approaching a normal bowel habit was with a self-administered phosphate enema. Despite this, she frequently had intermittent, colicky abdominal pains, which occasionally became severe.

She complained of dyspareunia – which was attributed, in part, to the forward projection of faecal 'rocks' from an impacted rectum. She also complained of dizzy spells which proved, on investigation, to be due to classical *grand-mal* epilepsy. Fortunately, her fits responded well to treatment with phenobarbitone, although this enzyme-inducing agent was withdrawn for the special bile-acid studies (see below).

Investigations

The intestinal bile acid deficiency was confirmed by aspirating duodenal fluid before and after intravenous CCK stimulation of gallbladder contraction when dark, pigment-rich 'bile' was obtained. Although it looked entirely normal, its total bile acid concentration was markedly reduced, with most of the samples having total bile acid concentrations in the 0.5–1.0 mmol/l range. In fact, the highest bile acid concentration in her bile-rich duodenal juice was 4 mmol/l, which was well below the corresponding values found in our gallstone patients, where the mean was 64 mmol/l. We also documented bile acid deficiency in the serum – as evidenced by a 14 h profile of the serum conjugates of CDCA measured by radioimmunoassay. With few exceptions, the values in the patient's serum were below the normal range found in control subjects taking the three conventional meals of the day.

Because of constipation, faecal collection and analysis were difficult, but we estimated that faecal bile acid output was also grossly diminished at about 40 mg/day – as opposed to the normal of some 500 mg/day[10].

Having confirmed bile acid deficiency in the intestine, and having shown bile acid deficiency in serum, bile and faeces, we went on to exclude common diseases of the liver and intestine which might have affected the two active transport mechanisms for bile acids – in the distal ileum and at the sinusoidal membrane of the liver. There was no evidence of disease at these sites. We therefore went on to measure the pool sizes and synthesis rates of the two primary bile acids, cholic acid and CDCA, using the classical Lindstedt isotope dilution technique[36]. The results in the patient were compared with published results in normal controls and in patients with gallstones who are known to have a reduced bile acid pool size[37] (this seemed appropriate since our patient too was shown to have developed cholesterol gallstones which were subsequently removed during elective cholecystectomy). Analysis of the isotope dilution results showed that there was a gross deficiency of both primary bile acids, but particularly a deficiency in the cholic acid pool[7]. This was confirmed by a GLC tracing of the trifluoroacetate derivatives of the patient's biliary bile acids where cholic acid accounted for only 17% of the bile acid total.

There were corresponding changes in the synthesis of the two primary bile acids. The synthesis of both was diminished but this particularly affected cholic acid synthesis which was markedly reduced[7]. This led us to postulate that there must have been a defect in hepatic bile acid synthesis – presumably affecting mainly cholic acid production which is largely rate-limited by the enzyme cholesterol 12α hydroxylase[38]. Later, when the patient came to elective cholecystectomy, a small wedge biopsy of liver was taken, and with the help of Dr Kostos Mitropoulis at the Royal Postgraduate Medical School we measured the activity of the rate-limiting enzymes for cholesterol

(HMGCoA reductase) and bile acid and cholic acid (cholesterol 7α and 12α hydroxylase) synthesis. The results showed that there was a reduced level of HMGCoA reductase, a low-normal 7α hydroxylase activity but a marked deficiency in the 12α hydroxylase enzyme. It seems, therefore, that this unique patient had a presumed congenital bile acid deficiency associated with marked constipation. While we cannot conclusively prove a cause-and-effect relationship between the low faecal bile acid output and her constipation, in the absence of other colonic disease, it is tempting to speculate that the two might be related.

Conclusions

This, then, is a brief review of the relationship between bile acids and the colon with a particular emphasis on constipation and diarrhoea. The role of bile acids in promoting hyperabsorption of dietary oxalate[39] in patients with enteric hyperoxaluria[40] has not been discussed, nor has the controversial question of bile acids and colon cancer[41] been addressed. However, these topics have been fully discussed elsewhere[42].

Acknowledgements

Thanks are due to many colleagues from our unit, whose work formed the basis for this review. In particular, I would like to thank Doctors N. R. Breuer, V. S. Chadwick, J. H. Iser, G. M. Murphy, M. T. Podesta, D. S. Rampton, G. E. Sladen and N. Tanida. Miss Kate Teasdale kindly typed the script.

References

1. Lind, L. R. (1969). Translator of *The Epitome of Andreas Vesalius*. p.44, (Cambridge, Ma.: MIT Press)
2. Hofmann, A. F. (1972). Bile acid malabsorption caused by ileal resection. *Arch. Intern. Med.*, **130**, 597
3. Rowe, G. G. (1968). Control of tenesmus and diarrhoea by cholestyramine administration. *Am. J. Med. Sci.*, **255**, 84
4. Hess Thaysen, E. and Pedersen, L. (1973). Diarrhoea associated with idiopathic bile acid malabsorption. Fact or fantasy? *Dan. Med. Bull.*, **20**, 174
5. Heubie, J. E., Balistreri, W. F., Fondacaro, J. D., Partin, J. C. and Schubert, W. K. (1982). Primary bile acid malabsorption: defective *in vitro* active bile acid transport. *Gastroenterology*, **83**, 804
6. Iser, J. H., Dowling, R. H., Murphy, G. M., Ponz de Leon, M., and Mitropoulos, K. A. (1977). Congenital bile salt deficiency associated with 28 years of intractable constipation. In Paumgartner, G. and Stiehl, A. (eds.) *Bile Acid Metabolism in Health and Disease*. pp.231-234. (Lancaster: MTP Press)
7. Ross, C. A. C., Frazer, A. C., French, J. M., Gerrard, J. W., Sammons, H. G. and Smellie, J. M. (1955). Coeliac disease. The relative importance of wheat gluten. *Lancet*, **i**, 1087
8. Chadwick, V. S., Gaginella, T. S., Carlson, C. L., Debongnie, J. C., Phillips, S. F. and Hofmann, A. F. (1978). Effect of molecular structure on bile acid induced alteration in absorption function, permeability and morphology in the perfused rabbit colon. *J. Lab. Clin. Med.*, **74**, 661

9. Iser, J. H., Dowling, R. H., Mok, H. Y. I. and Bell, C. D. (1975). Chenodeoxycholic acid treatment of gallstones – a follow-up report and analysis of factors influencing response to therapy. *N. Engl. J. Med.*, **293**, 378

10. Podesta, M. T., Murphy, G. M., Sladen, G. E., Breuer, N. F. and Dowling, R. H. (1982). Fecal bile acid excretion in diarrhoea: effect of sulfated and non-sulfated bile acids on colonic structure and function. In Paumgartner, G., Stiehl, A. and Gerok, W. (eds.) *Biological Effects of Bile Acids*. pp.245-256. (Lancaster: MTP Press)

11. Subbiah, M. T. P., Tyler, N. E., Buscaglia, M. D., Marai, L. (1976). Estimation of bile acid excretion in man: comparison of isotopic turnover and faecal excretion methods. *J. Lipid Res.*, **17**, 78

12. McJunkin, B., Fromm, H., Sarva, R. P. and Amin, P. (1981). Factors in the mechanism of diarrhoea in bile acid malabsorption: faecal pH – a key determinant. *Gastroenterology*, **80**, 1454

13. Salvioli, G. and Salati, R. (1979). Faecal bile acid loss and bile acid pool size during short-term treatment with ursodeoxycholic and chenodeoxycholic acid in patients with radiolucent gallstones. *Gut*, **20**, 698

14. Tanida, N., Hikasa, Y., Hosomi, M., Satomi, M., Oohama, I. and Shimoyama, T. (1981). Faecal bile acid analysis in healthy Japanese subjects using a lipophilic anion exchanger, capillary column gas chromatography and mass spectrometry. *Gastroenterol. Jap.*, **16**, 363

15. Breuer, N. F., Rampton, D. S., Tammar, A., Murphy, G. M. and Dowling, R. H. (1983). Effect of sulphated and non-sulphated bile acids on colonic structure and function in the rat. *Gastroenterology*, **84** (in press)

16. Kirwan, W. D., Smith, A. N., Mitchell, W. D., Falconer, J. D., and Eastwood, M. A. (1975). Bile acids and colonic motility in the rabbit and the human. *Gut*, **16**, 894

17. Falconer, J. D., Smith, A. N. and Eastwood, M. A. (1978). Effects of bile salts and prostaglandins on colonic motility in the rabbit. In Duthie, H. L. (ed.) *Gastrointestinal Motility in Health and Disease*. pp.607-617. (Lancaster: MTP Press)

18. Flynn, M., Darby, C., Hyland, J., Hammond, P. and Taylor, I. (1979). The effect of bile acids on colonic myoelectrical activity. *Br. J. Surg.*, **66**, 776

19. Binder, H. J., Filburn, C. H. and Volpe, B. T. (1975). Bile salt alteration of colonic electrolyte transport: Role of cyclic adenosine monophosphate. *Gastroenterology*, **68**, 503

20. Conley, D. R., Coyne, M. J., Bonorris, G. G., Chung, A. and Schoenfield, L. J. (1976). Bile acid stimulation of colonic adenylate cyclase and secretion in the rabbit. *Am. J. Dig. Dis.*, **21**, 453

21. Coyne, M. J., Bonorris, G. G., Chung, A., Conely, D. and Schoenfield, L. J. (1977). Propranolol inhibits bile acid and fatty acid stimulation of cyclic AMP in human colon. *Gastroenterology*, **73**, 971

22. Corazza, G. R., Ciccarelli, R., Caciagli, F. and Gasbarrini, G. (1979). Cyclic AMP in human colonic mucosa before and during chenodeoxycholic acid therapy. *Gut*, **20**, 489

23. Feinstein, J. D., Coyne, M. J., Bonorris, G. G., Chung, A. and Schoenfield, L. J. (1977). Bile acid and fatty acid effect on intestinal cylic–AMP, $Na^+–K^+$–ATPase and secretion. *Gastroenterology*, **72**, 1183 (abstract)

24. Nell, G., Forth, W., Freiburger, T. Rummel, W. and Wanitschke, R. (1975). Characterisation of permeability changes by test molecules in rat colonic mucosa under the influence of sodium deoxycholate. In Matern, S., Hackenschmidt, J., Back, P. and Gerok, W. (eds.) *Advances in Bile Acid Research*. pp.419-424. (Stuttgart: FK Schattauer-Verlag)

25. Saunders, D. R., Hedges, J. R., Sillery, J., Esther, L., Matsumura, K. and Rubin, C. E. (1974). Morphological and functional effects of bile salts on rat colon. *Gastroenterology*, **68**, 1236

26. Rampton, D. S., Breuer, N. F., Vaja, S. G., Sladen, G. E. and Dowling, R. H. (1981). Role of prostaglandins in bile salt-induced changes in rat colonic structure and function. *Clin. Sci.*, **61**, 641

27. Pierce, N. F., Carpenter, C. C. J., Elliot, H. L. and Greenough, W. B. (1971). Effects of prostaglandins, theophylline and cholera toxin upon transmucosal water and electrolyte movement in the canine jejunum. *Gastroenterology*, **60**, 22

28. Matuchansky, C. and Bernier, J. J. (1973). Effect of prostaglandin E_1 on glucose, water and electrolyte absorption in the human jejunum. *Gastroenterology*, **64**, 1111

29. Mize, B. F., Wu, W. C. and Whalen, G. E. (1974). The effect of Prostaglandin E_2 on net jejunal transport and mean transit time. *Gastroenterology*, **66**, 747 (abstract)
30. Bukhave, K. and Rask-Madsen, J. (1980). Saturation kinetics applied to *in vitro* effects of low prostaglandin E_2 and $F_{2\alpha}$ concentrations on ion transport across human jejunal mucosa. Gastroenterology, **78**, 32
31. Taub, M., Coyne, M. J., Bonorris, G. G., Chung, A., Coyne, B. and Schoenfield, L. J. (1978). Inhibition by propranolol of bile acid- and PGE-stimulated cAMP and intestinal secretion. *Am. J. Gastroenterol.*, **70**, 129
32. Waldman, D. B., Gardner, J. D., Zfass, A. M. and Makhlouf, C. M. (1977). Effects of vasoactive intestinal peptide, secretin and related peptides on rat colonic transport and adenylate cyclase activity. *Gastroenterology*, **73**, 518
33. Gordon, S. J., Kinsey, M. D., Magen, J. S., Joseph, R. E. and Knowlessar, O. D. (1979). Structure of bile acids associated with secretion in the rat cecum. *Gastroenterology*, **77**, 38
34. Conley, D., Coyne, M., Chung, A., Bonorris, G. and Schoenfield, L. (1976). Propranolol inhibits adenylate cyclase and secretion stimulated by deoxycholic acid in the rabbit colon. *Gastroenterology*, **71**, 27
35. Binder, H. J., Dobbins, J. W., Racusen, I. C. and Whiting, D. S. (1978). Effect of propranolol on ricinoleic acid and deoxycholic acid-induced changes of intestinal electrolyte movement and mucosal permeability: evidence against the importance of altered permeability in the production of fluid and electrolyte accumulation. *Gastroenterology*, **75**, 668
36. Lindstedt, S. (1957). The turnover of cholic acid in man. *Acta Physiol. Scand.*, **40**, 1
37. Vlahcevic, Z. R., Bell, C. C. Jr., Buhac, I., Farrar, J. T. and Swell, L. (1970). Diminished bile acid pool size in patients with gallstones. *Gastroenterology*, **59**, 165
38. Danielsson, H. (1969). Formation and metabolism of bile acids. In Bittar, A. B. and Bittar, C. D. (eds.) *The Biological Basis of Medicine.* Chapter 8
39. Chadwick, V. S., Elias, E., Bell, C. D. and Dowling, R. H. (1974). The role of bile acids in the increased intestinal absorption of oxalate after ileal resection. In Matern, P., Hackenschmidt, J., Back, P. and Gerok, W. (eds.) *Advances in Bile Acid Research.* pp. 435–440. (Stuttgart: Schattauer-Verlag)
40. Smith, I. H. and Hofmann, A. F. (1974). Acquired hyperoxaluria, urolithiasis, and intestinal disease: a new digestive disorder. *Gastroenterology*, **66**, 1257 (Editorial)
41. Hill, M. J. and Aries, V. C. (1971). Faecal steroid composition and its relationship to cancer of the large bowel. *J. Pathol.*, **104**, 129
42. Malt, R. A. and Williamson, R. C. W. (eds.) (1982). *Colonic Carcinogenesis.* (Lancaster: MTP Press)

11
Bile acid malabsorption

L. BARBARA

The bile acid (BA) pool size is preserved in the enterohepatic circulation (EHC) by means of an efficient intestinal absorption[1].

The BA, which enter the small intestine after gallbladder emptying, take part in the digestion and absorption of fat and fat-soluble vitamins in the jejunum and proximal ileum; then they are absorbed, mainly in the distal ileum[2,3].

Two modalities of bile acid absorption have been identified: passive absorption and active absorption, the former mechanism operating in the proximal small intestine and the colon, the latter accounting for the absorption in the distal ileum.

As far as the passive absorption mechanism is concerned, this inversely correlates with the number of hydroxyl groups and the degree of ionization[4,5].

The hydroxyl groups increase the binding of BA to water; therefore, the partition coefficient of the BA into the lipid membranes of the cells is decreased.

Passive ionic diffusion now is thought to account for little of the total BA absorption, while the protonate molecule, i.e. non-ionized, is considered the major determinant of the passive absorption.

Therefore, since the pK_a of unconjugated BA present as 'monomers' is about 5, i.e. more similar to the pH of the intestinal lumen than that of the conjugated forms, unconjugated BA, mainly dihydroxy, are candidates for passive absorption.

The active BA intestinal transport is operating in the terminal ileum, though the exact mechanism is not yet known and its histochemical localization is still to be fully determined.

Active absorption follows Michaelis–Menten kinetics[6]: V_{max} increasing with the number of OH groups, K_m being, on the contrary, related to conjugation, either with taurine or glycine[7].

The colon helps maintain the enterohepatic circulation of BA by means of passive absorption[8]: its contribution to the total absorption may be important in cases of BA malabsorption (BAM) in the small intestine[9].

In health, only about 10–15% of the total BA pool is lost daily in the faeces; in presence of interruption of the EHC, with or without mucosal damage, the BA are malabsorbed[10].

Various conditions have been so far described in association with BAM, though a cause–effect relationship has not been identified for each of them; three types of BAM have been listed[11]: the first is due to ileal resection or disease[10,12,13]; the second is regarded as a primary BAM; the third is found in association with clinical conditions, such as cholecystectomy, fenformine treatment, or renal failure[11].

The first type of BAM, which is pathognomonical for the disease, is related either to Crohn's disease or to ileal resection: the severity of the malabsorption depends on the extent of the ileal involvement.

The second type of BAM, firstly described by Thaysen and Pedersen[14,15] and later studied by us[16], seems to be related either to an increased BA synthesis rate, overloading the ileal transport system or to impaired intestinal absorption of a normal BA load, due probably to a defect in the carriers in the ileal mucosa.

The third type has been found in uraemic patients[17], patients on biguanydes therapy, though this second case has not been confirmed, and in cholecystectomy, possibly because of the increased recycling frequency of the BA pool.

Since ileal resection has been almost always found in association with changes in the enterohepatic circulation of bile acids at the level of intestinal absorption, two syndromes have been described, depending upon the length of the resection[10]:

(1) Bile acid diarrhoea: the increased concentration of bile acids in the colon induces diarrhoea in resections under 100 cm. In this syndrome usually none or slight steatorrhoea is present (8–20 g/day); BAM is present, and hepatic bile acid synthesis is increased[18] to maintain a normal or only slightly decreased jejunal bile acid concentration. The concentration of the bile acids in the faecal water is increased; in particular, dihydroxy bile acids are present in concentrations similar to those which have been shown to cause water and electrolyte secretion during colonic perfusion in man[19]. Cholestyramine[20] is considered to have abolished diarrhoea by binding BA, thus preventing their secretory effect in the colon. Although a cholestyramine-induced steatorrhoea may develop, this is usually of no caloric or symptomatic consequence[2].

(2) Fatty acid diarrhoea: in cases of resection over 100 cm, steatorrhoea is usually severe (〉20 g/day); bile acid malabsorption is severe and jejunal bile acid concentration is usually decreased, despite an increased BA synthesis rate. Because of a decreased bile acid secretion, the concentration of the BA in the faecal water of colonic content is normal and bile acids do not induce water secretion in the colon. In this case, hydroxy fatty acids may induce water and electrolyte secretion in the colon[22,23]. Cholestyramine treatment is of no sympto-

matic benefit; it increases steatorrhoea, causing significant caloric loss; long-chain triglycerides/medium-chain triglycerides exchange decreases both diarrhoea and steatorrhoea and is probably of caloric benefit[24,25].

The development of a bile supersaturated in cholesterol and hyperoxaluria are further disturbances in the syndrome of broken enterohepatic circulation of bile acids.

The reduced return of bile acids to the liver leads to a decreased bile acid secretion into bile; the hepatic BA synthesis rate increases, but, when the interruption of the EHC is severe (large ileal resections), it is not increased enough to maintain a secretion of BA able to solubilize biliary cholesterol: a lithogenic bile and cholesterol gallstones may develop.

As far as the high incidence of urinary oxalate stones in patients with ileal resection is concerned, several possible mechanisms for hyperoxaluria have been proposed. So far, the most reliable mechanism seems to be related to the amount of fatty acids malabsorbed in the colon, which bind calcium ions, leaving oxalate in solution available for absorption.

The two syndromes described by Hofmann do not seem, so far, completely separated, and results from our laboratory[26] seem to suggest that, in cases of very short ileal resection (40–50 cm), little, if any, BAM is present; in resection of about 100 cm, BAM is accounted for by almost only trihydroxy BAM, possibly because of the better intestinal conservation of dihydroxy BA, due to passive absorption in the small intestine and the colon. In these cases, a bile-acid mediated diarrhoea does not seem always possible, because few dihydroxy bile acids are malabsorbed.

When the EHC is more severely interrupted, i.e. in large resections, the malabsorbed dihydroxy BA may induce water and electrolyte secretion in the colon, and, when the jejunal concentration of the BA is reduced, fatty acid diarrhoea simultaneously develops.

In even larger ileal resections, both bile acids and fatty acids precipitate for the low intestinal pH and the diarrhoea is due to the great amount of fluids entering the colon.

Different techniques are so far available for measuring BAM.

BAM may be assessed by measuring the *fraction of ring-labelled bile acid* (usually taurocholate), excreted in stools, 24–48 hours after intravenous administration in fasting conditions[27-29].

Usually, only about 10% of the labelled trihydroxy BA is recovered from healthy subjects; this amount is severely increased in cases of interruption of the EHC. Since a trihydroxy BA, conjugated with taurine, is used, the test gives information about the impairment of active absorption; in fact, the very low taurocholic acid pK_a (1.8) makes the passive absorption of this moiety very unlikely.

The use of ring-labelled glycochenodeoxycholic acid may give information about the interruption of the dihydroxy BA circulation.

Principle of the test

The fraction of the ring-labelled BA is related to the fraction of the same endogenous BA not absorbed in the ileum.

If a ^{3}H-ring-labelled BA is used, a small part of radioactivity is removed by bacteria and converted to H_2O, which is absorbed and enters the body water[30]. Part of the labelled BA is deconjugated, and cholic acid or its bacterial product, deoxycholic acid, may be in part absorbed and in part reconjugated with glycine. The remaining [3H] radioactivity is lost with stools, the amount of which depends upon the completeness of colonic emptying.

The use of a non-absorbable faecal marker (usually $^{51}CrCl_3$) can assess the recovery of the test substance.

VALUE OF THE RING-LABELLED BA IN THE DIAGNOSIS OF BA MALABSORPTION

The test seems[31] to be sensitive and accurate, provided a faecal marker is used.

In fact, patients with diarrhoea, but not ileal disease, do not have BAM and the ratio of the BA radioactivity to the marker radioactivity differentiates them from patients with BAM.

$^{51}CrCl_3$ does not seem to behave ideally as a faecal marker, since it may precipitate, forming insoluble salts.

Polyethylene glycol (PEG 4000), a marker of the watery phase of stools, may be a better choice[32].

In most patients with BAM, *bile acid pool size* is reduced[33] and the fractional turnover rate is increased; it is technically difficult to measure the efficiency of the reabsorption in patients with BAM, because of the high fractional turnover rate, but the evaluation of the pool size by Lindstedt's technique may be successful, provided the duodenal bile sampling is obtained at very short time intervals.

BAM is also assessed by the [1-14] glycocholic acid test. The amide bond linking the steroid moiety to glycine may be cleaved by bacteria present in the small intestine, in cases of bacterial overgrowth, and in the colon, in healthy subjects.

The ^{14}C-glycine moiety, when released, is converted to $^{14}CO_2$, which promptly diffuses through the intestinal wall and is expired.

Increased deconjugation may occur both in cases of bacterial colonization of the small intestine and in cases of BAM in the small intestine, when great amounts of bile acids enter the colon.

The test, usually performed according to the method of Fromm and Hofmann[34] distinguishes between bacterial overgrowth and BAM, provided the combined breath $^{14}CO_2$ and faecal ^{14}C excretion test is performed (Figure 11.1).

The test is rapid, simple and safe, the radiation dose involved is comparable with that of a routine X-ray of the colon; it is less than that of a Shilling test.

175

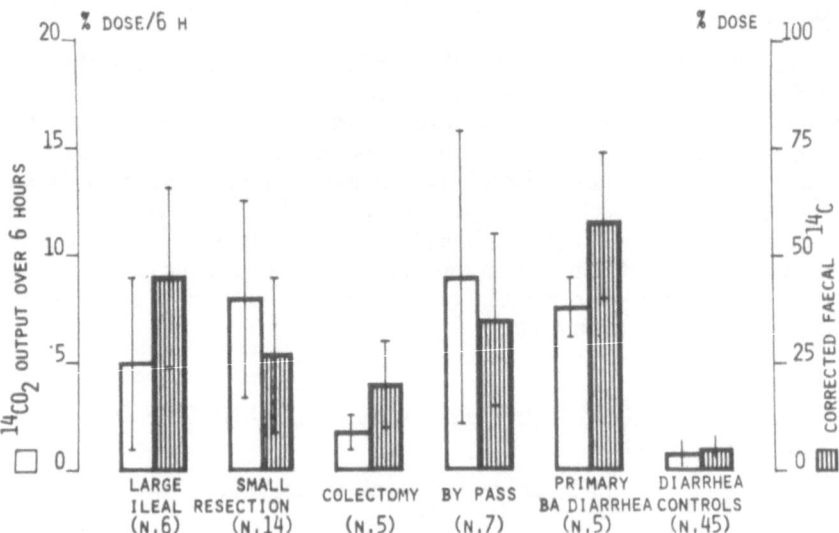

Figure 11.1 Cholyl-1-^{14}C glycine test in different groups of patients. N=No. of patients

Moreover, the biological half-life of [1-^{14}C] glycocholic acid is less than 5 days.

The breath-test, as well as the Shilling test, is influenced both by the mucosal function and by the interaction of the test substance with intestinal bacteria.

While a negative breath-test in cases of bacterial overgrowth must always be interpreted with caution and considered together with the ^{14}C faecal excretion. According to Fromm[35], the cholyl-1-^{14}C-glycine assay with combined measurements of breath and faecal ^{14}C is as sensitive as the ring-labelled taurocholic acid faecal excretion and more sensitive in detecting BAM, and more sensitive than the Shilling test in assessing ileal dysfunction.

In order to avoid as much as possible the influence of variations in the colonic emptying in the interpretation of the ^{14}C results, the use of a faecal marker is recommended[36]. Thaysen[36] suggested the use of carmine red, which is the best choice for out-patients. The marker can be used together with the test meal[37] or 24 hours after the beginning of the study[38].

Since the intestine is the major determinant of *serum bile acid levels*[39,40], in patients with normal liver function, and since the hepatic clearance seems independent from fasting and postprandial condition[39], serum BA levels have been regarded as a possible test of bile acid malabsorption[41].

The development of sensitive 'Radioimmunoassay techniques specific for classes of bile acids (conjugates chenodeoxycholic and cholic acids) made the easy determination of these BA in fasting and postprandial conditions possible as well as a better understanding of the two different enterohepatic circulation dynamics of tri- and dihydroxy bile acids[42] and their different extent of EHC interruption in ileal resections.

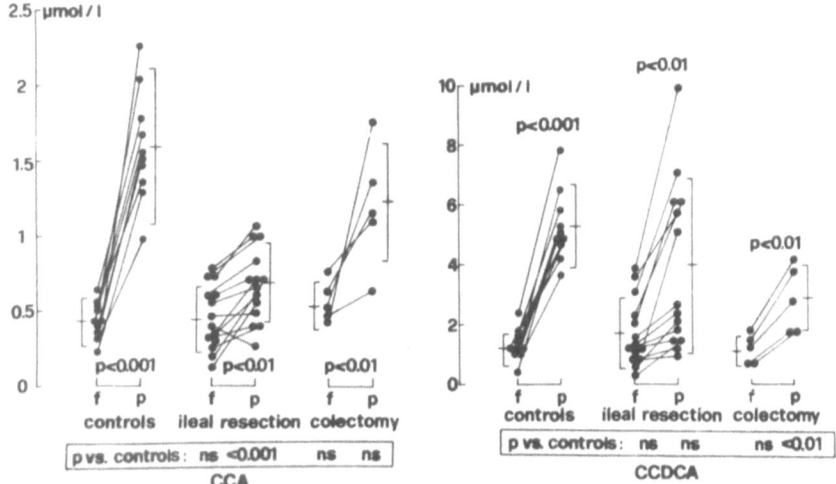

Figure 11.2 Diurnal variations of serum levels of cholic (CCA) and chenodeoxycholic (CCDCA) acid conjugates in patients with ileal resection

Cholic acid conjugates have been reported to be low in fasting patients with BAM[1] and their postprandial rises were found to be low and progressively diminishing with each meal[1]. Chenyl-conjugate value peaks after meals[43], however, were found lower but constant throughout the day in patients with BAM.

Data from our laboratory[41] seem to indicate that, in patients with BAM (positive 1-^{14}C-glycocholic acid test), serum fasting levels of chenodeoxycholic acid conjugates are normal, while cholic acid conjugates are low, mainly in patients with large ileal resection and more severe BAM.

Chenodeoxycholic acid postprandial peaks were found to be almost normal in patients with BAM, while cholic acid peaks were severely reduced, if not abolished by malabsorption (Figure 11.2); both cholic and chenodeoxycholic conjugates postprandial peaks inversely correlate with the respective acid faecal excretion. Moreover, recent studies indicate that a positive correlation is present between cholic acid pool size and cholic acid peaks after meals[44] in children with ileal resections.

These data further support the concept of a better intestinal absorption of dihydroxy BA in cases of ileal resections and indicate that cholic acid rises after meals closely parallel the degree of intestinal absorption impairment, and prove to be a more sensitive index of terminal ileum involvement than chenodeoxycholic acid ones, whilst chenodeoxycholic acid peaks may have a diagnostic significance in detecting colonic dysfunction.

Perfusion studies in the human colon[9] in fact have demonstrated that the rate of chenodeoxycholic acid absorption in the colon averages nine times that of cholate and that the colon may contribute significantly to the conservation of the dihydroxy bile acid pool, mainly in condition of BAM in the small intestine.

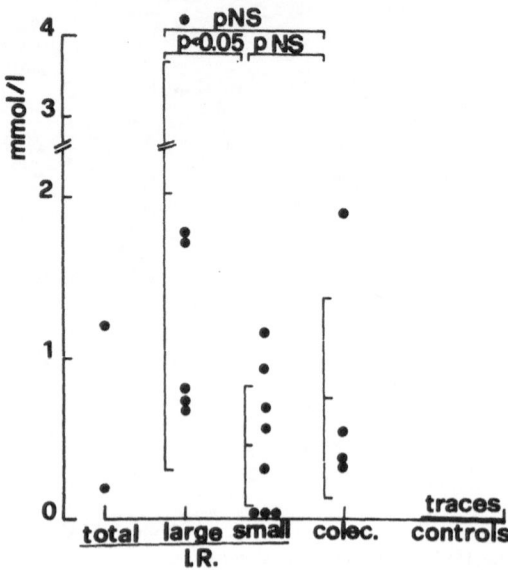

Figure 11.3 Faecal bile acids in patients with ileal resections and colectomy

Futhermore, recent studies[45,46] indicate that the determination of the *serum rises of glycocholic acid* after the oral administration of 1 g glycocholic acid may be clinically useful, the patients with BAM having very little or absent peaks within 5 hours from the ingestion of the BA.

The sensitivity and the specificity of the test, however, is still to be better evaluated. Similarly the serum ursodeoxycholic acid determination[47] after an oral load of the bile acid has been also proposed as a test of intestinal absorption, in patients without liver disease.

As well as the diagnosis of liver disease, also in the detection of intestinal malabsorption, the use of an exogenous BA oral load seems so far preferable to the endogenous BA load because such variables as gallbladder emptying intestinal transit, hepatic blood flow can be avoided.

Since the *daily bile acid faecal excretion* represents the hepatic daily synthesis of bile acids from cholesterol[1], the degree of interruption of the EHC of bile acids is paralleled by an increase in the hepatic synthesis rate and faecal bile acid excretion.

In healthy subjects, cholic acid synthesis is about twice that of chenodeoxycholic acid, because of the better intestinal conservation of the latter BA. In intestinal resections, the enterohepatic circulation of cholic acid is more severely interrupted than that of chenodeoxycholic acid and the daily synthesis of the former becomes about ten-fold higher than the latter one[26].

The daily bile acid faecal excretion is determined usually by gas–liquid chromatographic analysis[48], which provides quantitative and qualitative information of total and single faecal bile acids (Figure 11.3).

BAM does not mean bile acid diarrhoea: prerequisites of the occurrence of a bile acid mediated diarrhoea are: the presence of high amounts of secretory BA in the faecal content (dihydroxy BA malabsorption) and a pH value keeping these BA in solution[26].

The faecal pH is so far considered the major determinant of the dihydroxy BA concentrations in the faecal water[49]: from colonic intubation studies, chenodeoxycholic and cholic acid solubility in the faecal water has been found[26] to be quite similar to that reported by *in vitro* studies[50-52] and cheno appears slighty more soluble than deoxy.

Since small ileal resection appears to be associated with an alkaline pH, while in large resections the pH appears to become acidic, in large resections faecal bile acid precipitation prevents the bile acid diarrhoea[48].

Therefore, in large resections, the large amounts of fluids in the colon, *per se*, cause diarrhoea. Data from our laboratory[26] failed to find a close correlation between the pH value and the length of the resection; large resections were not always found associated with acidic pH; therefore in these cases, high amounts of dihydroxy bile acids were found in the faecal water.

The concentration of dihydroxy BA reported to have cathartic properties in man has been shown of the order of 1.5 mmol/l (1–3 mmol/l)[19]: this may be not exactly the same that is eventually found in the faecal water, since the actual concentration in the faecal water is the result of the dilution of the bile acids by the colonic secretion.

In spite of alkaline faecal pH, cheno and deoxy are in solution in a smaller percentage than should be expected: this may be accounted for by absorption of BA to fibres, nutrients or organic materials[48]. Once the bile acid malabsorption has been demonstrated, the evaluation of the dihydroxy BA in the faecal water is needed as well as the faecal BA pattern in order to ascertain the presence of a BA diarrhoea.

This information is usually achieved by the enzymatic determination of total BA in the faecal water, after ultracentrifugation at $100\,000\,g$[13] for 3 hours, combined with gas–liquid chromatography.

In healthy subjects, only deoxycholic and lithocholic acid are found in stools; in patients with BAM, primary BA are also present in large amounts.

Since primary BA are also present in patients with diarrhoea, without BAM, their presence has no diagnostic significance.

In patients with bile acid diarrhoea, cholestyramine administration abolishes diarrhoea, by binding the BA; though it is effective in the treatment of the diarrhoea, it induces fat maldigestion. Moreover, the EHC interruption may become more severe, leading to cholesterol gallstone formation.

In cases of fatty acid diarrhoea, the administration of medium-chain triglycerides instead of long-chain triglycerides improves steatorrhoea and is of metabolic benefit.

Neither of these therapies correct the bile acid deficiency in these patients[53,54], therefore a bile acid replacement therapy has been proposed.

Ursodeoxycholic acid, the 7-beta-epimer of chenodeoxycholic acid decreases cholesterol saturation in bile[55], is passively absorbed in the small intestine[56] and has no cathartic properties[57].

Therefore, when chronically administered to patients with ileal resection, it may reduce the diarrhoea by replacing the cathartic chenodeoxycholic acid, and meanwhile it may improve the cholesterol solubility in bile[58].

References

1. Small, D. M., Dowling, R. H. and Redinger, R. N. (1972). The enterohepatic circulation of bile salts. *Arch. Intern. Med.*, **130**, 552
2. Lack, L. and Weiner, I. M. (1936). Gastrointestinal bile salt transport: structure–activity relationships and other properties. *Am. J. Physiol.*, **210**, 1142
3. Schiff, E. R., Small, N. C. and Dietschy, J. M. (1972). Characterization of the kinetics of the passive and active transport mechanism for bile acid absorption in the small intestine and colon of the rat. *J. Clin. Invest.*, **51**, 1351
4. Hofmann, A. E. (1976). The enterohepatic circulation of bile acids in man. In Stolerman, G.H. (ed.) *Advances in Internal Medicine*. Vol. 21, p. 501. (Chicago: Yearbook Medical Publisher)
5. Wilson, F. A. and Dietschy, J. M. (1972). Characterization of bile acid absorption across the unstirred water layer and brush border of the rat jejunum. *J. Clin. Invest.*, **51**, 1351
6. Michaelis, L. and Menten, M. L. (1974). Der Kinetic der Invertinwirkung. *Biochemistry*, **249**, 333
7. Playoust, M. R. and Isselbacher, K. J. (1974). Studies on the transport and metabolism of conjugated bile salts by intestinal mucosa. *J. Clin. Invest.*, **43**, 467
8. Samuel, P., Saupol, G. M., Meilman, E., Mosbach, E. H. and Chafidazeh, M. (1968). Absorption of bile acids from the large bowel in man. *J. Clin. Invest.*, **47**, 2070
9. Mekhjian, H. S., Phillips, S. F. and Hofmann, A. F. (1979). Colonic absorption of unconjugated bile acids. Perfusion studies in man. *Dig. Dis. Sci.*, **24**, 545
10. Hofmann, A. F. (1972). Bile acid malabsorption caused by ileal resection. *Arch. Intern. Med.*, **130**, 597
11. Fromm, H. D., Farivar, H. and McJunkin, B. (1977). Type 3 bile acid malabsorption and diarrhoea. Evidence for a new clinical entity. *Gastroenterology*, **72**, 1060A.
12. Heaton, K.W. (1977). Disturbances of bile acid metabolism in intestinal disease. *Clin. Gastroenterol.*, **6**, 69
13. Hofmann, A. F. and Pooleu, J. R. (1972). Role of bile acid malabsorption in pathogenesis of diarrhoea and steatorrhoea in patients with ileal resection. I. response to cholestyramine or replacement of dietary long chain triglyceride. *Gastroenterology*, **62**, 918
14. Thaysen, E. H. and Pedersen, L. (1973). Diarrhoea associated with idiopathic bile acid malabsorption. Fact or fantasy? *Dan. Med. Bull.*, **20**, 174
15. Thaysen, E. H. and Pedersen, L. (1976). Idiopathic bile acid catharsis. *Gut*, **17**, 963
16. Aldini, R. *et al.* (1978). Primary cholerhoeic enteropathy. Presented at the *VI World Congress of Gastroenterology, Madrid, 1978.*
17. Gordon, S. J., Miller, L. J., Kinsley, M. D. and Kowlessar, O. D. (1976). Abnormal intestinal bile acid distribution in azotaemic man: a possible role in pathogenesis of uraemic diarrhoea. *Gut*, **13**, 415
18. Dowling, R. H., Mack, E. and Small, D. M. (1970). Effects of controlled interruption of the enterohepatic circulation of bile salts by biliary diversion and by ileal resection on bile salts, secretion, synthesis and pool size in the Rhesus monkey. *J. Clin. Invest.*, **49**, 232
19. Mekhjian, H. S., Phillips, S. F. and Hofmann, A. F. (1971). Colonic secretion of water and electrolytes induced by bile acids: perfusion studies in man. *J. Clin. Invest.*, **50**, 1569
20. Johns, W. H. and Bates, T. R. (1970). Quantification of the binding tendencies of cholestyramine, II. Mechanism of interaction with bile salt and fatty acid salt anions. *J. Pharm. Sci.*, **59**, 39
21. Hofmann, A. F. (1967). The syndrome of ileal disease and broken enterohepatic circulation: choleraic enteropathy. *Gastroenterology*, **52**, 752
22. James, A. T., Webb, J. P. W. and Kellock, T. D. (1961). The occurrence of unusual fatty acids in faecal lipids from human beings with normal and abnormal fat absorption. *Biochem. J.*, **78**, 333
23. Mastri, M. S., Goldblatt, L. A. and De Eds, F. (1962). Relation of cathartic activity to

structural modifications of ricinoleic acid of castor oil. *J. Pharm. Sci.*, **51**, 999

24. Greenberger, N. J., Ruppert, R. D. and Tzagaurnis, M. (1967). Use of medium chain triglycerides in malabsorption syndromes. *Ann. Intern. Med.*, **72**, 205

25. Zurier, R. B., Hashim, S. A. and Van Itallie, T. B. (1965). Effect of medium chain triglyceride on cholestyramine induced steatorrhoea in man. *Gastroenterology*, **49**, 490

26. Aldini, R. et al. (1981). Bile acid malabsorption and bile acid diarrhoea in intestinal resection. *Dig. Dis. Sci.* (in press)

27. Hofmann, A. F., Schoenfield, L. J. and Kohke, B. A. (1980). Method for the description of bile acid kinetics in man. *Meth. Med. Res.*, **12**, 149

28. Meihoff, W. E. and Kern, Fr. J. (1968). Bile salt malabsorption in regional ileitis, ileal resection, and mannitol induced diarrhoea. *J. Clin. Invest.*, **4**, 261

29. Stanley, M. M. and Memchausky, B. (1967). Faecal^{14}C bile acid excretion in normal subjects and patients with steroid-wasting syndromes secondary to ileal dysfunction. *J. Lab. Clin. Med.*, **70**, 627

30. Hepner, G. W. et al. (1973). Metabolism of steroid and aminoacid moieties of conjugated bile acids in man. III. Cholyltaurine (Taurocholic acid). *J. Clin. Invest.*, **52**, 433

31. Fromm, H., Thomas, P. J. and Hofmann, A. F. (1973). Sensitivity and specificity in tests of distal ileal function: prospective comparison of bile acid and vitamin B_{12} absorption in ileal resection patients. *Gastroenterology*, **64**, 1077

32. Wilkinson, R. (1971). Polyethylene glycol 4000 as a continuously administered nonabsorbable faecal marker for metabolic balance studies in human subjects. *Gut*, **12**, 654

33. Vantrappen, G., Ghoos, Y., Rutgeerts, P. and Janssens, J. (1977). Bile acid studies in uncomplicated Crohn's disease. *Gut*, **18**, 730

34. Fromm, H. and Hofmann, A. F. (1971). Breath-test for altered bile acid metabolism. *Lancet*, **ii**, 621

35. Fromm, H., Thomas, P. J. and Hofmann, A. F. (1973). Sensitivity and specificity in tests of distal ileal function: prospective comparison of bile acid and vitamin B_{12} absorption in ileal resection patients. *Gastroenterology*, **64**, 1077

36. Thaysen, E. H. (1977). Diagnostic value of the ^{14}C-cholylglycine breath-test. *Clin. Gastroenterol.*, **6**, 227

37. Roda, A. et al. (1977). Determination of ^{14}Co$_2$ in breath and ^{14}C in stool after oral administration of cholyl-l-^{14}C glycine: clinical application. *Clin. Chem.*, **23**, 2127

38. Lenz, K. (1975). An evaluation of the breath-test in Crohn's disease. *Scand. J. Gastroenterol.*, **10**, 655

39. LaRusso, N. F., Hoffman, N. E., Korman, M. G., Hofmann, A. F. and Cowen, A. E. (1978). Determinants of fasting and postprandial serum bile acid levels in healthy man. *Dig. Dis.*, **23**, 385

40. LaRusso, N. F., Korman, M. G., Hoffman, N. E. and Hofmann, A. F. (1974). Dynamics of the enterohepatic circulation of bile acids. *N. Engl. J. Med.*, **291**, 689

41. Aldini, R. et al. (1983). Diagnostic value of serum primary bile acids in detecting bile acid malabsorption. *Gut* (in press)

42. Angelin, B. and Bjokem, I. (1977). Postprandial serum bile acids in healthy man. Evidence for differences in absorptive pattern between individual bile acids. *Gut*, **18**, 606

43. Schalm, S. W. et al. (1978). Diurnal serum levels of primary conjugated bile acids. Assessment by specific radioimmunoassays for conjugates of cholic and chenodeoxycholic acid. *Gut*, **19**, 1006

44. Henbi, J. E., Balistrieri, W. F., Partin, J. C., Schubert, W. K. and Suchy, F. J. (1980). Enterohepatic circulation of bile acids in infants and children with ileal resection. *J. Lab. Clin. Med.*, **95**, 231

45. Matern, S. and Gerok, W. (1977). Specific radioimmunoassays for separate determination of unconjugated cholic acid, conjugated cholic acid and conjugated deoxycholic acid in serum and their clinical application. In *Radioimmunoassay and related procedures in medicine, 1977*, Vol. II, pp. 273-283. (Vienna: Internal Atomic Energy Agency)

46. Matern, S. and Gerok, W. (1979). Pathophysiology of the enterohepatic circulation of bile acids. *Rev. Physiol. Biochem. Pharmacol.*, **85**, 125

47. Ohkubo, H. (1981). Ursodeoxycholic acid tolerance test in patients with constitutional hyperbilirubinemias and effect of phenobarbital. *Gastroenterology*, **81**, 120

48. Grundy, S. M., Ahrens, E. H. and Miettinen, T. A. (1965). Quantitative isolation of

gas–liquid chromatographic analysis of total faecal bile acids. *J. Lipid Res.*, **6**, 3º7

49. Mejunkin, B., Fromm, H., Sarva, R. P. and Amin, P. (1981). Factors in the mechanism of diarrhoea in bile acid malabsorption: faecal pH. A key determinant. *Gastroenterology*, **60**, 1454

50. Small, D. M. (1971). The physical chemistry of cholanic acids. In Nairr, P. P. and Kritchevsky, D. (eds.) *The Bile Acids Chemistry, Physiology and Metabolism*, pp. 1-249. (New York-London: Plenum Press)

51. Hofmann, A. F. (1977). Bile acids, diarrhoea and antibiotics: data, speculation and a unifying hypothesis. *J. Infect. Dis.*, **135**, S126

52. Igimi, H. and Carey, M. C. (1980). pH solubility relations of chenodeoxycholic and ursodeoxycholic acids: physical–chemical basis for dissimilar solution and membrane phenomena. *J. Lipid Res.*, **27**, 72

53. Hofmann, A. F. and Grundy, S. M. (1965). Abnormal bile salt metabolism in a patient with extensive lower intestinal resection. *Clin. Res.*, **13**, 254 (Abstract)

54. Hardison, W. G. H. and Rosenberg, I. H. (1967). Bile salt deficiency in the steatorrhoea following resection of the ileum and proximal colon. *N. Engl. J. Med.*, **277**, 337

55. Makino, I., Shinozaki, K. and Yoshino, K. (1875). Dissolution of cholesterol gallstones by ursodeoxycholic acid. *Jpn. J. Gastroenterol.*, **72**, 690

56. Krag, G. and Phillips, S. F. (1974). Active and passive absorption in man: perfusion studies of the ileum and jejunum. *J. Clin. Invest.*, **53**, 1686

57. Chadwick, V. S., Gaginella, T. S. and Carlson, C. L. (1979). Effect of molecular structure on bile acid induced alterations in absorptive function, permeability and morphology in the perfused rabbit colon. *J. Lab. Clin. Med.*, **94**, 661

58. LaRusso, N. F. and Thistle, J. (1981). Ursodeoxycholic acid ingestion after ileal resection. Effect on biliary bile acid and lipid composition. *Dig. Dis. Sci.*, **26**, 705

12
The role of bile acids in intestinal absorption of cholesterol

NICHOLAS F. LaRUSSO

INTRODUCTION

Although chronic administration of chenodeoxycholic acid (CDCA) and ursodeoxycholic acid (UDCA) has been shown to dissolve cholesterol gallstones, the mechanism of this effect is unclear. Since diminished hepatic cholesterol secretion results from administration of each of these bile acids and is a prerequisite for their litholytic effect, any hypothesis explaining bile acid-induced gallstone dissolution must account for a diminution in hepatic cholesterol secretion. Possible explanations for suppression of hepatic cholesterol secretion by bile acids include inhibition of hepatic cholesterol synthesis and suppression of intestinal cholesterol absorption.

Studies addressing each of these hypotheses have generated data which often have little or only indirect relevance and, in some cases, are conflicting. For example, although both bile acids inhibit the hepatic activity of HMGCo-A-reductase, the rate-limiting enzyme of cholesterol synthesis, such inhibition may have little effect on the amount of cholesterol secreted in bile because most biliary cholesterol probably originates from a preformed pool of non-newly synthesized lipid. Moreover, large alterations in hepatic activity of this enzyme may not be accompanied by changes in biliary cholesterol secretion.

More relevant to the topic of this review are data concerning the effect of litholytic bile acids on cholesterol absorption. No effect of CDCA on cholesterol absorption has been observed in animals and man by some investigators, while other workers report that CDCA inhibits intestinal UDCA absorption of cholesterol. Two studies have evaluated the effect of UDCA on intestinal absorption of cholesterol; results of one showed significant inhibition, while results of the other showed no effect. Thus, although administration of CDCA and UDCA is known to dissolve cholesterol gallstones, the mechanism whereby these litholytic bile acids suppress hepatic cholesterol secretion continues to be obscure, and the role of altered cholesterol absorption in the dissolution process remains uncertain.

With this background, I will address the normal mechanisms whereby cholesterol is absorbed by the intestine, review the methods for measuring cholesterol absorption in man, survey the data relevant to the effect of bile acid administration on intestinal absorption of cholesterol, and discuss the complex relationships among cholesterol absorption, biliary cholesterol secretion, and gallstone dissolution.

CHOLESTEROL ABSORPTION

Cholesterol is a non-polar lipid that is insoluble in aqueous systems (Figure 12.1). Virtually all cells are capable of synthesizing cholesterol, but chemical degradation of cholesterol to bile acids occurs exclusively in the hepatocyte, and biliary excretion of cholesterol is the major mechanism by which the body disposes of excess cholesterol.

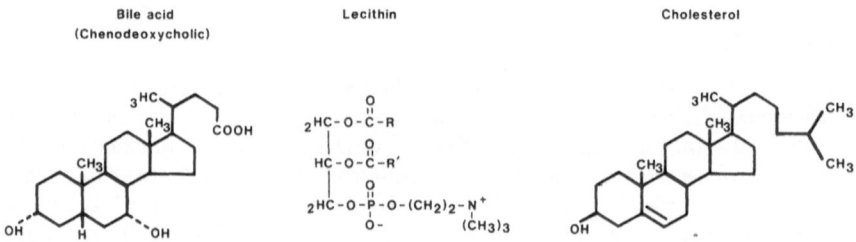

Figure 12.1 Chemical structure of biliary lipids

Cholesterol absorption occurs in the upper small intestine, and intestinal cholesterol is derived from exogenous and endogenous sources. Exogenous or dietary cholesterol has no nutritional value, and, although variable, the average dietary cholesterol intake in developed countries is 500–1000 mg/day. The proportion of dietary cholesterol present as free cholesterol or cholesterol ester is also variable but usually in the range of 90% free cholesterol and 10% cholesterol esterified with fatty acid. Endogenous cholesterol is derived from several sources, but biliary excretion provides the major input of endogenous cholesterol into the intestine. Secretion studies using marker-dilution techniques indicate that about 2 g/day of cholesterol is secreted by the liver into the intestine. Total cholesterol absorption appears to be directly related to the total (endogenous plus exogenous) input of cholesterol into the intestine. Increasing cholesterol intake results in greater cholesterol uptake although the percentage absorbed may be less. Thus cholesterol absorption is relatively, not absolutely, fixed.

Cholesterol absorption can conveniently be divided into four stages: intraluminal events, entry into absorptive cell, intracellular processing, and exit from mucosal cells.

Intraluminal events are initiated by the conversion of cholesterol esters to free cholesterol, a reversible enzymatic reaction catalysed by pancreatic cholesterol ester hydrolase (also called cholesterol esterase). This reaction requires bile acids, which probably act as co-factors, protect the enzyme against proteolysis, and favour the direction of de-esterification. Free cholesterol is then incorporated into micelles composed of bile acids and lipolytic products of triglyceride digestion (monoglyceride and fatty acids) (Figure 12.2). Bile acids are amphipathic molecules which facilitate cholesterol absorption by dispersing lipolytic products in micellar forms. For micellar solubilization, the bile acid concentration must be above their critical micellar concentration (CMC) which is approximately 2 mmol/l. Micellar dispersion increases the entry of fat into the absorptive cell by increasing the concentration of lipolytic products in the aqueous phase about 1000 times. Moreover, since the flux through the 'unstirred layer' on the mucosal surface of intestinal absorptive cells is a product of the concentration and the diffusion rate, micellar solubilization increases the flux through the aqueous phase at least 100 times. Cholesterol has low solubility in micelles composed of bile acids alone, but dissolves relatively well in bile-acid–fatty-acid–monoglyceride micelles, since it can pack between the liquid hydrocarbon chains of the lipolytic products. Indeed, at a fixed bile acid concentration the solubility of cholesterol increases in proportion to the concentration of lipolytic products.

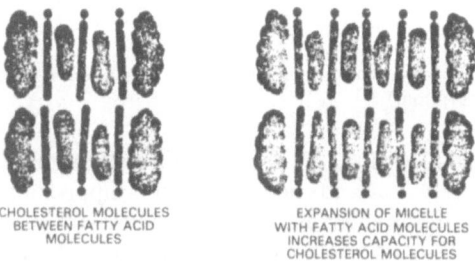

CHOLESTEROL MOLECULES
BETWEEN FATTY ACID
MOLECULES

EXPANSION OF MICELLE
WITH FATTY ACID MOLECULES
INCREASES CAPACITY FOR
CHOLESTEROL MOLECULES

Figure 12.2 Structure of mixed micelle (From AGA Undergraduate Teaching Project, Unit V, Lipid Digestion and Absorption.)

The precise mechanism whereby cholesterol enters the absorptive cell is not known. Uptake probably occurs from a true molecular solution which is kept saturated by cholesterol molecules moving out of the micelle (Figure 12.3). The micelle may also collide with the plasma membrane but is probably not absorbed.

After entry, intracellular processing of cholesterol occurs after free cholesterol is transported by an unknown mechanism, perhaps a cytosolic protein, to the endoplasmic reticulum for re-esterification by a mucosal cell cholesterol esterase with properties similar to those of pancreatic cholesterol ester hydrolase. Esterified cholesterol is then incorporated into chylomicrons (Figure 12.4) and very low density lipoproteins, probably within the Golgi.

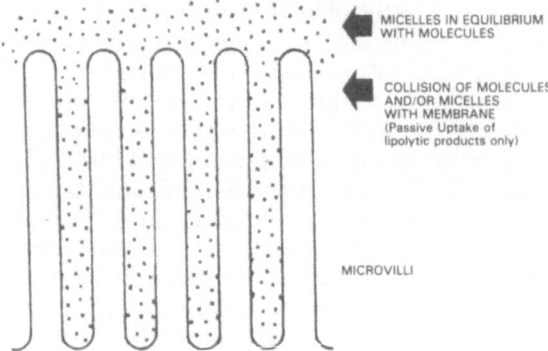

Figure 12.3 Uptake of lipolytic products (From AGA Undergraduate Teaching Project, Unit V, Lipid Digestion and Absorption.)

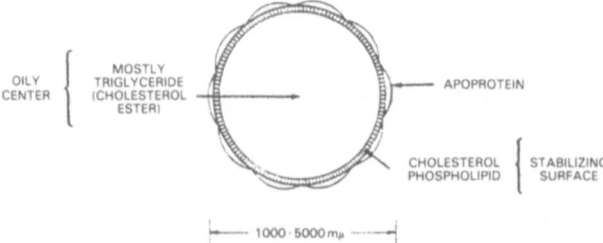

Figure 12.4 Structure of chylomicrons (From AGA Undergraduate Teaching Project, Unit V, Lipid Digestion and Absorption.)

The former are large (800–5000 Å), triglyceride-rich (approximately 90%), protein- (approximately 2%) and cholesterol-poor (approximately 5%) lipoproteins synthesized in the intestine, while the latter are smaller (30–80 Å), triglyceride-rich (60%) lipoproteins containing more protein (approximately 10%) and cholesterol (approximately 15%) and synthesized in both the intestine and liver.

Cholesterol exits from the mucosal cell via these lipoprotein vehicles which pass across the lateral borders of the enterocytes to enter intracellular spaces from which they diffuse into laterals. Chylomicrons travel via intestinal lymphatics into the cysterni chyli and then into the superior vena cava via the thoracic duct.

ROLE OF BILE ACIDS IN CHOLESTEROL ABSORPTION

Bile acids play a vital role in cholesterol absorption, probably at each of the steps outlined above. This is most dramatically demonstrated by the fact that complete bile diversion results in nearly complete cessation of cholesterol absorption.

During the intraluminal events of cholesterol absorption, bile acids, in conjunction with the lipolytic products of triglyceride digestion, solubilize free cholesterol into mixed-lipid micelles. In addition, bile acids are essential for the proper function of pancreatic cholesterol ester hydrolase, probably by at least two mechanisms. First, they may act as co-factors by enhancing the activity of this enzyme independently of their solubilizing properties. Moreover, different bile acids have different capacities for stimulating pancreatic cholesterol ester hydrolase; the trihydroxy bile acids are the most effective. Second, bile acids protect cholesterol ester hydrolase from proteolytic degradation by chymotrypsin.

Bile acids may also influence the intracellular processing of free cholesterol once it has entered the mucosal cell. For example, diversion of bile reduces the esterifying capacity of the intestine. Also, it has been suggested that bile acids may enhance the transport of mucosal chylomicrons into lymph.

METHODS FOR MEASURING CHOLESTEROL ABSORPTION IN MAN

There are a variety of established and validated methods for measuring cholesterol absorption in man, some of which are briefly summarized in Table 12.1. Most methods employ cholesterol radiolabelled with ^{3}H, ^{14}C or both. Other techniques have also been employed by particular investigators, but this table identifies those most commonly used. Each method has its strengths and weaknesses and no single method is clearly superior with respect to both accuracy and precision. The most appropriate method depends on the specific hypothesis being tested or the particular question being asked, the familiarity of the investigator with the individual techniques, and the facilities available. In many circumstances the precision or reproducibility of the method may be more important than the absolute accuracy, such as situations in which the effect of a particular drug or dietary regimen is being compared with a placebo. Ideally, more than one technique should be employed whenever conveniently possible.

CHOLESTEROL ABSORPTION AND GALLSTONE DISEASES

As reviewed earlier, bile acids clearly are major determinants of cholesterol absorption in man at a variety of levels. Moreover, everyone agrees that different bile acids may affect cholesterol absorption differently. For example, deoxycholic acid has been shown to inhibit cholesterol absorption by several groups of investigators, whereas cholic acid probably stimulates cholesterol absorption. Nevertheless, unresolved questions exist concerning the mechanism(s) whereby different bile acids affect cholesterol absorption differently, the relationships between alterations in intestinal cholesterol absorption and biliary cholesterol secretion induced by different bile acids, and the effect of litholytic bile acids on cholesterol absorption.

Little information is available on the possible mechanisms whereby bile acids might affect cholesterol absorption. As reviewed earlier, they could in-

BILE ACIDS IN GASTROENTEROLOGY

Table 12.1 Methods for measuring cholesterol absorption in man*

Designation	Material(s) administered	Administration regimen	Analyses	Determination	Representative results	Comments	References
I†	XOL	i.v., once	Faeces: neutral sterol mass and Plasma: XOL SA	Daily variation in mass absorbed	Mean: 250 mg/day Range:100–400 mg/day	Total stool collections required	1
II†	XOL	PO multiple	As above	As above	Mean: 580 mg/day Range: 300–700 mg/day	As above	1
III†	XOL	PO, multiple until 'steady-state'	As above	As above	Mean:≈ 175 mg/day ≈ 100 mg/day	Months to reach steady state	1
IV†	Radioactive beta-sitosterol	PO, once	Faeces: neutral sterol separation and isotope ratio	% absorption	Mean: 615 mg/day Range: 230–775 mg/day	Total stool collections required	1
V†	[³H]XOL [¹⁴C]XOL	i.v., once PO, multiple	Faeces: neutral sterol mass and SA	Daily variation in mass absorbed	—	Suitable only for specific situations (e.g., rapid XOL synthesis)	2
VI‡	[³H]XOL [¹⁴C]XOL	i.v., once PO, once	Plasma: radioactivity	% absorption	Mean: 42% Range: 16–63%	No indication of mass of XOL absorbed	3
VII†	XOL	Duodenal tube, hours	Bile: neutral sterol secretion	Mass absorbed	—	Quantitates endogenous and exogenous XOL absorbed	4
VIII†	XOL Radioactive beta-sitosterol	PO, multiple	Faeces: neutral sterol separation and isotope ratio	Daily variation in % absorbed	Mean: 54% Range: 47–65%		5

*Modified from Reference 5.
†Requires metabolic ward conditions.
‡Suitable for outpatient studies.
XOL = Radioactive cholesterol; PO = by mouth; SA = specific activity.

188

fluence cholesterol absorption at any one of the several steps involved in the intraluminal and intracellular phases of cholesterol absorption. Other possible mechanisms include direct mucosal damage, alterations in intestinal transit time modifying the duration of exposure of cholesterol to the mucosal cell, or the absolute amount of trihydroxy bile acids present in the intestinal lumen. However, considerable data are available on the effect of different bile acids on both intestinal cholesterol absorption and hepatic cholesterol secretion. The results suggest no direct or clear-cut relationship between bile acid induced alterations in cholesterol absorption and biliary cholesterol secretion. For example, deoxycholic acid inhibits intestinal cholesterol absorption but has no effect on biliary cholesterol secretion. Similarly, cholic acid stimulates cholesterol secretion but also does not affect biliary cholesterol secretion. These data suggest that, if a relationship does exist between bile acid induced changes in cholesterol absorption and biliary cholesterol secretion, the relationship is complex and other factors (e.g., direct effects of individual bile acids on hepatic lipoprotein and cholesterol metabolism) are probably involved.

At the present time, the effect of litholytic bile acids (CDCA and UDCA) on cholesterol absorption in man is controversial (Table 12.2). Most, but not all, investigators have observed no effect of CDCA on cholesterol absorption when given in doses sufficient to cause both decreased cholesterol saturation in bile and gallstone dissolution. Less data exist on the effect of UDCA on intestinal cholesterol absorption in man; one study found no effect, while another found a significant diminution of cholesterol absorption after UDCA administration. The reasons for these differences are not apparent; different methodology, different dose regimens, and different patient populations may all contribute.

Although the relationships among absorption of cholesterol, secretion of biliary cholesterol, and plasma cholesterol levels are complex and although

Table 12.2 Effect of litholytic bile acids on cholesterol absorption in man

Reference	Results
Chenodeoxycholic acid:	
6	Inconclusive
7	No effect
8	Decreased
9	No effect
10	No effect
11	No effect
12	No effect
Ursodeoxycholic acid:	
13	Decreased
12	No effect

controversy continues regarding the effect of litholytic bile acids on absorption of cholesterol, several generalizations seem appropriate. First, it seems likely that at least some agents that lower serum cholesterol levels by inhibiting absorption of cholesterol do not concurrently alter secretion of biliary cholesterol. This suggests that such drugs, compared with agents that decrease serum lipid levels by different mechanisms (for example, clofibrate), are unlikely to be associated with bile saturated with cholesterol or with an increased incidence of cholesterol cholelithiasis. Second, attempts at dissolution of cholesterol gallstones by agents whose only effect is to inhibit absorption of cholesterol are unlikely to be fruitful, in as much as no predictable correlation seems to exist between pharmacologically induced changes in the absorption of cholesterol and the concentration of cholesterol in bile. Finally, a thorough description of the mechanism or mechanisms whereby litholytic agents unsaturate bile requires techniques that concomitantly measure secretion of biliary cholesterol, absorption of cholesterol, and synthesis of cholesterol in a homogeneous group of patients.

Further reading

Reviews
Treadwell, C. R. and Vanhouny, G. V. (1968). Cholesterol absorption. In *Handbook of Physiology – Alimentary Canal, III*, 1407
Freidman, H. I. and Nylund, B. (1980). Intestinal fat digestion, absorption and transport: A review. *Am. J. Clin. Nutr.*, **33**, 1108
Holt, P. R. (1972). The roles of bile acids during the process of normal fat and cholesterol absorption. *Arch. Intern. Med.*, **130**, 574

Bile Acids and Cholesterol Absorption
Andersen, J. M. (1979). Chenodeoxycholic acid desaturates bile – but how? *Gastroenterology*, **77**, 1146

References

1. Quintao, E., Grundy, S. M. and Ahrens, E. H. Jr. (1971). An evaluation of four methods for measuring cholesterol absorption by the intestine in man. *J. Lipid Res.*, **12**, 221
2. Sodhi, H. S., Kudchodkar, B. J., Varghese, P. and Duncan, D. (1974). Validation of the ratio method for calculated absorption of dietary cholesterol in man. *Proc. Soc. Exp. Biol.*, **145**, 107
3. Samuel, P., Crouse, J. R. and Ahrens, E. H. Jr. (1978). Evaluation of an isotope ratio method for measurement of cholesterol in man. *J. Lipid Res.*, **19**, 82
4. Grundy, S. M. and Mok, H. Y. I. (1977). Determination of cholesterol absorption in man by intestinal perfusion. *J. Lipid Res.*, **18**, 263
5. Crouse, J. R. and Grundy, S. M. (1978). Evaluation of a continuous isotope feeding method for measurement of cholesterol absorption in man. *J. Lipid Res.*, **19**, 967
6. Adler, R. D. Bennion, L. J., Duane, W. C. and Grundy, S. M..(1975). Effects of low dose chenodeoxycholic acid feeding on biliary lipid metabolism. *Gastroenterology*, **68**, 326
7. Tangedahl, T. N., Thistle, J. L., Hofmann, A. F. and Matseshe, J. W. (1979). Effect of β-sitosterol alone or in combination with chenic acid on cholesterol saturation of bile and cholesterol absorption in gallstone patients. *Gastroenterology*, **76**, 1341

8. Ponz de Leon, M., Carulli, N., Loria, P., Iori, R. and Zironi, F. (1979). The effect of chenodeoxycholic acid (CDCA) on cholesterol absorption. *Gastroenterology*, **77**, 223
9. Einarsson, K. and Grundy, S. M. (1980). Effects of feeding cholic and chenodeoxycholic acid on cholesterol absorption and hepatic secretion of biliary lipids in man. *J. Lipid Res.*, **21**, 23
10. Mok, H. Y. I. and Grundy, S. M. (1980). Cholesterol and bile acid absorption during bile acid therapy in obese subjects undergoing weight reduction. *Gastroenterology*, **78**, 62
11. Sama, C. and LaRusso, N. F. (1982). Effect of deoxycholic, chenodeoxycholic, and cholic acids on intestinal absorption of cholesterol in humans. *Mayo Clin. Proc.*, **57**, 44
12. LaRusso, N. F. and Thistle, J. (1983). The effect of litholytic bile acids on cholesterol absorption in gallstone patients. *Gastroenterology*, **84**, 265
13. Ponz de Leon. M., Carulli, N., Loria, P., Iori, R. and Zironi, F. (1980). Cholesterol absorption during bile acid feeding: effect of ursodeoxycholic acid (UDCA) administration. *Gastroenterology*, **78**, 214

13
Physiological immaturity of the enterohepatic circulation of bile acids

W. F. BALISTRERI, F. J. SUCHY, J. E. HEUBI AND W. M. BELKNAP

Biliary flow is directly dependent upon the adequate synthesis, conjugation, secretion, and recirculation of bile acids[1-3]. Efficient transport of bile acids is central to the biliary elimination of many endogenous and exogenous compounds since they are the main determinants of bile flow in the mature animal[4]. At birth the newborn can no longer depend upon placental excretory function, and during the transition from fetal to an extrauterine existence progressive maturation of the liver and gastrointestinal tract must occur. Inefficiency of normal physiological events such as bile secretion and fat digestion are the consequences of faulty adaptation to these new demands[5,6].

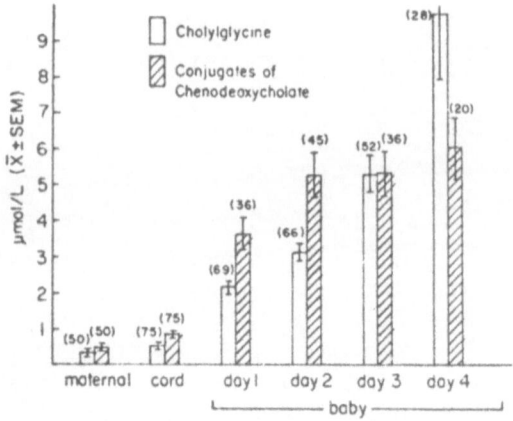

Figure 13.1 Serum concentrations of cholyglycine and conjugates of chenodeoxycholate in maternal and cord sera and from neonates during the first 4 days of life. (Numbers in parentheses indicate the number of subjects in each group.)

192

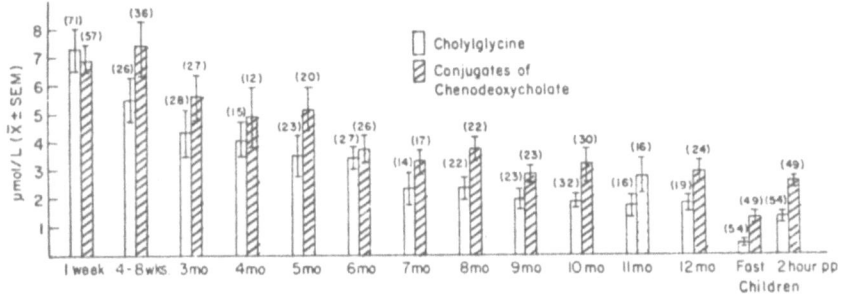

Figure 13.2 Serum concentrations of cholylglycine and conjugates of chenodeoxycholate during the first year of life.

Our previous investigation of the normal human adaptation of hepatic function to extrauterine life led to the observation that the serum concentrations of the conjugated primary bile acids are elevated in both the fasting and postprandial state in the human infant (Figures 13.1 and 13.2)[3]. This has provided indirect evidence of immature hepatic excretory function in normal infants.

In order to assess further the ontogeny of the enterohepatic circulation a suitable animal model was sought. It is known that in the rat there is a temporary period of morphological cholestasis in the first few days of life[7,8]. We therefore sought to define the interrelationship of the various steps of bile acid metabolism in the rat.

METHODS

Animal Model

The subject of our studies was the Sprague–Dawley rat killed throughout various phases of development into adult life. Fetal animals were obtained by Caesarean-section on day 21 and 22 of fetal life, and postnatal animals were studied at various intervals (e.g. 1, 4, 7, 10, 14, 21, 28, 42 and 56 days of age). This allowed us to measure and correlate with age several parameters of bile acid metabolism and the enterohepatic circulation.

Analyses

Serum bile acid concentration – Specifically, the concentration of total conjugates of cholic acid, the main bile acid found in this species, were measured in serum obtained from fetal, suckling, weaning and adult Sprague–Dawley rats using a sensitive and specific radioimmunoassay[9].

Bile acid pool size – The total pool of bile acids was estimated by excising the entire liver and gastrointestinal tract followed by homogenization, extraction and analysis of the bile acid content by gas chromatographic methods[10].

Bile acid uptake (hepatic) – Taurocholate uptake was assessed in hepatocytes isolated from rats of various ages throughout development. Hepatocytes were isolated by *in situ* collagenase perfusion. After preincubation (20 minutes at 37 °C), 2.0 ml of the cell suspension were incubated with [14C] taurocholate and varying concentrations of bile acids ranging from 5 to 200 μmol/l, and the uptake of taurocholate was assessed following microcentrifugation[11].

Bile Acid Conjugation – We studied conjugation of cholic acid in hepatocytes isolated by either collagenase digestion of fetal/neonatal rat liver slices or by *in vivo* collagenase perfusion in older rats[12,13]. Tracer unconjugated [14C] cholic acid was incubated with viable cells and the extent of conjugation measured at 30 minute intervals (for 3 hours) by TLC of the ethanol-NH_4 extract of the suspension. Biotransformation to the taurine (or glycine) conjugates was calculated from the fraction of the radioactivity eluted from each band.

Bile Acid Uptake (Intestinal) – Intestinal bile acid uptake was assessed using the villous technique developed by Heubi and Fondacaro[14]. Segments of jejunum and ileum were obtained from various aged animals and incubated for 2 minutes in Krebs–Ringer *bicarbonate* buffer with glucose (pH 7.4) at 37 °C with 14C-labelled taurocholate and various concentrations (0.1–3.5 mmol/l) of unlabelled bile acid. The segment was subsequently washed, freeze-dried and the villi chipped and weighed. The radioactivity was assessed and uptake per gram of dry weight was calculated.

RESULTS

Serum Bile Acids

The bile acid concentration obtained in serum from rats at various ages are shown in Figure 13.3[9]. Fetal serum bile acid levels were low, approximately 1–2 μmol/l, probably reflecting minimal enterohepatic circulation *in utero* and possible short circuiting by placental transport. The concentration of bile acids in serum rose abruptly with birth and the initiation of suckling, suggesting an inefficient hepatic extraction of the bile acids present in the increased portal blood flow in addition to an impairment of biliary secretion. There was a subsequent progressive rise in cholyl conjugate concentrations throughout the suckling and weaning phase, with levels approaching those noted in adult rats with induced cholestasis[12,15]. Following weaning at 21 days, there was a dramatic peak in bile acid concentrations to approximately 22 μmol/l; values then fell to achieve adult normal values by 56 days of age.

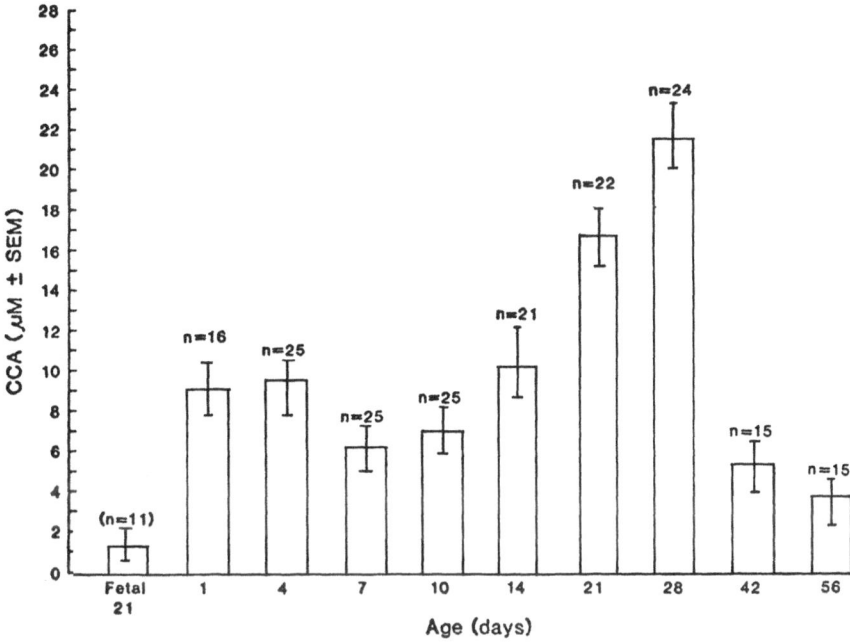

Figure 13.3 Serum concentration of conjugates of cholate (CCA) in developing rats (n = number of animals in each group)

Bile Acid Pool Size

The total bile acid pool size at various phases of development were found to increase directly with age, there was a progressive expansion of pool size from under 50 µg/(g body weight) to a value of over 500 µg/(g body weight) by the time adult life was reached (Figure 13.4).

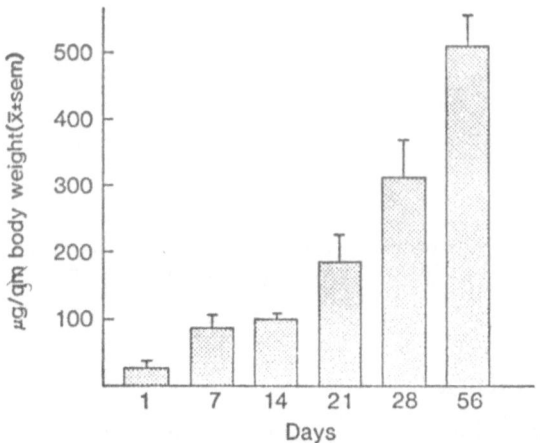

Figure 13.4 Bile acid pool size in developing rats

Hepatic Uptake

To define developmental changes in bile acid metabolism further, we determined the kinetics of taurocholate uptake by hepatocytes isolated from rats at 7, 14, 21, 28 and 56 days of age. There was a progressive increase in taurocholate uptake with age (Figure 13.5)[11]. The uptake process exhibited saturable kinetics in every age group with a maximum uptake velocity obtained above a taurocholate concentration of 200 μmol/l. There were no differences in K_m values but V_{max} increased progressively between 7 and 56 days of age (Figure 13.6). Comparable K_m values for the uptake process indicate that hepatocyte affinity for taurocholate remains constant during development whereas the rise in V_{max} with postnatal age may reflect an increase in the number of binding sites for bile acids.

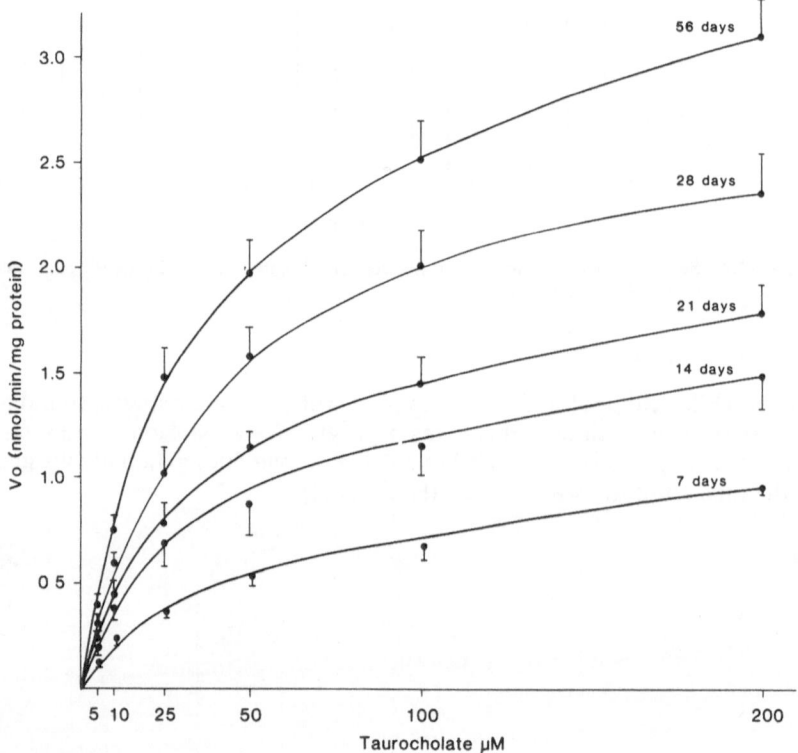

Figure 13.5 Initial velocity of taurocholate uptake (V_0) plotted against substrate concentration for hepatocytes isolated from developing rats. Each circle represents the mean ± SE of data obtained from six animals

Bile Acid Conjugation

The conjugation of bile acids favourably alters their physio-chemical properties, allowing optimal participation in bile flow, solubilization of dietary lipid and conservation by ileal active transport. The capacity to conjugate cholic acid was not fully developed in hepatocytes isolated from fetal and suckling rats[13]. Conjugation was most impaired in the fetal liver at a time when other metabolic processes such as protein synthesis were increased in comparison with the mature animal. There was a rapid maturation of conjugation at weaning. The increase was proportional to body weight and was fully developed by 2 months of age. Taurocholate was the predominant conjugate in every age group.

Intestinal Uptake

Jejunal uptake of taurocholate was linear with respect to bile acid concentration in the incubation media and was similar in all age groups studied. However, in ileal segments isolated from adult rats there was a demonstrable saturable process[16]. In contrast, in animals studied at 1 week of age both ileal and jejunal uptake were linear. Similar curves were obtained in 2-week-old animals. Active transport was not demonstrable until 3 weeks of age when saturation kinetics for ileal uptake were first observed (Table 13.1). Ileal active transport kinetics were determined by subtracting jejunal from ileal uptake. The K_m remained unchanged after 3 weeks; however, the V_{max} was highest at 3 weeks and declined thereafter. As was also demonstrated in the hepatocyte, binding affinity was constant; however, binding sites per unit ileal weight declined after 3 weeks. Age-related differences in permeability may not serve to facilitate bile acid recycling before the development of ileal active transport.

Table 13.1 Postnatal development of ileal bile acid transport in the rat

Age at time of study (weeks):	1 (n=18)	2 (n=26)	3 (n=19)	4 (n=15)	Adult (n=15)
Monomeric permeability coefficient (P_{app}) $(\mu mol\,min^{-1}(mg\,dry\,weight)^{-1}mmol^{-1}$	0.26	0.27	0.22	0.27	0.44
Maximal transport velocity (V_{app}) $(\mu mol\,min^{-1}mg\,(dry\,weight)^{-1}$	0	0	13.14	9.81	9.61
Michaelis constant (K_m) (mmol)	0	0	0.37	0.48	0.46

CONCLUSIONS

In early life there is an immaturity of the enterohepatic circulation. The serum bile acid concentration both in rats and in humans are elevated; these studies demonstrate that in the rat this occurs when bile acid pool size is diminished and ileal active transport is negligible (Table 13.2). This suggests that impaired hepatic clearance and/or impaired secretion is the major limit-

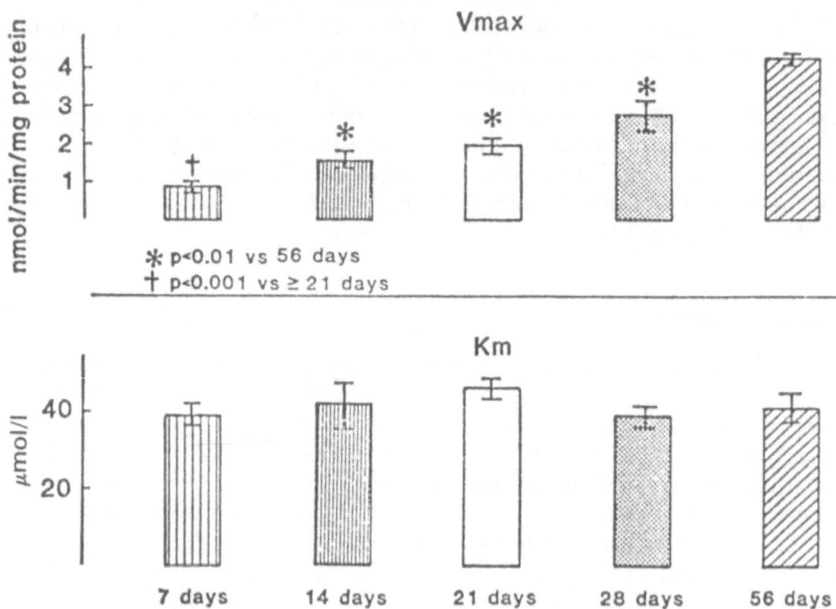

Figure 13.6 Rate constants for uptake of taurocholate by hepatocytes isolated from developing rats. Each bar represents the mean±SE of data obtained from six animals

ing factor at this time of life. This hypothesis has been confirmed by our data
which show impaired hepatic uptake of bile acids by hepatocytes in early
life. Later during maturation, at around the time of weaning, serum bile acid
levels increase further. There has been an expansion of the bile acid pool size
and the appearance of ileal active transport further suggesting that hepatic
uptake and/or secretion remain the limiting factor. With full maturation,
serum bile acid levels decrease, at a time when bile acid pool size has had a
ten-fold increase over fetal levels and ileal active transport is now efficiently
conserving the bile acid pool. These findings and the data obtained from our
study of isolated hepatocytes suggest that processes involved in hepatic bile
acid metabolism have progressively achieved adequate function.

It, therefore appears that developmental changes in the enterohepatic
circulation of bile acids are related to maturation of specific hepatic and intestinal cellular events which occur in a non-synchronous manner. Throughout development, the hepatic phase of bile acid metabolism seemingly limits
efficient cycling. The consequences of an impaired enterohepatic circulation
of bile acids are reflected in certain clinical consequences. An increased sus-
ceptibility to cholestasis is observed in infants with sepsis or during the use of
total parenteral nutrition; this may be due in part to a functional reduction of
bile flow related to 'physiologic cholestasis' and immaturity at several sites of
the enterohepatic circulation of bile acids[17]. In addition, the contracted bile
acid pool size and low intraluminal bile acid concentrations may place the
infant at a disadvantage since the critical micellar concentration required for

Table 13.2 Proposed sequence in the ontogeny of hepatic and intestinal events involved in bile acid metabolism

Early life (suckling phase)	Weaning	Adult
↑ Serum bile acid	↑ ↑ Serum bile acid	Serum bile acid
• ↓pool • ↓ileal transport	• ↑pool • ↑ ileal transport	• ↑↑pool • ↑↑ileal transport
∴ hepatic *Uptake* impaired (? regurgitation)	∴ hepatic phase remains limiting	∴ hepatic *Uptake*/ secretion efficient

fat digestion/absorption is not reached – a state of 'physiologic steatorrhoea' exists. The factors modulating the maturation of the various phases of the enterohepatic circulation of bile acids remain to be defined.

References

1. Hofmann, A. F. (1977). The enterohepatic circulation of bile acids. *Clin. Gastroenterol.*, **6**, 3
2. Boyer, J. L. (1980). New concepts of the mechanisms of hepatocyte bile formation. *Physiol. Rev.*, **60**, 303
3. Suchy, F. J., Balistreri, W. F., Heubi, J. E. *et al.* (1981). Physiologic cholestasis: elevations of the primary serum bile acid concentrations in normal infants. *Gastroenterology*, **80**, 1037
4. Forker, E. L. (1974). Mechanisms of hepatic bile formation. *Ann. Rev. Physiol.*, **39**, 323
5. Watkins, J. B. and Perman, J. A. (1977). Bile acid metabolism in infants and children. *Clin. Gastroenterol.*, **6**, 201
6. Andres, J. M., Mathis, R. K. and Walker, W. A. (1977). Liver disease in infants. I. Developmental hepatology and mechanisms of liver dysfunction. *J. Pediatr.*, **90**, 686
7. DeWolf-Peeters, C., DeVos, R. and Desmet, V. (1971). Histochemical evidence of cholestatic period in neonatal rats. *Pediatr. Res.*, **5**, 704
8. DeWolf-Peeters, C., DeVos, R. and Desmet, V. (1971). Electron microscopy and histochemistry of canalicular differential in fetal and neonatal rat liver. *Tissue & Cell*, **4**, 379
9. Belknap, W. M., Balistreri, W. F., Suchy, F. J. and Miller, P. C. (1981). Physiologic cholestasis II: Serum bile acid levels reflect the development of the enterohepatic circulation in rats. *Hepatology*, **1**, 613
10. Suchy, F. J., Heubi, J. E., Balistreri, W. F. and Belknap, W. M. (1981). The enterohepatic circulation of bile acids in suckling and weaning rats. *Gastroenterology*, **80**, 1351
11. Suchy, F. J. and Balistreri, W. F. (1982). Taurocholate uptake in hepatocytes from developing rats. *Pediatr. Res.* **16**, 282
12. Balistreri, W. F., Olinger, E. J., Yu, J. and Herker, E. (1978) Alterations in bile acid metabolism due to cholestasis in isolated hepatocytes. *Gastroenterology*, **75**, 953
13. Suchy, F. J. and Balistreri, W. F. (1980). Maturation of bile acid conjugation in hepatocytes from fetal and suckling rats. *Gastroenterology*, **78**, 1324
14. Heubi, J. E. and Fondacaro, J. D. (1982). Postnatal development of intestinal bile salt transport in the guinea pig. *Am. J. Physiol.* **243**, 6189
15. Balistreri, W. F., Zimmer, L., and Suchy, F. J. (1981). Ethinyl estradiol increases sulfotransferase activity with a concomitant elevation in serum bile acid levels. *Clin. Res.*, **29**, 710
16. Heubi, J. E., Rigney, J. L. and Suchy, F. J. (1982). Postnatal development of intestinal bile acid transport in the rat. *Pediatr. Res.* **16**, 432
17. Lester, R. (1980). Physiologic cholestasis. *Gastroenterology*, **78**, 864

14
Bile acids and bile flow

SERGE ERLINGER

According to current views, canalicular (hepatocytic) bile water transport is mostly an osmotic process: water and inorganic electrolytes flow into bile canaliculi along an osmotic gradient resulting from the extrusion of solutes by the hepatocytes into the canalicular lumen[1-3]. Although, over the past decade, much data has been generated, the overall understanding of the cellular and molecular events responsible for transepithelial transport in the liver is still poor and many aspects are controversial. In this paper, I will not attempt to provide a comprehensive review of the mechanisms of bile flow, since such reviews are available[3,4]. Rather, I will focus on those aspects which are most debated and on which further research is obviously needed. These include the mechanisms of bile salt transport by the liver, the localization and putative role of the sodium pump of hepatocytes, the relationship between bile salts and the sodium pump, the possible role of other inorganic ion 'pumps' (i.e. bicarbonate) and the respective roles of the transcellular and paracellular pathways.

CANALICULAR BILE FLOW

The maximal bile secretory pressure (about $30 \, cmH_2O$) exceeds the sinusoidal perfusion pressure (about $5-10 \, cmH_2O$). This simple observation is generally considered to rule out hydrostatic filtration as an important mechanism for canalicular bile secretion. Canalicular bile formation is therefore regarded as an osmotic water flow in response to active solute transport. Because of the excellent correlation between bile flow and bile-acid output in bile, bile acids are most probably one of the solutes generating bile flow: the term *bile-acid-dependent flow* is used to describe this fraction of bile flow. In contrast, flow that may be generated at low bile-acid outputs or in the absence of bile acids is described as *bile-acid-independent flow*[1-4]. Concepts regarding these two fractions are, however, changing and the cellular mechanisms are still controversial. The following discussion is an attempt to examine these concepts in the light of the observed facts and of mechanisms postulated in other transporting epithelia.

BILE-ACID-DEPENDENT FLOW

Because of the observation, in all species, of an excellent linear correlation between bile flow and bile-acid secretion into bile, it is not surprising that bile-acid secretion is regarded as a strong determinant of bile flow. The most widely accepted explanation for bile-acid induced choleresis is that the osmotic gradient created by ionized bile acids (or by their associated counter-ions) in the canalicular lumen provides a driving force for water and electrolytes. Other possibilities may, however, be considered, such as stimulation of transport of sodium or other ions. Two other questions regarding the mechanism of bile-acid-dependent choleresis have been discussed recently: what are the mechanisms of bile-acid transport by the liver cell; and what is the pathway of bile-acid-induced fluid movement?

Mechanism of bile-acid transport: role of Na^+,K^+-ATPase

The uptake of bile acids by the liver is a saturable, carrier-mediated process[5,6]. Furthermore, it exhibits a strong sodium dependence: uptake is considerably reduced when Na^+ is omitted from the external medium in the isolated rat liver[7,8] in isolated hepatocytes[9,10], in cultured hepatocytes[11] and, as shown more recently, in membrane vesicles prepared from rat liver[12-14]. Such Na^+ dependence is highly suggestive of a sodium-coupled transport: this type of transport is energized by the sodium gradient established by the Na^+ pump (or Na^+, K^+-ATPase). The postulated mechanism is thought to be a symport system transporting both Na^+ (along its electrochemical gradient) and a solute (in our case the bile acid), and allowing accumulation of the solute (the bile acid) against an electrochemical gradient. Because a system of this type allows such accumulation of the substrate against an electrochemical gradient, it is usually referred to as 'active'. Because it is not directly linked to an energy source (such as ATP), but rather to an ion gradient, it is referred to as 'secondary active'. Other well-characterized examples of secondary active transport systems using the Na^+ gradient provided by the Na^+,K^+-ATPase are glucose accumulation in the intestine and kidney tubule or transport of 'A' type amino acids in a variety of cells.

It is, therefore, reasonable to assume that bile-acid uptake by hepatocytes is a secondary active transport energized by the sodium gradient and hence, by the Na^+,K^+-ATPase. Once accumulated into the cell, the bile acid anion will tend to move out of the cell into the canalicular lumen along its chemical gradient (since, to start with, there is no bile acid in the lumen); this movement is favoured by the negative membrane potential, (approximately $-50\,mV$ in the mammalian liver) which tends to drive anions out of the cell. Since it is known that canalicular secretion of bile acids is limited by a transport maximum (T_m), one has to assume the existence of a canalicular carrier. A reasonable candidate is the bile-acid binding protein identified by Accatino and Simon[15]. It is not known, however, whether at this stage the carrier uses an additional source of energy or whether it is a passive carrier-mediated transport (e.g. facilitated diffusion). Using the Nernst equation, and assuming a hepatocyte bile-acid concentration of 0.1–0.3 mmol/l one

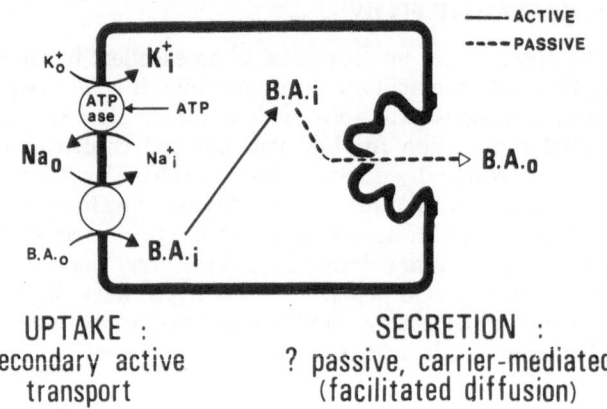

UPTAKE :
secondary active
transport

SECRETION :
? passive, carrier-mediated
(facilitated diffusion)

Figure 14.1 Hypothetical representation of bile-acid transport by hepatocytes. Blood bile acids ($B.A._o$) are taken up by the sinusoidal membrane by a symport system with Na^+, using the Na^+ gradient established by the Na^+,K^+-ATPase as its energy source. By this system (called a secondary active transport), bile acids may be accumulated into the cell against their electrochemical gradient ($B.A._i$). They can then move into the canalicular lumen down their electrochemical gradient, probably using a saturable canalicular 'carrier' ($B.A._o$). This excretory process may be passive (as depicted here) or may use an additional source of energy (not shown here). K^+_o = external K^+; K^+_i = internal K^+; Na_o = external Na^+; Na^+_i = internal Na^+ (from reference 21)

can calculate that hepatocyte to canaliculus concentration ratios of 1:5–1:10 could be achieved by a passive process. This could account for a canalicular non-micellar (monomeric) bile acid concentration in the vicinity of the critical micellar concentration. Higher concentrations could be achieved, in principle, by micellar sequestration.

In summary (Figure 14.1), bile acids are thought to be taken up from sinu-soidal blood by the hepatocyte by a secondary active transport system. Transport is probably energized by the Na^+ gradient created by the Na^+ pump (the Na^+,K^+-ATPase). Bile acids are then translocated to the canal-icular membrane and transported into bile canaliculi. It is not known whether canalicular transport is by a carrier-mediated process (facilitated diffusion), or if it requires an additional source of energy. However, the overall driving force for transport from blood to bile seems to be the Na^+,K^+-ATPase, using ATP as an energy source and the Na^+ gradient as the mode of coupling between transport itself and the energy source.

Bile-acid dependent flow movement: Transcellular or paracellular?

Because bile acids are transported through the canalicular membrane of the hepatocyte, it is often stated that the osmotic water flow in response to this transport also occurs through the canalicular membrane. However, the ionic composition of bile closely resembles that of the extracellular fluid. It is therefore necessary to postulate either an ionic equilibrium downstream along the biliary channels, or a paracellular water and ionic pathway from the intercellular space into the bile canaliculi. The first possibility seems unlikely, since, at least in the rat, the biliary channels seem relatively impermeable to ions.

We have already suggested, on structural grounds alone, that the liver could be a relatively 'leaky' epithelium. The fact that the bile-to-plasma concentration ratios for large solutes, such as inulin (mol wt 5000) or sucrose (mol wt 342) stabilized well before the hepatocyte-to-plasma concentration ratios has suggested a 'restricted' pathway which could be the intercellular route. More recent studies with polyethylene glycol-4000 support the view of a water flow through the intercellular junctions[16]. Experiments with the potent choleretics dehydrocholate or taurodehydrocholate have demonstrated a progressive increase in the bile-to-plasma concentration ratio of sucrose, a penetration of ionic lanthanum into the tight junctions and an increase in the number of intercellular 'blisters'. These observations have suggested that the paracellular pathway may be an important site for bile-acid induced water and ion movement into bile[17]. Consistent with this hypothesis is the rapid appearance in bile (approximately 10 minutes) of ferrocyanide (mol wt 484, hydrated form). In these elegant experiments, the biliary clearances of negatively charged solutes were consistently lower than those of the uncharged solutes of comparable molecular size, an observation suggesting that this pathway includes a barrier that selectively restricts passive anionic movement.

In summary, although the respective parts of the transcellular and paracellular pathways in bile-acid induced choleresis are not yet established, there are both structural and physiological arguments to consider that the paracellular pathway may be an important route for movement into bile of large solutes (such as inulin and sucrose) and, possibly, of smaller biliary electrolytes and water.

BILE-ACID-INDEPENDENT FLOW

Evidence

This postulated process has generated the greatest controversy. Plots of bile acid secretion rate against canalicular bile flow (as estimated by erythritol or mannitol clearance) display a positive intercept when extrapolated to the flow axis in all animal species studied, including man (for reviews, see references[1-4]). Although it is clear that the slope of such plots tend to increase at very low bile-acid secretion rates, possibly because bile-acid concentration falls below the critical micellar concentration, the extrapolated value in a given experiment does not change significantly and is generally regarded as the bile-acid independent fraction of canalicular bile flow. Whether the extrapolation procedure yields a correct quantitative estimation in all situatiuons is uncertain and quantitation should therefore be evaluated critically in any given experimental situation. Additional, and for some more convincing, evidence for canalicular flow-generating systems distinct from bile acids comes from the study of drugs which increase canalicular bile flow without

modifying bile salt secretion. Examples are phenobarbital and other barb-
iturates when given to rats for 3 or 4 days, theophylline, glucagon, hydrocortisone or the bicyclic anion SC-2644[1,3]. With the possible exception of
hydrocortisone, these drugs are not appreciably secreted into bile, so that
their choleretic effect cannot be attributed to an osmotic drive. Nor is there
any evidence that these compounds alter the osmotic activity of the bile acids
or the permeability of the biliary system to water or ions. The most appeal-
ing interpretation for canalicular bile-salt-independent bile formation is
therefore inorganic ion transport. Na^+ transport linked to the
Na^+,K^+-ATPase, and more recently, bicarbonate transport, have been
implicated.

Role of Na^+,K^+-ATPase

The role of Na^+,K^+-ATPase in bile-salt independent bile flow is, at present,
highly controversial. Evidence for a role of the Na^+-K^+-ATPase was
originally derived from studies of the effect of inhibitors of sodium transport
on bile flow (see reference 1). However, it has become clear that interpretation of the effect of such drugs as ouabain, ethacrynic acid and amiloride *in
vivo* is more complex than initially thought. Ouabain and ethacrynic acid
are themselves secreted into bile by concentrative processes and produce an
osmotic choleresis. This choleresis may mask, in part or in totality, their
possible inhibitory effect.

Thereafter, more direct evidence for a role of Na^+,K^+-ATPase has been
sought by studying the relationship between bile flow and Na^+,K^+ATPase
activity in liver cell plasma membranes. Experiments using oestrogens,
phenobarbital, other microsomal enzyme inducers, thyroid hormones and
chlorpromazine have, in general, shown excellent correlations between bile
flow (or its canalicular bile-acid-independent fraction) and
Na^+,K^+-ATPase activity measured in membrane preparations. The mechanism by which each agent modifies the enzyme activity differs probably
from one to the other. For example, oestrogens have been claimed to do so by
altering the lipid composition of the membrane, chlorpromazine and its
metabolites by modifying the local environment of the membrane (pH and
glutathione concentration; in both cases membrane fluidity may be
decreased), and phenobarbital by increasing enzyme synthesis. A major
problem, however, is to understand the mode of coupling between enzyme
activity and secretion. As seen before, the bulk of Na^+,K^+-ATPase activity
is located before, the bulk of Na^+,K^+-ATPase activity is located not on the
canalicular membrane (as would be expected for direct pumping of sodium
into the canaliculi) but on the sinusoidal and intercellular membrane. This
seems to be a general rule in transporting epithelia, Na^+ pump sites being
located on the basolateral site, regardless of the direction of net movement of
solute and water transport. There is little dispute, however, that the
Na^+,K^+-ATPase should ultimately be the agent of coupling between the
energy source and the transepithelial transport (we have already seen that it
is most probably true for the transhepatic transport of bile acids). At least

two ways in which Na+,K+-ATPase could drive ions (and subsequently water) through the liver can be proposed.

The first could be active transport of Na+ into the intercellular space followed by passive movement of the ion into the canalicular lumen through a tight junction cation channel. Considering a localization of the pump on the lateral (intercellular) membrane, it is clear that Na+ will be pumped into the long intercellular spaces. It will then tend to flow towards the extremities of these spaces (the one facing the sinusoids and the one facing the tight junctions and the canaliculi). The proportion of sodium flowing towards each end will depend on the resistances encountered along the way. We have already discussed the morphological and physiological evidence for permeability in the tight junctions. Admittedly sodium permeability of the liver tight junctions is unknown. But assuming a finite permeability for sodium and an even distribution of Na+ pump sites along the intercellular membranes, Na+ ions pumped near the tight junctions will flow through the junctions rather than through the long intercellular channels. The proportion of the total sodium pumped out of the hepatocyte which will, in this way, flow through the junctions may be small but still sufficient to drive water osmotically into the canalicular lumen.

The second possible way of coupling between Na+,K+-ATPase and secretion could be transport of an anion, such as Cl^- or HCO_3^- (or still another) using the Na+ gradient (in much the same way as bile acids themselves are transported). Sodium-driven Cl^- transport is widespread in many other epithelia. Although preliminary results do not support this view in the liver, it should certainly still be carefully examined. Bicarbonate transport by such a system has not been characterized but is also conceivable. In the next section a possible role of bicarbonate transport in bile-acid independent choleresis is discussed.

Role of bicarbonate transport

In the isolated, perfused rat liver, perfusion with a bicarbonate-free solution reduced the bile-acid independent flow by 50%[18]. Under this condition bicarbonate secretion was nearly eliminated, while sodium secretion was markedly reduced. In contrast, administration of SC-2644 to dogs increased canalicular bile flow and bicarbonate concentration in bile[19]. These observations have led to the conclusion that a bicarbonate transport mechanism may have a role in the elaboration of the bile-acid-independent flow. Ursodeoxycholate and 7-ketolithocholate increased canalicular bicarbonate secretion and bile flow in the rat[20], an effect possibly related to stimulation of the bicarbonate transport system by these bile acids. The cellular mechanism remains to be elucidated. Attempts to demonstrate a bicarbonate-sensitive ATPase in liver cell plasma membranes have been, as yet, unsuccessful[18], but other mechanisms (such as the Na+/H+ antiport of the kidney tubule or pancreas) are possible.

Relationship between bile acids and inorganic ion transport. Is the bile-acid independent flow really independent?

Several studies have suggested a link between bile acids and the so-called bile-acid independent flow. In particular, rats with a partial biliary obstruction had an increased bile-acid flux through the unobstructed liver, and, at the same time, an increased Na^+,K^+-ATPase activity and an increased bile-acid independent bile flow. Other examples are the decreased bile-acid secretion observed after oestrogen treatment in rats (when bile-acid-independent flow is mostly decreased), or still variations of the bile-acid independent flow at varying rates of bile-acid infusions. We have also seen the effect of ursodeoxycholate on what appears to be a canalicular bicarbonate transport.

If one postulates that bile-acid transport on the one hand and bile-acid-independent bile formation are both dependent on the Na^+,K^+-ATPase (as discussed above) such interrelationships are not surprising. Predictable consequences of such an hypothesis are:

(1) An increase in Na^+,K^+-ATPase activity will be associated with only an increase in bile-acid-independent bile flow, since the liver can only excrete the load of bile acids that is presented to it, and not more. This is observed after chronic (4 days) administration of phenobarbital in the rat (administration for a longer time might result in an increased synthesis, pool size, and hence, secretion).

(2) A decrease in Na^+,K^+-ATPase activity will be expected to result in a decrease of both bile salt transport (due to the decreased Na^+ gradient) and bile salt-independent flow. This dual decrease is usually observed with agents inhibiting Na^+,K^+-ATPase, such as ouabain in our earlier experiments, or oestrogens.

(3) An increased bile-acid uptake and flux by the hepatocyte might be expected to stimulate Na^+ entry into the cell (in the same way as glucose or amino acids do when they are transported in a Na^+-dependent fashion). This process could in turn activate Na^+,K^+-ATPase, since intracellular sodium is supposed to be one of the regulators of the Na^+ pump, and provide a mechanism by which the bile acids could act as regulators of the Na^+ pump.

Numerous other possibilities of interactions between the two processes (bile-acid dependent and independent) can be imagined. In this sense, bile-acid independent flow is not truly 'independent'. The term is, at present, however, the most commonly used and a better terminology might have to await a more accurate knowledge of the mechanisms involved.

CONCLUSION

We can now propose a revised two-component theory[21] of canalicular bile flow which has analogies with that recently proposed by Boyer[22]. Bile is an isotonic secretion deriving its energy from ATP, through the Na^+,K^+-ATPase. The Na^+,K^+-ATPase (the Na^+ pump) is located on the sinusoidal and/or lateral part of the plasma membrane (the basolateral membrane of other epithelia). It establishes a Na^+ gradient which is used to energize the uptake (by a Na^+ bile acid symport system) and accumulation of bile acids into the cells. Bile acids are subsequently transported into the canalicular lumen. They exert their choleretic effect either because of their own osmotic activity, or through that of associated counter-ions, or else by increasing sodium movement into the cell with subsequent activation of Na^+,K^+-ATPase. This process is responsible for the so-called bile-acid-dependent canalicular bile flow. Bile-acid-independent canalicular bile flow may be generated by one of two processes. One could be active Na^+ transport by the Na^+ pump into the intercellular space followed by passive movement of Na^+ through a caution-selective channel of the tight junction. The second could be movement of an anion (other than bile acid, such as Cl^- or HCO_3^-) using the sodium gradient generated by the Na^+,K^+-ATPase. Obviously, both bile-acid-dependent and bile-acid independent bile formation are ultimately linked to the activity of the Na^+,K^+-ATPase and inter-relationships may be anticipated between them. Terminology itself may have to be changed, because, according to this view, the two fractions are not truly independent.

In this way, the hepatic cell uses the activity of the Na^+,K^+-ATPase both to maintain a basal bile flow (bile-acid independent) and to drive the transport of bile acids. Such a dual mechanism makes sense from a teleological point of view because relying only upon bile acids to drive bile flow would be hazardous, since the bile acid load to the liver is subject to great variations which could lead, during the periods of very low bile acid secretion (i.e. between meals) to a dangerously low bile flow and eventually a blockage of secretion.

References

1. Erlinger, S. and Dhumeaux, D. (1974). Mechanisms and control of secretion of bile water and electrolytes. *Gastroenterology*, **66**, 281
2. Javitt, N. B. (1976). Hepatic bile formation. *N. Engl. J. Med.*, **295**, 1464, 1511
3. Forker, E. L. (1977). Mechanisms of hepatic bile formation. *Ann. Rev. Physiol.*, **39**, 323
4. Erlinger, S. (1982). Secretion of bile. In Schiff, L. and Schiff, E. (eds.) *Diseases of the Liver.* pp. 93–118. (Philadelphia: Lippincott)
5. Reichen, J. and Paumgartner, G. (1975). Kinetics of taurocholate uptake by the perfused rat liver. *Gastroenterology*, **68**, 132
6. Glasinović, J. C., Dumont, M., Duval, M. and Erlinger S. (1975). Hepatocellular uptake of taurocholate in the dog. *J. Clin. Invest.*, **55**, 419
7. Dietmaier, A., Gasser, R., Graf, J. and Peterlik, M. (1976). Investigations on the sodium-dependence of bile acid fluxes in the isolated perfused rat liver. *Biochem. Biophys. Acta*, **443**, 81
8. Reichen, J. and Paumgartner, G. (1976). Uptake of bile acids by the perfused rat liver. *Am. J. Physiol.*, **231**, 734
9. Schwarz, L. R., Burr, R., Schwenk, M., Pfaff, E. and Greim, H. (1975). Uptake of taurocholic acid into isolated rat-liver cells. *Eur. J. Biochem.*, **55**, 617
10. Anwer, M. S. and Hegner, D. (1978). Effect of Na^+ on bile acid uptake by isolated rat hepatocytes. *Hoppe-Seyler's Z. Physiol. Chem.*, **359**, 181
11. Schwarz, L. R. and Barth, C. A. (1979). Taurocholate uptake by adult rat hepatocytes in primary culture. *Hoppe-Seyler's Z. Physiol. Chem.*, **360**, 1117

12. Ruifrok, P. G. and Meijer, D. K. F. (1980). Sodium ion-coupled uptake of taurocholate by rat liver plasma membrane vesicles. *Liver*, **2**, 28
13. Inoue, M., Tran, T., Kinne, R. and Arias, I. M. (1981). Preparation of vesicles from rat liver sinusoidal and canalicular plasma membranes: mechanism of taurocholate uptake by sinusoidal membrane vesicles. *Hepatology*, **1**, 519 (abstract)
14. Duffy, M. C., Blitzer, R. L. and Boyer, J. L. (1981). Direct determination of the driving forces for taurocholate (TC) uptake into liver plasma membrane (LPM) vesicles. *Hepatology*, **1**, 507 (abstract)
15. Accatino, L. and Simon, F. R. (1976). Identification and characterization of a bile acid receptor in isolated liver surface membranes. *J. Clin. Invest.*, **57**, 496
16. Javitt, N. B., Dillon, D., Kok, E. and Wachtel, N. (1978). Mechanism of bile formation – Transcellular and paracellular pathways. In Preisig, R. and Bircher, J. (eds.) *The Liver. Quantitative Aspects of Structure and Function.* pp. 197-202. (Aulendorf: Cantor)
17. Layden, T. J., Elias, E. and Boyer, J. L. (1978). Bile formation in the rat. The role of the paracellular pathway. *J. Clin. Invest.*, **62**, 1375
18. Hardison, W. G. M. and Wood, C. A. (1978). Importance of bicarbonate in bile salt independent fraction of bile flow. *Am. J. Physiol.*, **235**, E158
19. Bernhart, J. L. and Combes, B. (1978). Characterization of SC-2644-induced choleresis in the dog. Evidence for canalicular bicarbonate secretion. *J. Pharmacol. Exp. Ther.*, **206**, 190
20. Dumont, M., Uchman, S. and Erlinger, S. (1980). Hypercholeresis induced by ursodeoxycholic acid and 7-ketolithocholic acid in the rat. Possible role of bicarbonate transport. *Gastroenterology*, **79**, 82
21. Erlinger, S. (1981). Hepatocyte bile secretion: current views and controversies. *Hepatology*, **1**, 352
22. Boyer, J. L. (1980). New concepts of mechanisms of hepatocytic bile formation. *Physiol. Rev.*, **60**, 303

15
Bile acid metabolism in liver disease

L. CAPOCACCIA, M. ANGELICO, A. ATTILI,
D. ALVARO, A. De SANTIS and M. MARIN

In this presentation, we will limit our interest to the modifications in bile acids (BA) during the course of liver cirrhosis (LC), thus excluding the behaviour in cholestasis. There is little doubt, on the other hand, that LC is the typical model of parenchymal chronic liver disease. Moreover, hepato-cellular disorders and cholestatic processes are often associated in LC and thus the major points of cholestasis will also be included.

BILE ACID POOL

The BA pool in normal subjects is 2–4 g, circulating 6–10 times a day. It comprises 40% cholic acid (CA), 40% chenodeoxycholic acid (CDCA) and 20% deoxycholic acid (DCA); lithocholic acid (LA) accounts for less than 1%.

In patients with LC the total BA pool is reduced to approximately half that in normal conditions. This reduction occurs essentially at the expense of CA and DCA, that of CDCA being negligible and therefore resulting in this BA becoming the major component of total BA pool. The CA/CDCA ratio, which is around 1 in the normal subject, appears in general reduced in LC[1].

The decrease in the CA pool is probably due to reduced synthesis of this BA, as will be discussed later. Conversely, much controversy exists as to why DCA is also reduced in LC. It has been demonstrated in fact that the formation of this BA in the intestine is actually reduced, despite substrate and micro-organisms being present in adequate amounts. It has also been hypothesized that the reaction may be inhibited in the colonic milieu of cirrhotics. Knodell et al.[2] suggested the induction of BA dehydrogenases in such patients, with formation of keto-bile acids, which in fact they found to be increased in the faeces of cirrhotics. A further reduction of DCA in bile has been demonstrated by us after portacaval shunt (PCS).

In normal subjects, more than 99% of the BA pool size is confined in the enterohepatic circulation (EHC). In LC a larger fraction of this pool is

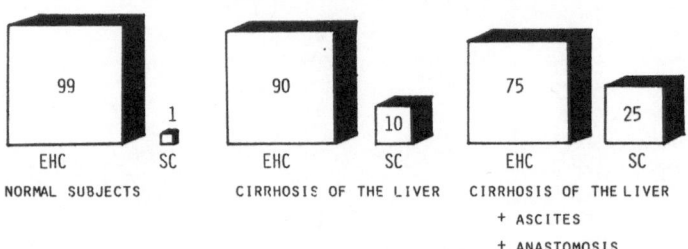

Figure 15.1 Percent distribution of total BA pool in the enterohepatic circulation (EHC) and in the systemic circulation (SC).

diverted into the systemic circulation (SC) and diffuses into the extracellular fluid (ECF). It may be grossly calculated that in normal subjects approximately 20 mg of BA are present in the 10 l ECF. In LC, approximately 150 mg of BA (i.e., about 10% of the total pool size) are present in the ECF. This increased presence of BA in the plasma of patients with LC occurs, as will be discussed later, for two main reasons: decreased hepatic cellular uptake; and increased hepatic blood by-pass. It is also conceivable that the percentage fraction of the pool size outside the EHC shows a further increase when ascites develop. Our data show that the quantity of BA outside the EHC is approximately doubled after surgical anastomosis (Figure 15.1).

BILE-ACID SYNTHESIS

In normal subjects, approximately 500 mg of BA are synthesized daily by the liver, 350 mg being CA and 150 mg CDCA.

In patients with LC the overall synthesis of primary BA is decreased, the reduction of CA accounting for the large majority. In fact, the synthesis of CA is reduced by about 70%, whilst that of CDCA is only slightly decreased. As already pointed out, the decreased synthesis of CA accounts for the reduction in the pool size of this BA. The synthesis ratio CA/CDCA approximates 1. Only in one study[3] was CDCA synthesis reduced by more than 50%. The reason why BA synthesis, especially that of CA, is depressed in LC is not known, even if selective impairment of 12 α-hydroxylase activity has been suggested since 1958 by Carey[4] and recently supported by Angelin et al.[5]. The latter authors, stimulating BA synthesis by cholestyramine administration in cirrhotic patients, observed that the increase in CA synthesis was lower than that normally occurring in normal subjects. More recently, Patteson et al.[3], administering various radiolabelled precursors of BA synthesis to advanced cirrhotics, failed to demonstrate any selective impairment in the BA synthesis pathway. Conversely, several steps were found to be slightly depressed, including the side-chain oxidation and the 12 α-hydroxylation step, and these authors therefore suggested that impaired 7 α-hydroxylation of cholesterol and/or lack of available cholesterol substrate are likely additional factors, which might explain the reduction also of CDCA synthesis. Halloran *et al.*[6] have demonstrated that HDL-free cholesterol is the prime source for BA synthesis and emphasize that in alcoholic liver disease HDL-cholesterol is markedly decreased and morphologically altered[7]. These alterations in plasma lipoproteins might be responsible for the decreased availability of cholesterol substrate for BA synthesis.

BILE-ACID TURNOVER

In normal conditions, CA presents a halflife of 2.2 days and CDCA of 3.1. In LC the fractional turnover rate (FTR) of CDCA remains unchanged, while that of CA is markedly slower ($t\frac{1}{2} = 4.1$ days). However, the prolonged halflife of CA only partially compensates its reduced synthesis: in fact, as mentioned above, the CA pool size is greatly decreased in this disease. The reason why the FTR of CA is more rapid in normal conditions than that of CDCA is not yet known but it is probably due to differences in the respective circulation of these BA within the enterohepatic system. The increased halflife of CA in LC is probably due to an overall reduction of BA conversion into degradation products, though a faecal increase of 7-keto products has been described in LC as already stated[2].

ENTEROHEPATIC CIRCULATION

Any substance to be taken as a model of EHC should have: efficient intestinal absorption, efficient hepatic uptake, and complete biliary secretion. BA represent such a substance.

Absorption

To our knowledge, no direct measurement of intestinal absorption of BA in LC is available. Even if intestinal malabsorption may be present in cirrhotics, much evidence has been forthcoming in support of the concept that BA absorption is not substantially reduced in these patients. In fact, the decreased FTR of CA and the rather efficient serum BA peak after a meal test or after an exogenous load provide indirect evidence in support of this statement. Furthermore, in moderately advanced LC, von Bergman *et al.*[8] found faecal excretion of acidic steroids to be within normal limits.

These points are obviously referred to the mechanism(s) of the intestinal absorption, whereas the overall quantity of absorbed BA is presumably lower than in normal conditions, intraluminal concentration of BA being lower in LC.

Hepatic uptake

The normal liver clears 92% of CA and 78% of CDCA on their first passage. This is another reason (together with the higher circulation rate of CDCA)

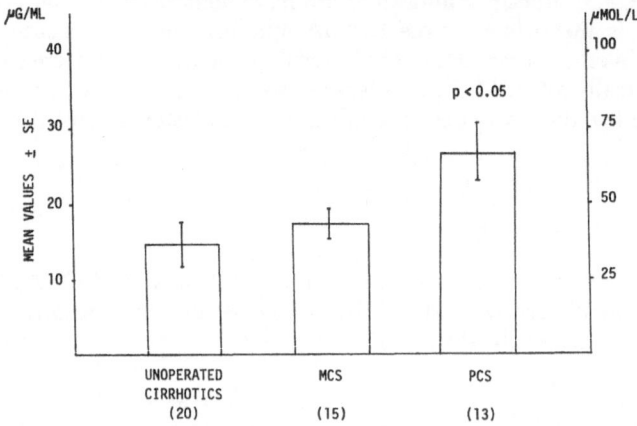

Figure 15.2 Total serum bile acid concentration in unoperated cirrhotics and in patients with mesocaval (MCS) or portacaval (PCS) shunt. Number in parentheses represents number of patients studied.

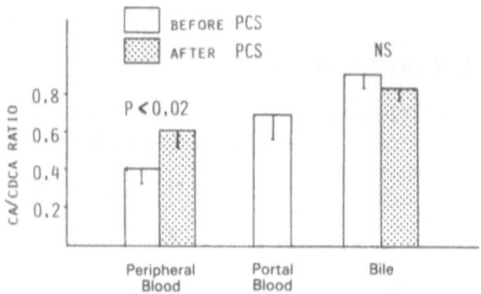

Figure 15.3 Bile acid ratios before and after portacaval shunt (PCS). (CA=cholic acid; CDCA=chenodeoxycholic acid.)

why the ratio CA/CDCA is lower in serum (approximately between 0.6 and 0.8) than in bile (about 1).

Hepatic clearance of BA in LC is clearly impaired, as demonstrated by the increase in serum BA both in fasting conditions and after exogenous or endogenous load. Moreover, in LC labelled BA injected intravenously are cleared from the peripheral circulation at a slower rate than in normal subjects. This principle is exploited clinically to assess hepatic function. The CA/CDCA ratio is lower (0.2–0.4) in LC than in normal subjects.

The two main reasons for the impaired BA clearance are decreased hepato-cellular clearing capacity and the presence of portal systemic shunting.

Which of these two mechanisms prevails is still not known. It is very difficult, on the other hand, to discriminate between the two. A model to evaluate the importance of blood liver by-pass is PCS. Obviously, also in this condition, the role played by the reduction of liver mass cell cannot be eliminated. However, all those studying this problem have described an increase in serum BA levels after PCS both in animals and in man. Poupon *et al.*[9] observed that the increase in serum BA levels was related to the time lapse after surgery and interpreted this finding as due to the progressive deterioration of hepatic function. Conversely, experimental data in dogs support the hypothesis that the serum BA increase is directly related to the hepatic blood flow[10].

Our findings[11] in a population of patients submitted to PCS or mesocaval shunt (MCS) seem to stress the importance of portal diversion in determining serum BA levels. In fact, these levels were found to be higher after PCS than after MCS. It is generally accepted that the latter procedure allows a better blood flow than the former[12]. It is also noteworthy that in MCS the CA/CDCA ratio was higher, as if CDCA would be allowed a somewhat effective hepatic uptake through the pancreatic veins[13]. The major role played by the diversion of liver blood flow is further demonstrated by a threefold increase in serum BA 2 months after PCS in the absence of any significant change in the liver function tests. In addition, the CA/CDCA ratio tends to increase, resembling more closely that of the portal levels (Figures 15.2 and 15.3).

Secretion

In patients with LC the overall secretion of BA is markedly reduced, the proportion of CA:CDCA becoming similar to that in the pool.

The relative reduction in the BA pool might have been expected to cause increased cholesterol saturation in gallbladder bile; on the contrary, fasting gallbladder bile in LC is not markedly supersaturated[8] and tends to unsaturation with evolution of the disease[14]. The secretion rate of the three biliary lipids shows that in LC secretion of cholesterol is more markedly reduced than that of BA and phospholipids[15], thus resulting in the rarity of cholesterol gallstones in this disease, though bile is markedly less concentrated than in normal subjects. Von Bergman *et al.*[8] suggested the presence, in moderately advanced LC (i.e. in patients with moderate supersaturation), of a much higher coupling of cholesterol to lecithin and BA at the levels of the canalicular membrane than in controls. Why the secretion of cholesterol is lower than the other two biliary lipids and/or cholesterol is more tightly coupled to BA is not known. In LC, Ponz de Leon *et al.*[16] observed a reduced activity of HMG-CoA reductase, the rate-limiting enzyme for cholesterol synthesis. They also showed that cholesterol absorption is significantly reduced in LC, the reduction being positively related to the severity of the disease and inversely related to the CA pool size.

CONJUGATION AND DECONJUGATION

Free BA present in the liver are conjugated with glycine or taurine before biliary secretion by a microsomal enzyme system (BA acyl CoA:amino-acid-

N-acyl transferase). No evidence exists that this enzymatic activity is altered in parenchymal liver damage. Biliary BA in LC as in normal subjects are all conjugated.

In normal conditions conjugation with taurine is limited by its low concentration in the liver. Thus the biliary glycine/taurine ratio is 3:1. When conjugation requirements increase (i.e., BA malabsorption, small-bowel contamination, treatment with cholestyramine or BA, etc.) the glycine/taurine ratio is markedly enhanced. Conversely, when synthesis of BA is decreased, such as in LC (i.e., fewer BA need to be conjugated) the glycine/taurine ratio decreases.

Glycine-conjugated BA are more readily deconjugated and have a more rapid turnover than taurine-conjugated BA[17]. It is not known whether the higher percentage of taurine-conjugated BA in LC with respect to that in normal subjects could account for the prolonged halflife of CA in LC.

SULPHATION

In normal subjects only a very small fraction of BA is sulphated and this is substantially of mono-hydroxylates (totally and approximately less than 1%) (3α, 5β-cholanic acid or lithocholic acid; 3β, 5Δ-cholanic acid).

The introduction of sulphate groups into the BA molecules modifies their physiochemical properties enhancing hydrosolubility and thus the renal and faecal excretion are thus increased. Conversely, much controversy exists as to whether sulphation represents a detoxifying process[18,19].

The sites of sulphation are the liver, kidneys and possibly also other organs. Monosulphates are poorly absorbed through the intestine.

Though cholestasis is the model for the metabolism of sulphates, a relevant fraction of BA sulphates is present in LC. This is probably related to the increased presence of BA outside the EHC in this disease. In LC, BA sulphates are increased in serum (between 5 and 30% according to various authors; around 25% in our patients), in urine (45–75%; 40% in our patients), but not in bile: the presence of measurable amounts of sulphated BA other than monohydroxylates was reported in only three cases in the series of patients studied by Stiehl[20] and by Makino *et al.*[21]. It is also noteworthy that in LC Stiehl *et al.*[20] calculated that less than 1% of the CA pool and 5% of the CDCA pool are sulphated. Synthesis of sulphated CA is 8% of the total synthesis of this BA; that of CDCA is 27%. The halflife of sulphated CA is 0.7 days and that of CDCA is 0.8 days; this rapid turnover is probably due to the high urinary excretion of sulphates.

Further data on the metabolism of sulphates may be deduced from studies on patients submitted to PCS, i.e.:

(1) BA sulphates are present in minimal quantities in bile.
(2) Portal levels of BA sulphates, although not significantly, are higher than peripheral levels. This difference suggests the existence of intestinal sulphation[22].
(3) Serum BA levels after PCS are significantly increased, those of sulphates being only slightly and not significantly increased with

respect to preoperative levels (Figure 15.4).
(4)   BA sulphates have a rather poor EHC.

BILE ACID METABOLISM IN PRIMARY BILIARY CIRRHOSIS

Some aspects of BA metabolism have been studied by Raedsch *et al.*[23] in patients with primary biliary cirrhosis (PBC) and varying degrees of cholestasis: PBC offers a good model of both cholestasis and hepatocellular disease. Essentially they found serum BA to be increased several fold (up to $300\,\mu mol/l$) and highly correlated with urinary BA excretion. About one third of urinary BA were found to be unsulphated, one third monosulphated and one third polysulphated and/or glucuronated. They also found that CA and CDCA were both sulphated at either the 3 position and/or the 7 position. BA pool size, turnover rate and synthesis were found to be essentially similar to those reported in patients with LC without cholestasis. 4–38% of CDCA synthesis was sulphated. These authors concluded that the main abnormalities of BA metabolism in cholestasis secondary to BLC were marked increase in BA sulphation and a shift to renal excretion as a primary route of BA elimination.

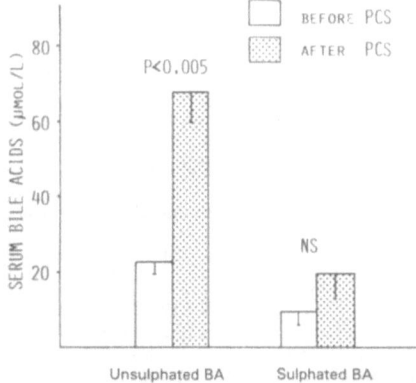

Figure 15.4   Serum bile acid (BA) levels before and after portacaval shunt (PCS).

References

1. Vlahcevic, Z. R., Prugh, M. F., Gregory, D. H. and Swell, L. (1977). Disturbances of bile acid metabolism in parenchymal liver cell disease. *Clin. Gastroenterol.*, **6**, 25
2. Knodell, R. G., Dean Kinsey, M., Boedeker, E. C. and Collin, D. P. (1976). Deoxycholate metabolism in alcoholic cirrhosis. *Gastroenterology*, **71**, 196
3. Patteson, T. E., Vlahcevic, Z. R., Schwartz, C. C., Gustafsson, J., Danielsson, H. and Swell, L. (1980). Bile acid metabolism in cirrhosis. VI. Sites of blockage in the bile acid pathways to primary bile acids. *Gastroenterology*, **79**, 620
4. Carey, J. B. Jr. (1958). Serum trihydroxy-dihydroxy bile acid ratio in liver and biliary tract disease. *J. Clin. Invest.*, **37**, 1494
5. Angelin, B., Einarsson, K. and Hellström, K. (1978). Effect of cholestyramine on bile and acid kinetics in portal cirrhosis of the liver: Evidence of a selective defect in the formation of cholic acid. *Am. J. Dig. Dis.*, **23**, 1115

6. Halloran, L. G., Schwartz, C. C., Vlahcevic, Z. R. et al. (1978). Evidence for high density lipoprotein free cholesterol as the primary precursor for bile acid synthesis in man. Surgery, 84, 1
7. Sabesin, M. S., Hawkins, L. H., Kuiken, L. and Ragland, B. J. (1977). Abnormal lipoproteins and lecithin-cholesterol acyltransferase deficiency in alcoholic liver disease. Gastroenterology, 72, 510
8. Von Bergman, K., Mok, H. Y., Hardison, W. G. M. and Grundy, S. M. (1979). Cholesterol and bile acid metabolism in moderately advanced, stable cirrhosis of the liver. Gastroenterology, 77, 1183
9. Poupon, R. E., Poupon, R. Y., Grosdemouge, M. L. and Erlinger, S. (1977). Effect of portacaval shunt on serum bile acid concentration in patients with cirrhosis. Digestion, 16, 138
10. Horak, W., Gangl, A., Funovics, J. and Grabner, G. (1975). Effect of portacaval shunt and arterialization of the liver on bile acid metabolism. Gastroenterology, 69, 338
11. Angelico, M., Attili, A. F., Cantafora, A., Lombardi, M., Thau, A. and Capocaccia, L. (1979). Differences in serum bile acid composition between unoperated cirrhotic patients with portacaval or mesocaval shunt. Digestion, 19, 126
12. Harmon, G. W., Zinner, M. L. and Reynolds, D. G. (1977). Comparison of portal flow distribution after portacaval and mesocaval shunts. J. Surg. Res., 22, 343
13. Angelin, B., Einarsson, K. and Hellström, K. (1976). Evidence for the absorption of bile acids in the proximal small intestine of normo- and hyper-lipidaemic subjects. Gut, 17, 420
14. Vlahcevic, Z. R., Yoshida, T., Juttijudata, P., Bell, C. C. and Swell, L. (1973). Bile acid metabolism in cirrhosis. III. Biliary lipid secretion in patients with cirrhosis and its relevance to gallstone formation. Gastroenterology, 64, 298
15. Schwartz, C. C., Almond, H. R., Vlahcevic, Z. R. and Swell, L. (1979). Bile acid metabolism in cirrhosis. V. Determination of biliary lipid secretion rates in patients with advanced cirrhosis. Gastroenterology, 77, 1177
16. Ponz de Leon, M., Loria, P., Iori, R. and Carulli, N. (1981). Cholesterol absorption in cirrhosis: the role of total and individual bile acid pool size. Gastroenterology, 80, 1428
17. Hepner, G. W., Hofmann, A. F. and Thomas, P. J. (1972). Metabolism of steroid and aminoacid moieties of conjugated bile acid in man. I. Cholyl glycine (glycocholic acid). J. Clin. Invest., 51, 1889
18. Stiehl, A. (1974). Sulfation of bile salts: a new metabolic pathway. Digestion, 11, 406
19. Yousef, I. M. B., Tuchweber, B., Vank, R. J., Massé, D., Audet, M. and Roy, C. C. (1981). Lithocholate cholestasis – sulfated glycolithocholate-induced intrahepatic cholestasis in rats. Gastroenterology, 80, 233
20. Stiehl, A., Ast, E., Czygan, P., Frohling, W., Raedsh, R. and Kommerell, B. (1978). Synthesis and turnover of sulfated and non sulfated cholic acid and chenodeoxycholic acid in patients with cirrhosis of the liver. Gastroenterology, 74, 572
21. Makino, I., Hashimoto, H., Shinozaki, K., Yoshino, K. and Nakagawa, S. (1975). Sulfated and unsulfated bile acid in urine, serum and bile of patients with hepatobiliary disease. Gastroenterology, 68, 545
22. Podesta, M. T., Murphy, G. M., Sladen, G. E., Beuer, N. F. and Dowling, R. H. (1979). Fecal bile acid excretion in diarrhea: Effect of sulfated and non-sulfated bile acids on colonic structure and function. In Paumgartner, G., Stiehl, A. and Gerok, W. (eds.) Biological Effects of Bile Acids, pp. 245–256. (Lancaster: MTP Press)
23. Raedsch, R., Lanterburg, B. H. and Hofmann, A. F. (1981). Altered bile acid metabolism in primary biliary cirrhosis. Dig. Dis. Sci., 26, 394

16
Serum bile acids and bile acid tolerance tests in liver disease

G. PAUMGARTNER, G. A. MANNES and F. STELLAARD

It has been recognized for many years that elevated concentrations of bile acids in serum are markers of hepatobiliary disease. The availability of commercial kits for enzymatic and radioimmunological determination of serum bile acids has made it feasible to determine serum bile acids in clinical routine. For optimal use and interpretation of serum bile acid measurements in clinical practice it is important to know the determinants of bile acid concentrations in serum.

DETERMINANTS OF BILE ACID CONCENTRATIONS IN SERUM

In healthy subjects the bile acid pool of about 6 mmol is almost completely confined within the enterohepatic circulation[1]. Less than half a percent of the pool is present in the peripheral blood. This is accomplished by an extremely efficient active transport mechanism located in the sinusoidal plasma membrane of the hepatocyte[2,3] which removes about 88% of conjugated cholate from portal blood during one passage[4]. Extraction of unconjugated cholate is somewhat less, namely about 70%[4], and extraction of unconjugated chenodeoxycholate is about 62%[5]. Renal elimination of bile acids is so small under normal conditions that it can be neglected. Consequently, bile acids are eliminated from peripheral blood almost exclusively by hepatic clearance.

In healthy subjects and in patients with mild to moderate liver disease, hepatic bile acid transport operates far below saturation[2]. Therefore, hepatic extraction of bile acids remains practically constant over the whole range of physiological bile acid loads to the liver[6-8]. Thus, for the diurnal changes of the bile acid concentrations in peripheral blood intestinal input of bile acids is the major determinant[8].

Input of bile acids from the intestine may occur via two pathways: firstly, via the hepatic circulation; and secondly – in certain disease states – via portal–systemic shunts. Thus, the degree of first-pass elimination of bile acids by the liver is an important determinant of bile acid concentration in systemic blood. A decrease of first-pass elimination of bile acids can result from diminished hepatic extraction of bile acids or from increased portal–systemic shunting. It should be noted that a reduction of first-pass elimination from 90 to 80% will increase the spillover of bile acids into the systemic circulation by 100%.

First-pass elimination will influence bile acid levels in serum not only after exogenous oral bile acid loads and after meals, but also in the fasting state, since bile acid delivery into the duodenum continues in the interdigestive state[9].

After meals serum bile acids increase 2–6-fold because of considerably increased delivery of bile into the intestine and transport of bile acids towards the terminal ileum[10-13]. Chenodeoxycholic acid shows the most rapid and largest increase followed by deoxycholic acid and cholic acid. This is mainly due to the fact that chenodeoxycholic acid is absorbed more rapidly from the intestine and is extracted by the liver less efficiently than deoxycholic and cholic acid[13].

Whereas bile acid concentrations in the fasting state, after meals and after an oral bile acid load are influenced by hepatic first-pass elimination of portal bile acids, the bile acid concentrations after an intravenous bile acid load are mainly determined by hepatic clearance of systemically circulating bile acids. A similar situation is present in patients with a surgical end-to-side portacaval shunt. In these patients portal blood is diverted into the systemic circulation and serum bile acids distribute in the systemic circulation before undergoing elimination by the liver. The blood supply of the liver in these patients is only arterial. Poupon et al.[14] have found that the decrease of hepatic clearance of bile acids in these patients with cirrhosis and portacaval shunt was mainly caused by a reduction of the inherent ability of the liver to remove bile acids from the blood rather than by the reduction of liver blood flow.

The determinants of the bile acid concentration in serum are as follows:

(1) Intestinal absorption;
(2) Hepatic elimination;
    (a) First-pass elimination (from portal blood);
    (b) Systemic clearance (from peripheral blood)
       – intrinsic clearance
       – liver blood flow.

The concentration of bile acids in serum of peripheral blood at any moment is determined by the instantaneous balance between input of bile acids from the intestine and elimination of bile acids by the liver. Hepatic elimination of bile acids occurs during their first hepatic passage from portal blood and after their recirculation from the systemic circulation both from portal and arterial blood. The clearance of bile acids from the peripheral blood depends on the inherent ability of the liver to remove bile acids (intrinsic clearance of bile acids) and on liver blood flow. In subjects with a normal liver, intestinal input of bile acids is the major determinant of serum bile acid concentrations. In patients with liver disease diminished hepatic elimination is responsible for the elevations of serum bile acids. The reduced hepatic elimination of bile acids in liver disease results from a diminished hepatic clearance, from porto-systemic shunting or from a combination of both.

SENSITIVITY OF ELEVATED SERUM BILE ACIDS FOR DETECTION OF LIVER DISEASE

Diagnostic use of serum bile acids requires information on the relative sensitivities of fasting and postprandial bile acid determinations for detection of liver disease. The serum concentration of bile acids in the fasting state and 2 hours after a standardized test meal has therefore been compared with various tests of liver function[15]. Total bile acids in serum were determined by an enzymatic–fluorimetric method in various groups of patients with histologically verified liver disease[15]. In this study the determination of postprandial serum bile acids proved to be nearly as sensitive for detection of liver disease (unselected patients with alcoholic cirrhosis, chronic hepatitis) than BSP-retention and more sensitive than transaminases. Fasting serum bile acids were less sensitive than postprandial bile acids.

On the basis of the concepts discussed above, it is difficult to explain the increased sensitivity of postprandial serum bile acids found by some authors[15-18] but not others[19,20]. If first-pass elimination of bile acids is reduced after meals, it should also be reduced in the fasting state. The smaller sensitivity of fasting serum bile acids, found by workers using the enzymatic method, could simply reflect methodological difficulties of measuring small changes of bile acid concentrations by the enzymatic assay at low concentrations. In other words, the signal to noise ratio could be too small in the fasting state to detect small to moderate deviations from normal.

Consequently, we have compared fasting and postprandial serum bile acids using both the enzymatic assay and a sensitive radioimmunoassay in the same patients[21]. For the enzymatic test the kit from Nygaard, for the radioimmunoassay the kit from Becton Dickinson was used. We have performed this comparison in a group of patients with liver cirrhosis who had normal transaminases, because it is this group of patients which often poses diagnostic difficulties.

Again the postprandial bile acids were a more sensitive parameter than fasting serum bile acids when the enzymatic assay was used (Figure 16.1). By contrast, the sensitivity of fasting and postprandial bile acids was equal, namely 93% when the radioimmunoassay was used. The sensitivities obtained with conventional liver function tests were 69% for γ-glutamyl-transferase or less. These data demonstrate that fasting serum bile acids were as sensitive for detection of liver disease as postprandial bile acids provided that an assay with high sensitivity and accuracy is used.

When the serum bile acid concentrations are correlated with other tests of liver function there is no significant correlation with serum enzymes, serum albumin or prothrombin time. However, a significant correlation was found between postprandial serum bile acids and BSP-retention[15]. This may be

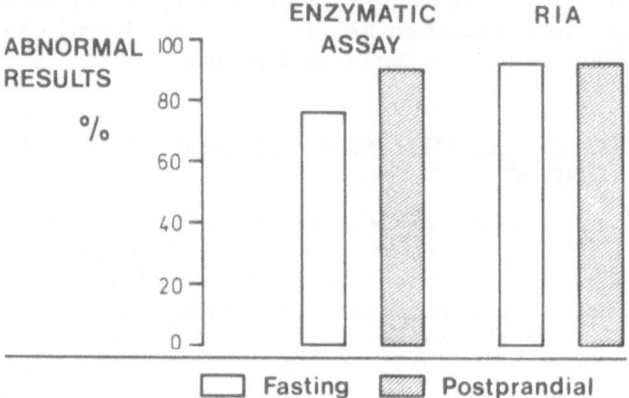

Figure 16.1 Percentage of abnormal results (sensitivity) of enzymatic and radioimmuno-logical serum bile acid determinations in the fasting and in the postprandial state in patients ($n=29$) with cirrhosis of the liver (documented by histology and/or peritoneoscopy) and normal serum transaminases (SGOT and SGPT)

explained by the fact that BSP and bile acid elimination have common determinants. Both depend on excretory function of the liver and on liver blood flow. However, considerable deviations of postprandial serum bile acid levels from this correlation in individual patients occur. This must be expected because of numerous variables involved in the endogenous bile acid loading test. In contrast to the BSP-test, postprandial serum bile acids are not only dependent on hepatic removal, but also on delivery of bile acids into the duodenum, on intestinal motility and on intestinal absorption of bile acids.

To eliminate the variations in intestinal input of bile acids, intravenous bile acid tolerance tests have been developed[22]. However, the sensitivity of these i.v. tests for detection of liver disease was unsatisfactory[23-25]. Oral bile acid tolerance tests employing cholate[26] or ursodeoxycholate[27,28] met with more success but have so far not gained wide acceptance.

To elucidate the factors which contribute to the higher sensitivity of oral as compared with intravenous tolerance tests, oral and intravenous tolerance tests have been performed with ursodeoxycholic acid[29]. This bile acid is absorbed in proximal parts of the small intestine by passive non-ionic diffusion.

After oral administration of ursodeoxycholic acid (1.5 mg (kg body weight)$^{-1}$) to healthy subjects, serum concentrations of this bile acid increased to peak levels within 15–30 minutes. Thereafter a decrease compatible with first-order kinetics followed in all subjects. When the same dose of ursodeoxycholic acid (1.5 mg/kg) was ingested by patients with mild liver disease or with cirrhosis, the peak concentrations were increased up to two-fold in mild liver disease and up to three-fold in patients with cirrhosis[29]. While the plasma disappearance rate constants of patients with mild liver disease showed practically complete overlap with those of the healthy controls, the disappearance rate constants of cirrhotics were decreased by an average of 40%. The increases of the area under the time–concentration curve in the patients were much more impressive than the decreases of the disappearance rate.

The finding of large changes in the area under the curve in the presence of relatively small changes in the disappearance rate may result from decreases in first-pass elimination which increase the systemic availability of urso-deoxycholic acid. This hypothesis was substantiated by studies in a small number of healthy subjects and cirrhotics who received the same dose of ursodeoxycholic acid orally and intravenously[29]. Systemic availability of ursodeoxycholic acid was calculated by dividing the area under the curve obtained after oral administration by the area under the curve obtained after intravenous administration of ursodeoxycholic acid. The results of this study support the pharmacokinetic concept that alterations of the systemic availability and the disappearance rate constant have a multiplicative rather than additive effect on the elimination of substances which are efficiently cleared by the liver[30].

In cirrhotics, a reduced first-pass extraction and a diminished systemic clearance of bile acids act together so that bile acids do not only enter the systemic circulation at increased rates but remain there for increased periods of time. The relative insensitivity of intravenous bile acid tolerance tests may be explained by the fact that disease-induced increases of systemic availability do not play a role in these tests.

References

1. Paumgartner, G. (1978). Hepatic synthesis and transport of bile acids. *Ital. J. Gastroenterol.*, **10**, Suppl. 1, 3
2. Reichen, J. and Paumgartner, G. (1976). Uptake of bile acids by the perfused rat liver. *Am. J. Physiol.*, **231**, 734
3. Reichen, J. and Paumgartner, G. (1980). Excretory function of the liver. In Javitt, N. B. (ed.) *Liver and Biliary Tract Physiology I. Internat. Rev. Physiol.* Vol. 21, p. 103. (Baltimore: University Park Press)
4. Gilmore, I. T. and Thompson, R. P. H. (1981). Direct measurement of hepatic extraction of bile acids in subjects with and without liver disease. *Clin. Sci.* , **60**, 65
5. van Berge Henegouwen, G. P. and Hofmann, A. F. (1977). Pharmacology of chenodeoxy-cholic acid. II. Absorption and metabolism. *Gastroenterology*, **73**, 300
6. LaRusso, N. F., Hoffman, N. E., Korman, M. G., Hofmann, A. F. and Cowen, A. E. (1978). Determinants of fasting and postprandial serum bile acid levels in healthy man. *Am. J. Dig. Dis* ., **23**, 385
7. Luey, K. L. and Heaton, K. W. (1979). Bile acid clearance in liver disease. *Gut*, **20**, 1083
8. Paré, P., Hoefs, J. C. and Ashcavai, M. (1981). Determinants of serum bile acids in chronic liver disease. *Gastroenterology*, **81**, 959
9. Peeters, T. I., Vantrappen, G. and Janssens, J. (1980). Bile acid output and the inter-digestive migrating motor complex in normals and in cholecystectomy patients. *Gastroenterology*, **79**, 678
10. LaRusso, N. F., Korman, M. G., Hoffman, N. E. and Hofmann, A. F. (1974). Dynamics of the enterohepatic circulation of bile acids. Postprandial serum conjugates of cholic acid in health, cholecystectomized patients, and patients with bile acid malabsorption. *N. Engl. J. Med.*, **291**, 689
11. Schalm, S. W., LaRusso, N. F., Hofmann, A. F., Hoffman, N. E., van Berge Henegouwen, G. P. and Korman, M. G. (1978). Diurnal serum levels of primary conjugated bile acids. Assessment by specific radioimmunoassays for conjugates of cholic and chenodeoxy-cholic acid. *Gut*, **19**, 1006

12. Roda, A. *et al.* (1977). Development, validation and application of a single tube radio-immunoassay for cholic and chenodeoxycholic conjugated bile acids in human serum. *Clin. Chem.*, **23**, 2107
13. Angelin, B. and Björkhem, I. (1977). Postprandial serum bile acids in healthy man. Evidence for differences in absorptive pattern between individual bile acids. *Gut*, **18**, 606
14. Poupon, R. Y., Poupon R. E., Lebrec, D., Le Quernec, L. and Darnis, F. (1981). Mechanisms for reduced hepatic clearance and elevated plasma levels of bile acids in cirrhosis. A study in patients with End-to-Side portacaval shunt. *Gastroenterology*, **80**, 1438
15. Grandjean, E. M., Paumgartner, G. and Preisig, R. (1979). Die Gallensäurenkonzentration im Serum nach einer Testmahlzeit bei hepatobiliären Erkrankrungen. Ein Vergleich mit quantitativen Tests der Leberfunktion. *Schweiz. Med. Wochenschr.*, **109**, 1280
16. Kaplowitz, N., Kok, E. and Javitt, N. B. (1973). Postprandial serum bile acid for the detection of hepatobiliary disease. *Am. Med. Assoc.*, **225**, 292
17. Barnes, S., Gallo, G. A., Trash, D. B. and Morris, J. S. (1975). Diagnostic value of serum bile acid estimations in liver disease. *J. Clin. Pathol.*, **28**, 506
18. Fausa, O. and Gjone, E. (1976). Serum bile acid concentrations in patients with liver disease. *Scand. J. Gastroenterol.*, **11**, 537
19. Pennington, C. R., Ross, P. E. and Bouchier, I. A. D. (1971). Serum bile acids in the diagnosis of hepatobiliary disease. *Gut*, **18**, 903
20. Barbara, L., Roda, A. and Roda, E. (1976). Diurnal variations of serum primary bile acids in healthy subjects and hepatobiliary disease patients. *Rendic. Gastroenterol.*, **8**, 194
21. Mannes, G. A., Stellaard, F. and Paumgartner, G. (1982). Increased serum bile acids in cirrhosis with normal transaminases. *Digestion*, **25**, 217
22. LaRusso, N. F., Hoffman, N. E., Hofmann, A. F. and Korman, M. G. (1974). Validity and sensitivity of an intravenous bile acid tolerance test in patients with liver disease. *N. Engl. J. Med.*, **292**, 1209
23. Ferguson, D. R., Calcraft, B. J., Hofmann, A. F. and Belobaba, D. T. A. (1976). Lack of sensitivity of a bile acid clearance test in the detection of liver disease (abstract). *Gastroenterology*, **71**, 905
24. Thjodleifsson B., Barnes, S., Chitranukroh, A., Billing, B. H. and Sherlock S. (1977). Assessment of the plasma disappearance of cholyl-1-^{14}C-glycine as a test of hepatocellular disease. *Gut*, **18**, 697
25. Gilmore, I. T. and Thompson, R. P. H. (1978). Kinetics of ^{14}C-glycocholic acid clearance in normal man and in patients with liver disease. *Gut*, **19**, 1110
26. Matern, S., Haag, M., Homs, Ch. and Gerok, W. (1977). Oral cholate tolerance test. An application of specific radioimmunoassays for the determination of serum conjugated cholic and deoxycholic acid. In Paumgartner, G. and Stiehl, A. (eds.) *Bile Acid Metabolism in Health and Disease*. pp. 253–261. (Lancaster: MTP Press)
27. Matern, S., Tietjen, K. G., Fackler, O., Hinger, K., Herz, R. and Gerok, W. (1979). Bioavailability of ursodeoxycholic acid in man: studies with radioimmunoassay for ursodeoxycholic acid. In Paumgartner, G., Stiehl, A. and Gerok, W. (eds.). *Biological Effects of Bile Acids*. pp. 109–118. (Lancaster: MTP Press)
28. Tashiro, H. (1979). Oral ursodeoxycholic acid tolerance test for patients with hepatobiliary disease. *Acta Hepatol. Jap.*, **20**, 369
29. Miescher, G., Paumgartner, G. and Preisig, R. (1983). Portal–systemic spill-over of bile acids: a study of mechanisms using ursodeoxycholic acid (In press)
30. Neal, E. A., Meffin, P. J., Gregory, P. B. and Blaschke, T. F. (1979). Enhanced bioavailability and decreased clearance of analgesics in patients with cirrhosis. *Gastroenterology*, **77**, 96

Index